T0362502

Urologic Pharmacology

Editor

CRAIG V. COMITER

UROLOGIC CLINICS
OF NORTH AMERICA

www.urologic.theclinics.com

Consulting Editor
KEVIN R. LOUGHLIN

May 2022 • Volume 49 • Number 2

ELSEVIER

1600 John F. Kennedy Boulevard • Suite 1800 • Philadelphia, Pennsylvania, 19103-2899

http://www.theclinics.com

UROLOGIC CLINICS OF NORTH AMERICA Volume 49, Number 2
May 2022 ISSN 0094-0143, ISBN-13: 978-0-323-84926-5

Editor: Kerry Holland
Developmental Editor: Diana Ang

© **2022 Elsevier Inc. All rights reserved.**

This periodical and the individual contributions contained in it are protected under copyright by Elsevier, and the following terms and conditions apply to their use:

Photocopying
Single photocopies of single articles may be made for personal use as allowed by national copyright laws. Permission of the Publisher and payment of a fee is required for all other photocopying, including multiple or systematic copying, copying for advertising or promotional purposes, resale, and all forms of document delivery. Special rates are available for educational institutions that wish to make photocopies for non-profit educational classroom use. For information on how to seek permission visit www.elsevier.com/permissions or call: (+44) 1865 843830 (UK)/(+1) 215 239 3804 (USA).

Derivative Works
Subscribers may reproduce tables of contents or prepare lists of articles including abstracts for internal circulation within their institutions. Permission of the Publisher is required for resale or distribution outside the institution. Permission of the Publisher is required for all other derivative works, including compilations and translations (please consult www.elsevier.com/permissions).

Electronic Storage or Usage
Permission of the Publisher is required to store or use electronically any material contained in this periodical, including any article or part of an article (please consult www.elsevier.com/permissions). Except as outlined above, no part of this publication may be reproduced, stored in a retrieval system or transmitted in any form or by any means, electronic, mechanical, photocopying, recording or otherwise, without prior written permission of the Publisher.

Notice
No responsibility is assumed by the Publisher for any injury and/or damage to persons or property as a matter of products liability, negligence or otherwise, or from any use or operation of any methods, products, instructions or ideas contained in the material herein. Because of rapid advances in the medical sciences, in particular, independent verification of diagnoses and drug dosages should be made.

Although all advertising material is expected to conform to ethical (medical) standards, inclusion in this publication does not constitute a guarantee or endorsement of the quality or value of such product or of the claims made of it by its manufacturer.

Urologic Clinics of North America (ISSN 0094-0143) is published quarterly by Elsevier Inc., 360 Park Avenue South, New York, NY 10010-1710. Months of issue are February, May, August, and November. Business and Editorial Offices: 1600 John F. Kennedy Blvd., Suite 1800, Philadelphia, PA 19103-2899. Periodicals postage paid at New York, NY and additional mailing offices. Subscription prices are $403.00 per year (US individuals), $1054.00 per year (US institutions), $100.00 per year (US students and residents), $459.00 per year (Canadian individuals), $1075.00 per year (Canadian institutions), $100.00 per year (Canadian students/residents), $530.00 per year (foreign individuals), $1075.00 per year (foreign institutions), and $240.00 per year (foreign students/residents). Foreign air speed delivery is included in all *Clinics* subscription prices. All prices are subject to change without notice. **POSTMASTER:** Send address changes to *Urologic Clinics of North America*, Elsevier Health Sciences Division, Subscription Customer Service, 3251 Riverport Lane, Maryland Heights, MO 63043. **Customer Service: 1-800-654-2452 (US). From outside the United States, call 1-314-447-8871. Fax: 1-314-447-8029. E-mail: JournalsCustomerServiceusa@elsevier.com (for print support)** and **JournalsOnlineSupport-usa@elsevier.com (for online support)**.

Reprints. For copies of 100 or more, of articles in this publication, please contact the Commercial Reprints Department, Elsevier Inc., 360 Park Avenue South, New York, New York 10010-1710. Tel.: 212-633-3874; Fax: 212-633-3820; E-mail: reprints@elsevier.com.

Urologic Clinics of North America is covered in MEDLINE/PubMed (*Index Medicus*), *Excerpta Medica, Current Contents/Clinical Medicine, Science Citation Index,* and *ISI/BIOMED.*

Contributors

CONSULTING EDITOR

KEVIN R. LOUGHLIN, MD, MBA
Emeritus Professor of Surgery (Urology),
Harvard Medical School, Visiting Scientist,
Vascular Biology Research Program at Boston
Children's Hospital, Boston, Massachusetts,
USA

EDITOR

CRAIG V. COMITER, MD
Professor, Department of Urology, Professor
(by courtesy), Department of Obstetrics and
Gynecology, Stanford University School of
Medicine, Stanford, California, USA

AUTHORS

NITYA ABRAHAM, MD
Associate Professor, Department of Urology,
Montefiore Medical Center, Albert Einstein
College of Medicine, Bronx, New York, USA

OSHORENUA AIYEGBUSI, MBChB
Nephrology Registrar, The Glasgow Renal and
Transplant Unit, Queen Elizabeth University
Hospital, Glasgow, United Kingdom

MARWAN ALKASSIS, MD
Department of Urology, Hôtel Dieu de France,
Université Saint Joseph, Beirut, Lebanon

KHALID ALKHATIB, MD
Division of Urological Surgery, Center for
Surgery and Public Health, Brigham and
Women's Hospital, Harvard Medical School,
Boston, Massachusetts, USA

DAVID BOSONI, MD
Research Center for Reproductive Medicine,
Gynecological Endocrinology and Menopause,
IRCCS S. Matteo Foundation, Department
of Clinical, Surgical, Diagnostic and
Pediatric Sciences, University of Pavia, Pavia,
Italy

LOGAN BRIGGS, BA
Division of Urological Surgery, Center for
Surgery and Public Health, Brigham and
Women's Hospital, Harvard Medical School,
Boston, Massachusetts, USA

TONY CHEN, MD
Clinical Assistant Professor of Urology, Stanford
University School of Medicine, Center for
Academic Medicine, Palo Alto, California, USA

**CHRISTOPHER J. CHERMANSKY, MD,
FPMRS**
Chief of Urology, UPMC Magee-Womens
Hospital, Department of Urology, Pittsburgh,
Pennsylvania, USA

RAUL I. CLAVIJO, MD
Assistant Clinical Professor, Department of
Urology, University of California, Davis,
Sacramento, California, USA

WHITNEY CLEARWATER, MD, MPH
Department of Obstetrics and Gynecology and
Women's Health, Fellow, Female Pelvic
Medicine and Reconstructive Surgery, Albert
Einstein College of Medicine, Montefiore
Medical Center, Bronx, New York, USA

ALEXANDER P. COLE, MD
Division of Urological Surgery, Center for Surgery and Public Health, Brigham and Women's Hospital, Harvard Medical School, Boston, Massachusetts, USA

SIMON CONTI, MD, MEd
Department of Urology, Stanford University School of Medicine, Stanford, California, USA

LAURA CUCINELLA, MD
Research Center for Reproductive Medicine, Gynecological Endocrinology and Menopause, IRCCS S. Matteo Foundation, Department of Clinical, Surgical, Diagnostic and Pediatric Sciences, University of Pavia, Pavia, Italy

MICHAEL L. EISENBERG, MD
Professor of Urology, Stanford University School of Medicine, Center for Academic Medicine, Palo Alto, California, USA

CALYANI GANESAN, MD
Division of Nephrology, Stanford University School of Medicine, Stanford, California, USA

MEERA GANESH, BA
Northwestern University Feinberg School of Medicine, Chicago, Illinois, USA

MARINA O. GUIRGUIS, MD
Fellow, Female Pelvic Medicine and Reconstructive Surgery, UPMC Magee-Womens Hospital, Pittsburgh, Pennsylvania, USA

NICOLE HANDA, MD
Department of Urology, Northwestern University Feinberg School of Medicine, Chicago, Illinois, USA

DUANE HICKLING, MD, MSc
Urology Staff, Department of Surgery, Division of Urology, Female Pelvic Medicine and Reconstructive Surgery, University of Ottawa, Ottawa, Ontario, Canada

ADAM S. KIBEL, MD
Division of Urological Surgery, Center for Surgery and Public Health, Brigham and Women's Hospital, Harvard Medical School, Boston, Massachusetts, USA

STEPHANIE KIELB, MD
Professor of Urology, Medical Education, and OB/GYN, Divsion Chief, Reconstructive Urology, Neurourology, and Pelvic Medicine, Residency Program Director, Department of Urology, Northwestern University Feinberg School of Medicine, Chicago, Illinois, USA

BENJAMIN KING, MD
Assistant Professor of Surgery, Department of Urology, University of Vermont Medical Center, Burlington, Vermont, USA

MUHIEDDINE LABBAN, MD
Division of Urological Surgery, Center for Surgery and Public Health, Brigham and Women's Hospital, Harvard Medical School, Boston, Massachusetts, USA

JUSTIN LOLOI, MD
Resident PGY2, Department of Urology, Montefiore Medical Center, Albert Einstein College of Medicine, Bronx, New York, USA

SRINIWASAN B. MANI, MD
Department of Urology, University of California, Davis, Sacramento, California, USA

ELLIS MARTINI, MD
Research Center for Reproductive Medicine, Gynecological Endocrinology and Menopause, IRCCS S. Matteo Foundation, Department of Clinical, Surgical, Diagnostic and Pediatric Sciences, University of Pavia, Pavia, Italy

ELLON MCGREGOR, MBChB, MD
Nephrology Consultant, Honorary Senior Lecturer, The Glasgow Renal and Transplant Unit, Queen Elizabeth University Hospital, School of Medicine, Dentistry and Nursing, The University of Glasgow, Glasgow, United Kingdom

SIOBHAN K. MCMANUS, MBChB, PhD
Nephrology Consultant, The Glasgow Renal and Transplant Unit, Queen Elizabeth University Hospital, Glasgow, United Kingdom

MARK A. MOYAD, MD, MPH
Jenkins/Pokempner Director of Complementary and Alternative Medicine, University of Michigan Medical Center, Department of Urology, Ann Arbor, Michigan, USA

EVAN A. MULLOY, MD
Urology Fellow in Male Reproductive Medicine, Stanford University School of Medicine, Center for Academic Medicine, Palo Alto, California, USA

ROSSELLA E. NAPPI, MD, PhD
Professor of Obstetric and Gynecology, Chief, Research Center for Reproductive Medicine, Gynecological Endocrinology and Menopause, IRCCS S. Matteo Foundation, Department of Clinical, Surgical, Diagnostic and Pediatric Sciences, University of Pavia, Pavia, Italy

FARNOOSH NIK-AHD, MD
Urology Resident Physician, Department of Urology, University of California, San Francisco, California, USA

ALEXANDER PLOCHOCKI, MD, MPH
Resident, Department of Urology, University of Vermont Medical Center, Burlington, Vermont, USA

ALESSANDRA RIGHI, MD
Research Center for Reproductive Medicine, Gynecological Endocrinology and Menopause, IRCCS S. Matteo Foundation, Department of Clinical, Surgical, Diagnostic and Pediatric Sciences, University of Pavia, Pavia, Italy

JAMES ROSS, MD
Urology Fellow, Department of Surgery, Division of Urology, Functional and Reconstructive Urology, University of Ottawa, Ottawa, Ontario, Canada

ALISON SCHULZ BS
Medical Student, Albert Einstein College of Medicine, Bronx, New York, USA

ALAN W. SHINDEL, MD, MAS
Professor, Department of Urology, University of California, San Francisco, San Francisco, California, USA

KYLE SPRADLING, MD
Department of Urology, Stanford University School of Medicine, Stanford, California, USA

KATE I. STEVENS, MBChB, PhD
Nephrology Consultant, Honorary Senior Lecturer, The Glasgow Renal and Transplant Unit, Queen Elizabeth University Hospital, Glasgow, United Kingdom

SYLVIA O. SUADICANI, PhD
Associate Professor, Department of Urology, Montefiore Medical Center, Albert Einstein College of Medicine, Bronx, New York, USA

LARA TIRANINI, MD
Research Center for Reproductive Medicine, Gynecological Endocrinology and Menopause, IRCCS S. Matteo Foundation, Department of Clinical, Surgical, Diagnostic and Pediatric Sciences, University of Pavia, Pavia, Italy

QUOC-DIEN TRINH, MD
Associate Professor, Division of Urological Surgery, Center for Surgery and Public Health, Brigham and Women's Hospital, Harvard Medical School, Boston, Massachusetts, USA

ALEKSANDRA WALASEK, MD
Department of Urology, Massachusetts General Hospital, Boston, Massachusetts, USA

DIMITAR V. ZLATEV, MD
Department of Urology, Massachusetts General Hospital, Boston, Massachusetts, USA

Contents

Medical Treatment of Hypogonadism in Men   197

Sriniwasan B. Mani and Raul I. Clavijo

Urologists may commonly diagnose hypogonadism in adult men experiencing an age-related decline in serum testosterone. Low serum testosterone in conjunction with symptoms such as decreased libido, fatigue, memory deficit, or decreased vitality is described as testosterone deficiency syndrome. There are numerous therapeutic options, although each is unique in its formulation, administration, and side-effect profile. For this reason, treatment can prove to be challenging for each unique patient case. The clinician must carefully monitor key serum markers before and during treatment. With careful dosing and monitoring, therapeutic benefit can be achieved reliably and sustainably.

Pharmacotherapy for Erectile Dysfunction in 2021 and Beyond   209

Farnoosh Nik-Ahd and Alan W. Shindel

Erectile dysfunction (ED), defined as the inability to develop or maintain an erection firm enough for satisfactory sexual intercourse, is a common urologic condition that increases in prevalence with age but can affect men of any age. There have been numerous pharmacologic advancements for the treatment of ED over the past 40 years. Here, we will review the mainstays of the pharmacologic treatment of ED: OTC/herbal supplements, phosphodiesterase type V inhibitors (PDE5I), intraurethral suppositories (MUSE), and intracorporal injections (ICI).

Medical Treatment of Disorders of Ejaculation   219

Tony Chen, Evan A. Mulloy, and Michael L. Eisenberg

Ejaculation and orgasm are complex phenomena within the male sexual response cycle. Disordered ejaculation commonly presents as premature or delayed ejaculation, although issues with painful ejaculation, retrograde ejaculation, or postorgasmic illness syndrome are also seen. This article will review the pathophysiology of these conditions as well as the current pharmacologic treatments available.

Medical Treatment of Benign Prostatic Hyperplasia   231

Alexander Plochocki and Benjamin King

In this article, we review the primary medical treatments of BPH-associated male LUTS, with a focus on physiology, indications, and side effects. We cover selective alpha-1 antagonists, anticholinergics, PDE5 inhibitors, 5-alpha reductase inhibitors, and beta-3 agonists. Through a review of the literature, we provide our clinical pathway for the medical management of BPH, generally starting with tamsulosin in most men and progressing to combination therapy based on patient's response and symptoms.

Patients using nutraceuticals represent a diverse patient population with a keen potential interest and/or adherence to healthy lifestyle changes. BPH nutraceuticals, including saw palmetto were as safe, but not more effective than placebo in the STEP and CAMUS clinical trials, but another high-quality saw palmetto product could be tested in a phase 3 trial. Several other BPH supplements need more recent robust clinical data, environmental oversight, or safety data. ED supplements, including Panax ginseng, and the notable nitric oxide (NO) enhancing amino acids arginine and citrulline have positive preliminary short-term efficacy data with and without PDE-5 inhibitors, but herbal quality control (QC) or safety signals with some of these agents in specific patient populations need to be resolved. "Less is more" should be the current mantra in the prostate cancer milieu, and potentially in some men with male infertility based on the FAZST trial because it is plausible some antioxidants are exhibiting prooxidant activity in some settings. Some prescription anthelmintic medications are being studied, others are being purchased over-the-counter (OTC), but their preliminary safety and efficacy against cancer have been concerning and questionable. In fairness, ongoing additional objective clinical trial data should become available soon, especially with mebendazole. DHEA or DHEA enhancing products have multiple concerns including HDL reductions, and their questionable use in men with BPH or prostate cancer based on the limited data. Some of these concerns should also be addressed in long-term robust clinical trials of prescription testosterone agents. Regardless, more attention should be directed toward heart-healthy lifestyle changes for most urologic men's health conditions, whether they are used in a preventive or synergistic setting with other acceptable clinical treatment options.

Overactive bladder is a disruptive urinary condition composed of urgency, frequency, and nocturia, which affects a large proportion of men and women. Symptoms are often associated with a decreased quality of life. After optimizing behavioral strategies, pharmacologic intervention is the next consideration for treatment. Therapeutic agents consist primarily of antimuscarinic and β-agonist medications, as well as off-label use of antidepressants in some cases. These medications, although effective, can be associated with considerable adverse side effects. Combination therapies along with novel therapeutics and drug targets are under investigation.

 Video content accompanies this article at http://www.urologic.theclinics.com.

Onabotulinumtoxin A is an effective therapeutic tool for urologic treatment. The toxin exerts multiple effects in the urinary tract system, which contributes to its utility. The toxin can be used to alleviate a variety of pathologic conditions if administered in the appropriate patient population.

Interstitial cystitis/bladder pain syndrome (IC/BPS) is defined as chronic discomfort perceived to be related to the urinary bladder accompanied by urinary urgency or frequency. Pharmacotherapies used to treat IC/BPS include oral and intravesical agents. Oral therapies include amitriptyline, hydroxyzine, cyclosporine A, and pentosan polysulfate sodium (PPS). CyA as treatment for IC/BPS demonstrates efficacy in patients with Hunners Lesions. The recent finding of pigmented maculopathy with chronic PPS is very concerning and must be discussed with patients. Intravesical therapies usually involve a mixture of multiple agents in a cocktail, most commonly alkalinized lidocaine and heparin.

Urinary tract infections (UTIs) are a common source of morbidity and require significant health care resources for diagnosis, treatment, and prevention. Antimicrobials represent the mainstay for the treatment of UTIs. Established guidelines exist for the antimicrobial treatment and prevention of uncomplicated UTIs; however, antimicrobial dependence and overuse have led to the emergence of antimicrobial resistance. Nonantimicrobial alternatives are an ongoing area of research and should be considered when clinically appropriate based on available evidence.

Female sexual dysfunction (FSD) comprises multiple overlapping sexual disorders with a multifaceted cause within the frame of the biopsychosocial model. Health care providers can screen for FSD according to their level of expertise and deliver at least basic counseling before eventually referring to sexual medicine specialists for specific care. The therapeutic algorithm comprises a multidisciplinary approach, including pharmacologic and nonpharmacologic management. Flibanserin and bremelanotide are psychoactive agents indicated for the treatment of generalized acquired hypoactive sexual desire disorder (HSDD) in premenopausal women, whereas transdermal testosterone is effective on HSDD in postmenopausal women. Menopause hormone therapy (systemic and local) is the mainstay for individualized management of women at midlife.

Androgen deprivation therapy, used alone or in combination, inhibits androgen activity either upstream at the level of the pituitary gland or downstream by disrupting the androgenesis pathway in the adrenal or androgen activity in prostate cells. Its appropriate utilization varies depending on disease stage, aggressivity, and resistance. Special consideration should be given to side effects, as it can affect patients' quality of life and might interact with their treatment for other conditions.

Cancer immunotherapy has transformed urologic oncology by expanding the arsenal of available treatment options and improving outcomes. The number of patients eligible for immune-based cancer treatment continues to increase as indications for currently approved therapies expand with new agents being developed and studied. In this review the authors discuss the major recent clinical developments in immunotherapy for the treatment of urologic cancers.

UROLOGIC CLINICS OF NORTH AMERICA

SERIES OF RELATED INTEREST
Surgical Clinics of North America
https://www.surgical.theclinics.com/

Foreword

Urologic Pharmacology: Its Debt to Teddy Roosevelt and the Founding of the Food and Drug Administration

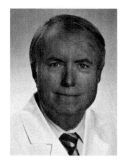

Kevin R. Loughlin, MD, MBA
Consulting Editor

In the late 1800s, there was essentially no government supervision of the food and drug industries. Upton Sinclair exposed the sickening conditions of the meat-packing industry in his book, *The Jungle*.[1] This served to initiate more public and government awareness for the regulation of food products and drugs.

Harvey W. Wiley, MD was a young physician from Indiana who became one of the early champions of greater government oversight in these areas.[2] He met a kindred spirit in the person of Theodore Roosevelt. Through their efforts, Congress became aware of the problem, and this resulted in the Food and Drug Act, which was signed into law on June 30, 1906, by Roosevelt. This legislation was administered by the Bureau of Chemistry, which gave rise to the Food and Drug Administration, or FDA, in 1930. Without the passion of Wiley and the unwavering support of Roosevelt, this legislation would likely have been postponed for decades.

A few years ago, I was in conversation with the CMO of our institution, who happened to be a general surgeon. The hospital was introducing more pharmacologic tracking into the Electronic Medical Record. He commented to me that as a general surgeon, he routinely had to deal with only two classes of drugs: antibiotics and narcotics, whereas urologists prescribed a pharmacopeia of drugs for a variety of conditions.

Dr Craig Comiter has assembled a group of experts for this issue of the *Urologic Clinics* to address this important area of urologic pharmacology. The topics covered in this issue are expansive and range from the treatment for hypogonadism to benign prostatic hyperplasia to urinary tract infections to immunotherapy.

Urology is perhaps the most unique of all the surgical specialties in its blend of both medicine and surgery to treat patients. This comprehensive issue will serve the reader well, as it provides both a current and a comprehensive review of the subject.

Kevin R. Loughlin, MD, MBA
Vascular Biology Program at
Boston Children's Hospital
300 Longwood Avenue
Boston, MA 02115, USA

E-mail address:
kloughlin@partners.org

REFERENCES

1. Pure Food and Drug Act. Available at: https://en.wikipedia.org/wiki/Pure_Food_and_Drug_Act. Accessed January 15, 2022.
2. Harvey W. Wiley/FDA. Available at: https://www.fda.gov/about-fda/fda-leadership-1907-today/harvey-w-wiley. Accessed January 15, 2022.

Urol Clin N Am 49 (2022) xiii
https://doi.org/10.1016/j.ucl.2022.03.002
0094-0143/22/© 2022 Published by Elsevier Inc.

Foreword

Urologic Pharmacology: Its Debt to Teddy Roosevelt and the Founding of the Food and Drug Administration

Kevin R. Loughlin, MD, MBA
Consulting Editor

Preface
Pharmacology in Urology

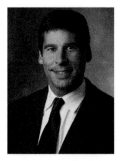

Craig V. Comiter, MD
Editor

Pharmacology is the branch of medicine concerned with the effects, modes of action, and uses of drugs. Urology was foundational in the establishment of pharmacotherapeutic treatment for cancer. Eighty years ago, Charles Huggins published his ground-breaking research, demonstrating that the course of prostate cancer can be affected by hormonal manipulation, which ultimately won him the Nobel Prize in Physiology. Amazingly, this nearly century-old treatment with hormonal manipulation remains at the forefront of our treatment for metastatic prostate cancer. This was the first demonstration that chemicals can control cancer. Shortly thereafter, in 1948, Sidney Farber studied the anticancer effects of antifolates and demonstrated that methotrexate can lead to remission in pediatric acute lymphoblastic leukemia.

Urologic pharmacology is not limited to oncologic indications. Rather, pharmaceuticals are indicated for the treatment of virtually all urologic conditions, ranging from urinary tract infections to voiding dysfunction to disorders of male and female sexual function. Urology continues to be a leader in the field of pharmacology, with fifteen drugs topping $100 million annually for Medicare part B and D spending.

Pharmacologic treatment of urologic disease will most certainly continue to change over time, but unlike the often "one-and-done" surgeries that we successfully perform, pharmacotherapy is often chronically administered, and even successful treatment can have both short-term and long-term side effects. In this issue of the *Urologic Clinics*, I have selected fourteen areas of urologic pharmacology that we feel play an important role in daily urologic care and have undergone substantial refinement over the past several years. Each author has taken a very broad topic and expertly narrowed it down, using scientific evidence to give best-practice recommendations. And lest we not forget the importance of nonprescription neutriceuticals, which are not only popular but also efficacious for treating a variety of urologic conditions.

I would like to thank the authors who have dedicated their time and expertise to this important publication. I expect the readers will agree that it is because of the generosity of our academic colleagues that we can quickly reference these topics that we encounter frequently in our urologic practice.

Poisons and medicine are often the same substance given with different intents.
— Peter Mere Latham, 19th-century English physician and educator

Craig V. Comiter, MD
Department of Urology
Department of Obstetrics and Gynecology
Stanford University School of Medicine
Stanford, CA, USA

Center for Academic Medicine
Urology 5656
453 Quarry Road
Palo Alto, CA 94304, USA

E-mail address:
ccomiter@stanford.edu

Urol Clin N Am 49 (2022) xv
https://doi.org/10.1016/j.ucl.2022.03.001
0094-0143/22/© 2022 Published by Elsevier Inc.

urologic.theclinics.com

Medical Treatment of Hypogonadism in Men

Sriniwasan B. Mani, MD, Raul I. Clavijo, MD*

KEYWORDS

- Testosterone • Hypogonadism • Estradiol • Polycythemia • Andropause

KEY POINTS

- Treatment of hypogonadism can help ameliorate medical conditions that may be exacerbated by testosterone deficiency including anemia, a decrease in bone mineral density, and a decrease in sexual function.
- The choice for treatment of hypogonadism largely should be tailored to a patient's risk factors for adverse effects, lifestyle, fertility status, and goals of care.
- Close monitoring of patients being treated for hypogonadism is essential to avoid potentially life-threatening side effects and ensure therapeutic changes to serum testosterone levels.

INTRODUCTION

Thorough understanding of the role of testosterone, both in its intrinsic role in the hypothalamic pituitary gonadal (HPG) axis and as a therapeutic agent, is necessary for both the andrology specialist and the practicing general urologist. Testosterone is ultimately an end product in the HPG axis, produced mostly by the testes in response to luteinizing hormone (LH). The entire cascade begins with the pulsatile release of gonadotrophin releasing hormone (GnRH) from the hypothalamus, which enters the hypophyseal portal system. From there, GnRH stimulates the anterior pituitary gland that secretes follicle-stimulating hormone (FSH) and LH, 2 hormones vital for reproduction.

Hypogonadism is defined as a deficiency of circulating testosterone in a genetic man. This deficiency can be further divided into primary and secondary hypogonadism. Primary hypogonadism is defined as lack of testosterone from the testes, otherwise known as primary testicular dysfunction, in which the hypothalamus and anterior pituitary gland are intact; this is also known as hypergonadotropic hypogonadism, due to the lack of feedback inhibition on the release of GnRH, FSH, and LH. Secondary hypogonadism is thus failure of either the hypothalamus or the anterior pituitary gland, also known as central hypogonadism or hypogonadotrophic hypogonadism.

Treating hypogonadism can be challenging for a urologist, especially in a landscape of ever-evolving therapeutic options. Optimal patient care entails rigorous diagnostic workup, as well as safe and judicious use of one or more of many methods of testosterone supplementation or manipulation of the HPG axis. In this article the authors' objective is to discuss the most current pharmacotherapy of hypogonadism and practical strategies for the care of these patients.

DEFINITIONS AND BACKGROUND

For the practicing urologist, hypogonadism will likely present as a constellation of symptoms such as a decreased libido, memory, and vitality; mood alterations; erectile dysfunction; changes in ejaculation; or decreased muscle strength, which may prompt evaluation of serum testosterone levels, ultimately leading to the diagnosis of testosterone deficiency syndrome (TDS)/hypogonadism. Although there is still no consensus on a laboratory definition for testosterone deficiency syndrome, several professional societies, including the American Urological Association,

Department of Urology, University of California, Davis, 4860 Y Street, Suite 2200, Sacramento, CA 95817, USA
* Corresponding author. 4860 Y Street, Suite 2200, Sacramento, CA 95817.
E-mail address: riclavijo@ucdavis.edu

Urol Clin N Am 49 (2022) 197–207
https://doi.org/10.1016/j.ucl.2021.12.008
0094-0143/22/© 2021 Elsevier Inc. All rights reserved.

agree that a diagnosis can be made if serum total testosterone is less than 300 ng/dL on 2 separate early morning serum tests[1]; this has ultimately been supported by a recent study performed to harmonize standard reference ranges of serum testosterone in several different longitudinal cohorts. In this study, a serum testosterone of 303 ng/dL corresponded to the fifth percentile of healthy, nonobese men aged 19 to 39 years.[2] This study also demonstrated that average serum testosterone also decreases with age. For example, the fifth percentile of nonobese subjects aged 80 to 89 years had an average serum testosterone of 218 ng/dL.[2]

When discussing causes of TDS, they can be generally divided into primary and secondary hypogonadism. An overt example of primary testicular failure as a cause for testosterone deficiency syndrome can be seen in Klinefelter syndrome, which affects up to 0.2% of newborns and is diagnosed in up to 4% of infertile men.[3] Other forms of primary testicular failure include testicular trauma, oncologic treatments that affect testicular function, and infectious processes (eg, mumps). Secondary hypogonadism is most commonly of irreversible origin such as in the case of inborn genetic mutations. A wide variety of genes have been identified for which mutations can lead to a spectrum of endocrine disorders that can result in hypogonadotrophic hypogonadism.[4] As new evidence emerges, we are increasingly aware of new genetic defects that ultimately contribute to the same phenotype of secondary hypogonadism. In a classic example of secondary hypogonadism, Kallmann syndrome is due to an interruption of migration of neurons that secrete GnRH, leading to a lack of LH and FSH resulting in low testosterone production.[4] As one may expect, genetic mutations that interfere with testosterone production are often diagnosed in adolescents who usually present with delayed puberty.

It is important to note that in addition to primary and secondary hypogonadism, we may further divide hypogonadism into reversible and irreversible causes. Irreversible causes may be due to inborn genetic defects or acquired dysfunction such as after a traumatic injury. Reversible causes are typically related to modifiable lifestyle factors. For example, a diagnosis of type 2 diabetes mellitus has been associated with hypogonadism, and it is suspected that insulin resistance and its impact on hypothalamic release of GnRH may be the root cause.[5]

Thus, comorbid conditions can have a significant influence on serum testosterone and thus further drive the natural decline that occurs with age. Platz and colleagues extracted serum testosterone data from men without comorbidities such as diabetes, congestive heart failure, cancer, or stroke and demonstrated that these healthy patients, although still experiencing age-related decline in testosterone, still had ultimately higher serum testosterone than their counterparts with the aforementioned comorbidities.[6] Even at the level of the testes, we see the impact of aging. Absolute Leydig cell number does not seem to change over time; however, their responsiveness to stimulation by LH does decrease. What is most telling is that although testosterone decreases with age, there does not seem to be a compensatory increase in LH, suggesting that the primary site of dysfunction lies in the pituitary response.[7]

Although an in-depth understanding of the varied causes of hypogonadism is essential, the most clinically relevant to the general urologist is late-onset or age-related hypogonadism. In fact, this is the cross-section of patients in which the general urologist may be able to intervene and help the most, given that there are both modifiable lifestyle factors and readily available therapeutic options. Testosterone supplementation, specifically in some of the aforementioned scenarios such as Klinefelter syndrome and Kallmann syndrome, presents as a logical therapeutic approach because the clinician is exogenously replacing that which the patient cannot natively produce—in essence, were it not for their genetic defect, one could safely assume testosterone production would proceed normally. Supplementation in the age-related hypogonadism category, however, poses a different type of challenge because there is no inherent inability to produce testosterone, and this subset of patients likely produced normal levels of testosterone throughout life. Thus, the approach to dosing, the side-effect profile, risk/benefit ratio, and the protocol for therapeutic monitoring is much more nuanced.

PHARMACOLOGIC MANAGEMENT OF TESTOSTERONE DEFICIENCY SYNDROME
Diagnosis

As previously mentioned, there is still no consensus on the absolute definition of TDS. However, the cutoff point of 300 ng/dL is a convenient clinical criterion that has ample evidence to support its use. When making the diagnosis, it is important to document 2 separate recordings of testosterone less than 300 ng/dL, ideally obtained as an early morning sample. In addition, the clinician is advised to thoroughly document symptoms such as a fatigue, decreased libido, memory deficits, decrease in muscle mass, depressed mood, or erectile dysfunction; this can be done by standardized templating by the clinician's preference or by using any readily available symptom survey. A thorough history must of course include any other past medical history (including previously resolved comorbid conditions that are no longer being treated) and a medication reconciliation.

Preassessment and Patient Counseling

Clinicians should thoroughly counsel patients on any potential risks and benefits before starting testosterone replacement (TRT); this is also an opportunity to risk stratify each patient and discuss with them how their medical history may affect the success of therapy. For example, a history of breast cancer precludes initiating therapy, as it is regarded as a contraindication. Similarly, known or suspected prostate cancer is also technically a strict contraindication, albeit with some controversy particularly in the setting of TRT in those on active surveillance for low-risk prostate cancer.[8,9]

While obtaining the past medical history, the urologist should pay particular attention to any history of myocardial infarction, deep venous thrombosis, or cerebral infarct, as these events have been identified by the Food and Drug Administration (FDA) to possibly occur at higher rates in patients who use exogenous testosterone.[10–12] In fact, despite the controversy about study quality and patient populations studied, the publication of manuscripts associating TRT with cardiovascular risk led to a notable decrease in new testosterone prescriptions in 2013.[13]

The presence of obstructive sleep apnea, lower urinary tract symptoms, and benign prostatic hypertrophy is not necessarily a contraindication to TRT according to a current summary of evidence showing no clinically significant aggravation of symptoms, but it is worth mentioning to patients that these symptoms have been shown to worsen in some individual studies.[14–16] Finally, discerning a patient's desire for fertility is of utmost importance, as TRT can result in infertility by inhibiting FSH/LH production via negative feedback, drastically affecting spermatogenesis.[17]

It is necessary to obtain a baseline set of laboratories before initiating TRT to assist in both diagnostic workup and monitoring for side effects. Prostate-specific antigen (PSA) should be obtained, especially if the patient is older than 40 years, as there is a theoretic risk of diagnosing occult prostate cancer.[10] Complete blood count must be documented, as polycythemia is a known

risk of TRT. Baseline estradiol should be drawn, as it may increase during treatment and reveal an underlying imbalance of testosterone to estradiol ratio. Obtaining prolactin and LH is also highly recommended, especially because modifiable conditions such as prolactinoma can be diagnosed and intervention could potentially treat secondary hypogonadism. A ferritin level may also be useful for diagnosing hemochromatosis in the setting of very low testosterone values with evidence for secondary hypogonadism.

In addition, clinicians must consider the side effects of the drug delivery method itself. Injections carry the risk of pain and bruising and thus require ample patient education to ensure they are performed correctly. Transdermal gels must be applied carefully, specifically to hairless and moist patches of skin, as any contact with any other individual can result in direct transfer of the medication and incorrect application can exacerbate risk of allergic response.

What follows is a detailed discussion of the many available therapeutic options for testosterone replacement. Regardless of the mechanism of delivery, the goal of TRT is to reestablish circulating serum testosterone to physiologic levels, as much as reasonably possible.

Short- and Medium-Acting Injectable Formulations

Testosterone can be injected in depot form when formulated as a testosterone molecule bonded to an ester carbon chain. Variance in the size and conformation of the carbon chain will affect the half-life of the resultant active testosterone molecule. These formulations are administered via intramuscular (IM) injection, the most common being testosterone cypionate (TC) and enanthate (TE). Given the long half-life of up to 9 days, these formulations are dosed weekly or biweekly, and per the FDA can even be administered monthly although we do not recommend that time interval.[18] The caveat with such infrequent dosing regimens is a "peak and valley" effect in which the concentration of available medication diminishes toward the end of the dosing cycle. The high initial availability of testosterone at the time of dosing could potentiate polycythemia, hyperestrogenemia, or mood disturbances.[19] In a series of 11 hypogonadal men, supratherapeutic levels of testosterone (1112 ± 297 ng/dL) could be measured up to 5 days after the initial injection of TC, 200 mg, IM with levels dropping to an average of 400 ng/dL by the end of 2 weeks. Thus, desirable testosterone levels could be achieved during the entire dosing period, albeit within a wide range.[20] To avoid such wide fluctuations, we tend to recommend self-administered testosterone IM at weekly intervals in our practice. Our preferred starting dose is 100 mg weekly of testosterone cypionate (eg, 0.5 mL of a 200 mg/mL solution) delivered through the IM route. Other routes, such as self-administered subcutaneous injection and twice weekly injections at lower doses are mentioned in the literature and used in our clinic, but have not been approved by the FDA.[21] For biweekly injections our preference is to use testosterone enanthate given its slightly shorter half-life. Ultimately, short-acting injections offer patients a reliable method of attaining physiologic testosterone levels when compared with other popular formulations such as transdermal topical medications. Side effects of the injectable form include pain and inflammation at the injection site, difficulties with viscosity of oil carriers, as well as allergic reactions to the inactive ingredients used in the formulation solution.

Long-Acting Injections

Testosterone undecanoate (TU) is a long-acting injectable formulation, whose half-life of 21 days is greater than that of TE and TC. The FDA has approved a starting dose of 750 mg of TU injected IM initially, then at week 4, and then every 10 weeks thereafter. Patients can expect to achieve peak testosterone levels at 7 days after each injection. A reliable therapeutic steady state is usually reached after the third injection administered at week 14[22]; this is an ideal option for patients who want to minimize the number of injections needed for sustained treatment but does put the burden of compliance on the patient, given that the initial treatment period requires careful adherence to the dosing regimen to reach steady state levels. TU still carries the side effect of pain and inflammation at the injection site, which may be more noticeable when compared with short-acting injectables, as a larger volume of medication is needed for a full TU dose. Although rare, pulmonary oil microembolism and anaphylaxis have been reported with TU use.

Transdermal Testosterone Delivery

Most of the men on TRT, approximately two-thirds, use gel or cream preparations. The most common brand-name formulations of transdermal testosterone are Testim and AndroGel. In the gel or cream formulation, the testosterone molecule is suspended in a hydroalcoholic gel than can be readily absorbed via the skin in a time-dependent manner.[23] Pharmacokinetic studies show systemic exposure to testosterone is highly variable following topical applications of either Testim and AndroGel with several peaks occurring throughout the day and average max testosterone concentrations ranging from 368 to 480.[24] We recommend administration of transdermal testosterone onto hairless, moist areas of skin such as the shoulders, upper arms, and abdomen, ranging from 40 to 100 mg of delivered testosterone daily. An effect can be detected as soon as 18 to 24 hours after administration, but steady state levels are more reliably reached after the third day of administration.[23,24] Gels and creams are preferred among patients given their simplicity, eliminating the use for needles. Side effects include skin irritation. There is always the risk of poor compliance (in maintaining a regular dosing regimen as well as appropriately administering the medication in the correct location), which can lead to subtherapeutic testosterone levels. It may behoove the provider to physically identify ideal locations of administration for the patient during physical examination to improve compliance. Patients should also be counseled on the risks of skin-to-skin contact with others.

Androderm is another transdermal formulation administered as a daily patch. This product can closely mimic the physiologic circadian variation of testosterone, as it is applied at night, with peak testosterone levels seen the following morning. Although peak levels range from 412 to 498 ng/dL, even with appropriate use trough levels have been recorded well less than 300 ng/dL.[25] The side effect of skin irritation seems to the be the biggest challenge with this medication, as up to one-third of patients will discontinue it for this reason.[26]

Intranasal Testosterone

Intranasal testosterone gel (Natesto) is a more recent advance in testosterone formulation and delivery. The high permeability of the nasal mucosa allows for enhanced absorption of testosterone, as the drug is able to bypass first pass metabolism, thus increasing its bioavailability. An appropriate starting dose is 1 actuation (5.5 mg of testosterone) per nostril 2 or 3 times per day. Pharmacokinetic studies in hypogonadal men shows an average testosterone of 386 ng/dL when used 3 times per day with a range of 200 to 935 ng/dL during an administration period.[27]

There is emerging evidence that use of Natesto may have a limited effect on LH and FSH, thus preserving semen parameters such as total motile sperm count at 3 and 6 months after initiating treatment.[28,29] Intranasal testosterone may thus be an excellent option for patients who wish to maintain fertility while undergoing TRT, assuming they are monitored closely with serial pituitary hormone and semen analyses. Natesto is FDA approved and thus allows patients to avoid off-label use of medications such as human chorionic gonadotropin (hCG) or clomiphene citrate, which we typically reserve mostly for those of fertile age. Common side effects include headache, sinusitis, runny or stuffy nose, nosebleed, and nasal discomfort.

Implantable Testosterone Pellets

The implantable testosterone pellet (name brand Testopel, 75 mg testosterone per pellet) is another long-acting formulation of testosterone. These can be inserted in the outpatient setting directly into the subcutaneous tissue in the upper buttocks or lower back through a small incision under local anesthesia. After administration, mean peak testosterone levels can typically be achieved at 4 weeks postimplantation. In pharmacokinetic studies, mean total testosterone tended to be maintained greater than 300 ng/dL for 4 months regardless of pellet number (range 6–10). However, higher pellet numbers were associated with levels closer to mid-normal of testosterone throughout the entire treatment period of 3 months in one retrospective study.[30] In general, these pellets can be inserted every 3 to 4 months but close monitoring of testosterone levels during treatment may dictate a modified schedule, as patient factors such as body mass index can affect absorption and thus efficacy.[31] This method of TRT can lead to side effects such as pain/discomfort at insertion site, hematoma, infection, skin rash, and pellet extrusion. With the exception of pain, the aforementioned side effects are all quite rare, occurring at a rate of less than 1%. In the ideal case, a patient would only need 4 treatments per year, rendering this a desirable option for patients who are unable to inject themselves and want to minimize procedures. More recently, insurance coverage changes have limited pellet coverage to 6 pellets in many patients, thus limiting the use of this product in certain populations such as clinics with no access to compounded testosterone pellets or patients unable to afford the cash price of additional pellets.

Oral Testosterone Formulations

Oral formulations of TU have been available outside of the United States for some years but have only been recently approved by the FDA. The oral TU available in Europe and some parts of Asia is marketed as Andriol Testocaps. Classically, oral testosterone formulations such as methyltestosterone, which undergoes first pass metabolism in the liver, posed a significant risk of hepatotoxicity, which prevented its approval by the FDA.[10] Even with safer oral testosterone options available, metabolism of testosterone when administered orally has often led to a difficulty in achieving reliable eugonadal testosterone levels. Thus came the development of oral formulations that would avoid first pass hepatic metabolism and raise testosterone levels reliably to therapeutic levels. Jatenzo, a relatively new formulation of oral TU and the first approved by the FDA, is consumed in capsule form in a self-emulsifying vehicle that uses a lipoprotein shell to shield TU from first-pass metabolism, taking advantage of intestinal lymphatic absorption to deliver a more consistent and reliable amount of testosterone into the circulation, with low potential for hepatotoxicity. The pharmacokinetic profile of Jatenzo allows for BID dosing, as peak concentrations of testosterone are reached 2 hours after administration, falling to nadir levels at around 12 hours. The largest clinical trial studying Jatenzo reports average testosterone concentrations at 489 ± 158 ng/dL. This phase III study demonstrated that 87% of hypogonadal men were able to achieve normal serum testosterone levels consistently, most reaching steady-state levels 7 days after initiating treatment.[32,33] Although many practices have not yet incorporated this medication mostly due to lack of insurance coverage for aging related/idiopathic hypogonadism, the manufacturer recommends twice daily dosing at a starting dose of 237 mg. Serum testosterone can be monitored within a week of initiating therapy, ideally drawn at a time in between doses. Unique side effects include headache, decreased high-density lipoprotein (HDL) cholesterol, and nausea. Other brands currently under FDA review include Tlando and Kyzatrex.

Human Chorionic Gonadotropin

Endogenous LH, under the influence of GnRH, stimulates Leydig cells in the testicle to produce most of a man's circulating testosterone. The hCG molecule is morphologically similar to LH and shares the same cellular receptor. Thus, hCG can be used to stimulate endogenous testosterone production. An example of this is in the setting of hypogonadotrophic hypogonadism where hCG has been demonstrated to stimulate sperm production by directly increasing intratesticular testosterone.[34] In studies on men with normal testosterone, hCG can increase testosterone levels almost 2-fold 2 days after receiving a 1500 IU dose of hCG.[35] Although relatively scant, current literature supports the effectiveness of hCG in patients with age-related or idiopathic TDS, with the added benefit of preserving semen parameters and testicular volume compared with exogenous testosterone formulations.[36] Although studies are promising, hCG is not FDA approved for the treatment of TDS and thus is typically used "off-label." There are no established dosing guidelines, but extrapolating from prior studies it would follow that low-dose hCG given in more frequent doses may be more effective at improving testosterone as opposed to less frequent larger doses.[35] It has also been shown that hCG can induce a biphasic response in serum testosterone, resulting in a peak at 2 to 4 hours and a higher one at 48 to 72 hours after one administration of hCG.[37] This translates to an ideal dosing regimen of a single dose every third or fourth day. In our practice we prefer starting with 2000 IU of hCG via intramuscular or subcutaneous injection 2 times per week. Without larger studies in the treatment of age-related/idiopathic TDS, however, it is difficult to ascertain any unique side effects associated with hCG in our typical TDS population.

Clomiphene Citrate

Another option for treating TDS, also used "off-label" by many andrologists, is clomiphene citrate (Clomid). Clomiphene is a selective estrogen receptor modulator that is prepared as a racemic mixture of 2 isoforms (enclomiphene and zuclomiphene), thus possessing both receptor antagonist and agonist activities. It competitively binds to estrogen receptors in the hypothalamus and pituitary gland and decreases the effect of estrogen's negative feedback. This results in increased LH production and subsequently an increase in testosterone. It then follows that clomiphene has the potential to preserve LH and FSH production and thus spermatogenesis as well. Given its impact on fertility preservation, younger men have been the target population in clinical research studying clomiphene. One particular study examined 86 healthy young men (mean 29 years of age) taking clomiphene at either 25 mg or 50 mg every other day. This study demonstrated an increase in total testosterone from a mean of 192 to 485 ng/dL after 6 months of treatment. No patients in this cohort experienced any side effects.[38] In general, side effects of clomiphene citrate that have been reported include headaches, gastrointestinal symptoms, hot flushes, nausea, dizziness, visual disturbance, weight gain, and fluid retention. There have been rare reports of central retinal vein occlusion (in a patient with factor V Leiden) as well as intracranial venous thrombosis.[39] More recently, an isolated enclomiphene isomer,

marketed as Androxal, was developed to avoid the side-effect profile of the zuclomiphene isomer.[11] It should be noted that neither formulation has been approved by the FDA for the purpose of increasing serum testosterone. There is no standardized clomiphene dose but its half-life is around 10 to 14 days. Given this, we recommend starting at 25 mg 2 times per week. The clinician can titrate up from this dose while following serum testosterone and monitoring for side effects.

Selective Androgen Receptor Modulators

Although not yet clinically available, there is ample research to suggest that a new class of drugs, selective androgen receptor modulators (SARM), could potentially provide therapeutic benefit to men with hypogonadism. SARMs are any nonnative steroid molecule that bind to the androgen receptor with both agonist and antagonist behavior. The androgen receptor is itself a nuclear receptor that promotes transcription of targeted DNA sequences. The androgen receptor is found in many tissue types, and studies have shown that SARMs can be modified to have more tissue-specific sites of action.[40] In experimental trials, SARMs have been shown to have benefit in treating cachexia, muscular dystrophy, and osteoporosis, further highlighting the broad tissue-specific prevalence of the androgen receptor.[41] With respect to hypogonadism, it is yet to be seen how SARMs may play a specific role in symptom management. Decreased libido may be a potential therapeutic target in the eventual use of SARMs for hypogonadism, as animal models have shown promising results in increasing sexual behavior in rats.[42] The most common side effects noted in studies evaluating SARMs are headache, increased serum alaine aminotransferase levels, and decreased HDL levels.[41] These side effects, however, will vary based on the particular SARM that is being investigated, as they all have varied agonist and antagonist activity. Concerning to a practicing urologist is the growing popularity in the bodybuilding and physique circles of these compounds. Thus, it is prudent to ask about its use when evaluating a man for TDS or infertility.[43]

Monitoring

It is advisable to monitor several serum markers while a patient is on testosterone replacement therapy. Depending on the therapeutic agent, it is recommended to at the very least obtain serum testosterone anywhere from 1 to 3 months after initiating treatment; this is detailed further in **Table 1**. Obtaining a serum testosterone value at the suggested early time-point can facilitate

Table 1
Testosterone replacement therapy

	Brand/Name	Starting Dose	Advantages	Disadvantages	Monitoring
Potential for pituitary suppression: moderate to high					
Short-Acting Injectables	Testosterone cypionate, Testosterone enanthate, Testosterone propionate	100 mg, IM, administered weekly (TE and TM)	• Weekly + dosing • Consistent absorption	• "Peak and valley" effect • Injection pain/reactions • Polycythemia/hyperestrogenemia risk	• 1st lab: 4–6 wk after initiation • Subsequent: every 3 to 6 mo
Long-Acting Injectables	Testosterone undecanoate (Aveed)	750 mg IM initially and at 4 wk, then 750 mg IM every 10 wk	• Infrequent administration • Reliable absorption	• Injection pain/reactions • Pulmonary oil microembolism • Initial dosing intervals necessary to achieve steady state	• 1st lab: end of first 10-wk interval (steady state) • Subsequent: end of dosing intervals
Gels/Creams	Testim and AndroGel	40–100 mg, topical	• Noninvasive • Lower polycythemia/hyperestrogenemia risk	• Transference potential • Variance in absorption • Compliance • Rash	• At least 1 wk after initiation, 2–8 h after administration
Patches	Androderm	1 patch daily, topical	• Noninvasive • Lower polycythemia/hyperestrogenemia risk	• Dermatitis in up to 1/3 • Variance in absorption	• At least 1 wk after initiation, 3–12 h after administration
Pellets	Testopel	6–14 pellets every 3–4 mo Subcutaneous	• Infrequent administration • Reliable absorption	• Procedure site reactions: infection, pellet extrusion, hematoma	• 4–6 wk after administration to evaluate peak • Alternatively at the end of dosing interval
Oral	Jatenzo	237 mg twice a day	• Avoids first-pass hepatic metabolism • Least invasive/burdensome (oral route)	• Headache, diarrhea, nausea, decreased HDL	• At least 1 wk after initiation, timed in between doses (trough)

(continued on next page)

Table 1
(continued)

	Brand/Name	Starting Dose	Advantages	Disadvantages	Monitoring
Potential for pituitary suppression: low					
Intranasal	Natesto	1 actuation (5.5 mg of testosterone) per nostril 2 or 3 times per day	• Noninvasive (mucosa) • Clinically insignificant impact on spermato-genesis (short term)	• Requires at least twice-a-day administration • Variable absorption levels	• At least 1 wk after initiation
Potential for pituitary suppression: none to low					
Clomiphene	Clomid	25–50 mg every other day	• Noninvasive • Inexpensive • No pituitary suppression (spermatogenesis preserved)	• Potential estrogenic side effects • Case reports of blood clots	• Not established • Consider 2–6 wk postinitiation
Human chorionic gonadotropin (hCG)	Pregnyl	2000 IU every other day or BIW	• Preservation of quali-tative spermatogenesis	• Expensive • May lead to decreased FSH (feedback) without clomiphene support	• Not established • Consider 2–6 wk postinitiation

Abbreviations: BIW, twice per week; IM, intramuscular; IU, international units; mg, milligrams; TC, testosterone cypionate; TE, testosterone enanthate.

titration of the drug. Overall, along with side effects noted later, patients should be evaluated for the common side effects of acne, hair loss, and testicular atrophy (when using exogenous testosterone).

There is considerable risk of polycythemia, mostly associated with testosterone injections. Thus, it is important to monitor hematocrit and hemoglobin.[44] This risk is likely directly proportional to the dose, as has been demonstrated in one study investigating weekly dosing of testosterone enanthate.[45] For routine monitoring, it is most convenient to obtain a hematocrit value every time serum testosterone is checked. If polycythemia occurs, it can be treated by decreasing the dose or referring the patient for phlebotomy or blood donation. Whether phlebotomy or dose adjustment is required to treat polycythemia, subsequent hematocrit values should be checked as well to assess for resolution.

Hepatotoxicity is of concern when using oral testosterone due to hepatic metabolism, as described earlier.[46] Some formulations do carry a lower risk however, such as oral testosterone undecanoate (Jatenzo). Elevated liver enzymes are observed in patients taking more traditional oral testosterone formulations, which are not available in the United States. Routine monitoring of liver enzymes is not recommended otherwise. Although Jatenzo was shown to be associated with decreased HDL cholesterol, monitoring of lipid profiles while using this medication or any other testosterone formulation is still not supported by current evidence.[47,48]

It is also advisable to monitor estradiol levels routinely. Maintenance of normal estradiol levels is a goal of TRT, as estradiol has been shown to play a key role in maintenance of libido and body fat composition.[49] Furthermore, estradiol is a key hormone in the maintenance of bone mineral density, as aromatization of testosterone to estradiol has been shown to be key in preserving bone health.[50] On the other side, hyperestrogenemia has been associated with symptoms of water retention, weight gain, irritability, and gynecomastia and may potentially increase risk of cardiovascular adverse events. Aromatase inhibitors such as anastrozole can be judiciously used in hyperestrogenemic men undergoing TRT to maintain estradiol at normal levels if a decrease in testosterone dose is not possible for therapeutic reasons. Overall, although no consensus exists as to what optimal estradiol levels are in men, we strive for a level between 20 and 60 pg/mL based on appearance of symptoms in our patient population.

We have mentioned that there is a theoretic risk of prescribing testosterone replacement therapy with a patient harboring occult prostate cancer.

Thus, most society guidelines recommend measuring PSA in age-appropriate men (>40 years of age in the setting of TRT), along with performing a digital rectal examination at least annually.[51,52]

In addition to laboratory test monitoring, it is essential to adopt a reliable measurement of symptoms to document and track patient improvement while on testosterone replacement therapy. The clinician's goal should be to both achieve eugonadal levels of testosterone as well as address the patient's most concerning symptoms. There are several available patient surveys and questionnaires, including the Androgen Deficiency in the Aging Male questionnaire, which we suggest as a basic clinical monitoring tool.[53] If a patient does not derive any benefit from testosterone replacement, then it is not advisable to continue due to potential risks in the absence of any therapeutic improvement.

Lastly, certain populations who are being monitored not only for improvements in testosterone but also for fertility potential warrant regular measurement of pituitary-derived LH and FSH and occasionally semen analyses.

SUMMARY

Hypogonadism in the adult men is often encountered by the practicing urologist as an age-related decline in serum testosterone. It is generally agreed on that testosterone less than 300 ng/dL, in conjunction with symptoms associated with TDS warrant some form of treatment, most commonly by testosterone supplementation. Every practitioner should counsel patients thoroughly on the challenges of treating hypogonadism and the clinical ambiguity surrounding its management. However, in this comprehensive review we provide key data to inform management of such patients, which can provide some concrete guidance. While treating a patient for testosterone deficiency, it is of utmost importance to closely monitor both symptoms and laboratory values of interest. Side effects vary with respect to different medications but are largely benign and reversible. Ultimately it is up to the clinician to pay careful attention to their patients and tailor care to the individual, using this guide as a framework.

CLINICS CARE POINTS

- TDS can be diagnosed in men who have a measured serum testosterone of less than 300 ng/dL on 2 separate mornings in conjunction with a range of clinical symptoms.

- Several therapeutic options are available for testosterone supplementation or pituitary stimulation in different formulations such as injections, gels/creams, patches, or oral medications.
- Close monitoring of several different serum markers must be performed for any patient treated for TDS to monitor for both therapeutic impact and side-effect prevention.

DISCLOSURE

The authors report no conflicts of interest in this work.

REFERENCES

1. Mullhall JP, Trost LW, Brannigan RE, et al. Evaluation and management of testosterone defiency: AUA guideline. J Urol 2018;200(2):423–32.
2. Travison TG, Vesper HW, Orwoll E, et al. Harmonized reference ranges for circulating testosterone levels in men of four cohort studies in the United States and Europe. J Clin Endocrinol Metab 2017;102(4): 1161–73.
3. Bonomi M, Rochira V, Pasquali D, et al. Klinefelter syndrome (KS): genetics, clinical phenotype, and hypogonadism. J Endocrinol Invest 2017;40(2): 123–34.
4. Viswanathan V, Eugster EA. Etiology and Treatment of Hypogonadism in Adolescents. Pediatr Clin North Am 2011;58(5):1181–200.
5. Crisostomo L, Pereira SC, Monteiro MP, et al. Lifestyle, metabolic disorders and male hypogonadism – a one-way ticket? Mol Cell Endocrinol 2020;516: 110945.
6. Platz EA, Barber JR, Chadid S, et al. Nationally representative estimates of serum testosterone concentration in never-smoking, lean men without aging-associated comorbidities. J Endocr Soc 2019;3(10):1759–70.
7. Mulligan T, Iranmanesh A, Veldhuis JD. Pulsatile IV infusion of recombinant human LH in leuprolide-suppressed men unmasks impoverished Leydig-cell secretory responsiveness to midphysiological LH drive in the aging male. J Clin Endocrinol Metab 2001;86(11):5547–53.
8. Snyder PJ, Bhasin S, Cunningham GR, et al. Lessons from the testosterone trials. Endocr Rev 2018; 39(3):369–86.
9. Snyder PJ, Bhasin S, Cunningham GR, et al. Effects of testosterone treatment in older men. N Engl J Med 2016;374:611–24.
10. Westaby D, Paradinas FJ, Ogle SJ, et al. Liver damage from long-term methyltestosterone. The Lancet 1977;310(8032):261–3.
11. Wiehle RD, Fontenot GK, Wike J, et al. Enclomiphene citrate stimulates testosterone production while preventing oligospermia: a randomized phase II clinical trial comparing topical testosterone. Fertil Steril 2014;102(3):720–7.
12. Wu C, Kovac JR. Novel uses for the anabolic androgenic steroids nandrolone and oxandrolone in the management of male health. Curr Urol Rep 2016; 17(10):72.
13. Baillargeon J, Kuo Y-F, Westra JR, et al. Testosterone prescribing in the United States, 2002-2016. JAMA 2018;320(2):200–2.
14. Marks LS, Mazer NA, Mostaghel E, et al. Effect of testosterone replacement therapy on prostate tissue in men with late-onset hypogonadism: a randomized controlled trial. JAMA 2006;296:2351–61.
15. Kohn TP, Mata DA, Ramasamy R, et al. Effects of testosterone replacement therapy on lower urinary tract symptoms: a systematic review and meta-analysis. Eur Urol 2016;69:1083–90.
16. Kim S-D, Cho K-S. Obstructive sleep apnea and testosterone deficiency. World J Mens Health 2019; 37(1):12–8.
17. World Health Organization Task Force on Methods for the Regulation of Male Fertility. Contraceptive efficacy of testosterone-induced azoospermia and oligozoospermia in normal men. Fertil Steril 1996;65: 821–9.
18. Palombi B. Depo®-Testosterone. 9 Available at: https://labeling.pfizer.com/ShowLabeling.aspx?id=548.
19. Dobs AS, Meikle AW, Arver S, et al. Pharmacokinetics, efficacy, and safety of a permeation-enhanced testosterone transdermal system in comparison with bi-weekly injections of testosterone enanthate for the treatment of hypogonadal men. J Clin Endocrinol Metab 1999;84:3469–78.
20. Nankin HR. Hormone kinetics after intramuscular testosterone cypionate. Fertil Steril 1987;47: 1004–9.
21. Spratt DI, Stewart II, Savage C, et al. Subcutaneous injection of testosterone is an effective and preferred alternative to intramuscular injection: demonstration in female-to-male transgender patients. J Clin Endocrinol Metab 2017;102:2349–55.
22. Wang C, Harnett M, Dobs AS, et al. Pharmacokinetics and safety of long-acting testosterone undecanoate injections in hypogonadal men: an 84-week phase III clinical trial. J Androl 2010;31: 457–65.
23. Wang C, Berman N, Longstreth JA, et al. Pharmacokinetics of transdermal testosterone gel in hypogonadal men: application of gel at one site versus four sites: a General Clinical Research Center Study. J Clin Endocrinol Metab 2000;85:964–9.
24. Marbury T, Hamill E, Bachand R, et al. Evaluation of the pharmacokinetic profiles of the new testosterone

topical gel formulation, Testim™, compared to AndroGel. Biopharm Drug Dispos 2003;24:115–20.

25. Swerdloff RS, Wang C, Cunningham G, et al. Long-term pharmacokinetics of transdermal testosterone gel in hypogonadal men. J Clin Endocrinol Metab 2000;85:4500–10.

26. Jordan WP, Atkinson LE, Lai C. Comparison of the skin irritation potential of two testosterone transdermal systems: an investigational system and a marketed product. Clin Ther 1998;20:80–7.

27. Rogol AD, Tkachenko N, Bryson N. Natesto™, a novel testosterone nasal gel, normalizes androgen levels in hypogonadal men. Androl 2016;4:46–54.

28. Masterson T, Molina M, Ibrahim E, et al. Natesto effects on reproductive hormones and semen parameters: results from an ongoing single-center, investigator-initiated phase IV clinical trial. Eur Urol Focus 2018;4(3):333–5.

29. Ramasamy R, Masterson TA, Best JC, et al. Effect of Natesto on reproductive hormones, semen parameters and hypogonadal symptoms: a single center, open label, single arm trial. J Urol 2020;204(3):557–63.

30. McCullough AR, Khera M, Goldstein I, et al. A multi-institutional observational study of testosterone levels after testosterone pellet (Testopel®) insertion. J Sex Med 2012;9:594–601.

31. Pastuszak AW, Mittakanti H, Liu JS, et al. Pharmacokinetic evaluation and dosing of subcutaneous testosterone pellets. J Androl 2012;33:927–37.

32. JATENZO® (testosterone undecanoate) [prescribing information]. Northbrook, IL: Clarus Therapeutics, Inc.; March 2019.

33. Data on file. Clinical Study Report: CLAR-18019. Clarus Therapeutics, Inc.Available at: https://www.accessdata.fda.gov/drugsatfda_docs/nda/2019/206089Orig1s000MedR.pdf.

34. Jarow JP, Zirkin BR. The androgen microenvironment of the human testis and hormonal control of spermatogenesis. Ann N Y Acad Sci 2005;1061:208–20.

35. Smals AG, Pieters GF, Boers GH, et al. Differential effect of single high dose and divided small dose administration of human chorionic gonadotropin on Leydig cell steroidogenic desensitization. J Clin Endocrinol Metab 1984;58:327–31.

36. Vignera SL, Condorelli RA, Cimino L, et al. Late-onset hypogonadism: the advantages of treatment with human chorionic gonadotropin rather than testosterone. Aging Male 2016;19:34–9.

37. Padrón RS, Wischusen J, Hudson B, et al. Prolonged biphasic response of plasma testosterone to single intramuscular injections of human chorionic gonadotropin. J Clin Endocrinol Metab 1980;50:1100–4.

38. Katz DJ, Nabulsi O, Tal R, et al. Outcomes of clomiphene citrate treatment in young hypogonadal men. BJU Int 2012;110:573–8.

39. Zahid M, Arshad A, Zafar A, et al. Intracranial venous thrombosis in a man taking clomiphene citrate. BMJ Case Rep 2016. https://doi.org/10.1136/bcr-2016-217403. bcr2016217403.

40. Handlon AL, Schaller LT, Leesnitzer LM, et al. Optimizing ligand efficiency of selective androgen receptor modulators (SARMs). ACS Med Chem Lett 2015;7(1):83–8.

41. Solomon ZJ, Mirabal JR, Mazur DJ, et al. Selective androgen receptor modulators: current knowledge and clinical applications. Sex Med Rev 2019;7(1):84–94.

42. Miner JN, Chang W, Chapman MS, et al. An orally active selective androgen receptor modulator is efficacious on bone, muscle, and sex function with reduced impact on prostate. Endocrinol 2007;148:363–73.

43. United States Food & Drug Adminstation. FDA in Brief: FDA Warns Against Using SARMs in Body-Building Products. 2017.

44. Jones SD, Dukovac T, Sangkum P, et al. Erythrocytosis and polycythemia secondary to testosterone replacement therapy in the aging male. Sex Med Rev 2015;3:101–12.

45. Coviello AD, Kaplan B, Lakshman KM, et al. Effects of graded doses of testosterone on erythropoiesis in healthy young and older men. J Clin Endocrinol Metab 2008;93:914–9.

46. Niedfeldt MW. Anabolic steroid effect on the liver. Curr Sports Med Rep 2018;17(3):97–102.

47. Bhasin S, Storer TW, Berman N, et al. The effects of supraphysiologic doses of testosterone on muscle size and strength in normal men. N Engl J Med 1996;335:1–7.

48. Whitsel EA, Boyko EJ, Matsumoto AM, et al. Intramuscular testosterone esters and plasma lipids in hypogonadal men: a meta-analysis. Am J Med 2001;111(4):261–9.

49. Finkelstein JS, Lee H, Burnett-Bowie SM, et al. Gonadal steroids and body composition, strength, and sexual function in men. N Eng J Med 2013;369:1011–22.

50. Dias JP, Melvin D, Simonsick EM, et al. Effects of Aromatase Inhibition vs. Testosterone in Older Men With Low Testosterone: Randomized-Controlled Trial. Androl 2016;4(1):33–40.

51. Alsina M, St Anna L. How should we monitor men receiving testosterone replacement therapy? J Fam Pract 2010;59(12):711–2.

52. Bhasin S, Brito JP, Cunningham GR, et al. Testosterone therapy in men with hypogonadism: an endocrine society clinical practice guideline. J Clin Endocrinol Metab 2018;103:1715–44.

53. Mohamed O, Freundlich RE, Dakik HK, et al. The quantitative ADAM questionnaire: a new tool in quantifying the severity of hypogonadism. Int J Impot Res 2010;22:20–4.

Pharmacotherapy for Erectile Dysfunction in 2021 and Beyond

Farnoosh Nik-Ahd, MD, Alan W. Shindel, MD, MAS*

KEYWORDS

- Penis • Erectile function • Erectile dysfunction • Pharmacotherapy • Sexuality • Sexual dysfunction

KEY POINTS

- Current understanding of the physiologic processes of penile erection has enabled the modern era of highly effective pharmacotherapy for ED.
- Understanding the pharmacologic and pharmacodynamics properties of available therapies helps practitioners optimize the care of individual patients.
- Novel therapeutics may be possible based on currently unexploited aspects of erectile physiology

INTRODUCTION

Erectile dysfunction (ED) is a common and vexing clinical problem that leads to the substantial disruption of quality of life and relationships.[1] Interest in facilitating and restoring erections is documented in ancient texts going back to the beginnings of recorded human history and probably extends back even further than that.[2] A variety of superstitions and herbal remedies have been touted; some of these ancient remedies have pharmacologic properties that are consistent with erectogenic effect and/or have been investigated in modern clinical trials.[2,3]

Despite millennia of interest in ED, it is only within the past 40 years that demonstrably and consistently effective pharmacologic treatments have been available for this common ailment. The arrival of effective pharmacotherapy for ED was heralded by the famous (or perhaps infamous) actions of Dr. Giles Brindley, who demonstrated his pharmacologically induced erection at a scientific session of the 1983 Annual Meeting of the American Urologic Association.[4] This dramatic presentation ushered in an era of effective pharmacotherapy for ED. Approximately 10 years later the fundamental role of nitrergic neurons (formerly known as nonadrenergic noncholinergic "NANC"

neurons) in mediating vascular responses was determined.[5] These discoveries paved the way for pharmacotherapies that modulated steps in the nitrergic pathway as treatments for ED, culminating in the release of the first highly effective and tolerable oral pharmacotherapy for ED in 1998.[6]

In this article, we review the current state of the art in pharmacotherapy for ED. An understanding of ED pharmacotherapy necessitates at least a brief review of the molecular mechanisms that mediate penile vasodilation. Our focus will be on agents currently approved for use by the United States Food and Drug Administration (US FDA) although we will also consider the commonly used (albeit not formally approved) agents used as injectable drugs for the induction of penile erection. The main classes of pharmacotherapy for ED are listed in **Table 1**. Brief consideration will be given to agents approved for use by regulatory bodies outside the United States. We will conclude with the consideration of directions for future research and development in medical therapy for ED.

MOLECULAR MECHANISMS OF ERECTION

A detailed discussion of the anatomic/tissue properties of the penis that allow for penile erection is

Department of Urology, University of California, 400 Parnassus Avenue, Suite A-610, San Francisco, CA 94143-0738, USA
* Corresponding author. 400 Parnassus Avenue, Suite A-610, San Francisco, CA 94143-0738.
E-mail address: alan.shindel@ucsf.edu

Urol Clin N Am 49 (2022) 209–217
https://doi.org/10.1016/j.ucl.2021.12.002
0094-0143/22/© 2021 Elsevier Inc. All rights reserved.

Table 1
Mainstays of pharmacotherapy for erectile dysfunction in the United States

Generic Name	Trade Name (TM)	FDA Approved Dosing	Mechanism
Sildenafil	Viagra Revatio	25–100 mg oral on-demand	Selective inhibitor of PDE5
Vardenafil	Levitra Staxyn	5–20 mg oral on-demand	Selective inhibitor of PDE5
Tadalafil	Cialis	5–20 mg oral on-demand 2.5–5 mg daily dose	Selective inhibitor of PDE5
Avanafil	Stendra	50–100 mg oral on-demand	Selective inhibitor of PDE5
Prostaglandin E1	Alprostadil Edex Caverject Constituent of "Trimix"	10–40 mcg intracavernous injection 125–1000 mcg intraurethral suppository	Activation of adenylyl cyclase
Phentolamine	Typically constituent of "Bimix/Trimix"	Variable concentration of intracavernous injection[a]	Inhibition of adrenergic vascular tone and adenylyl cyclase
Papaverine	Typically constituent of "Bimix/Trimix"	Variable concentration of intracavernous injection[a]	Non-selective inhibitor of PDE
Atropine	Typically constituent of "Quadmix"	Variable concentration of intracavernous injection[a]	Antimuscarinic (unclear efficacy)

[a] Phentolamine, papaverine, and atropine do not have formal FDA approval for ED.

beyond the scope of this article. The reader is referred to excellent historical and recent publications on this topic for more detail.[7,8] However, an understanding of the pharmacology of ED treatment requires some knowledge of the molecular mechanisms that regulate penile vasodilation.

The nitric oxide (NO) pathway has emerged as a fundamental and essential element of genital vasodilation.[7] NO is derived from neuronal and endothelial Nitric Oxide Synthase (nNOS and eNOS, respectively). NO is in turn responsible for activating Soluble Guanylate Cyclase, which catalyzes the conversion of Guanosine Triphosphate (GTP) to cyclic Guanosine Monophosphate (cGMP). cGMP plays a critical role in modulating a number of cellular processes via the activation of Protein Kinase G (PKG). The downstream effects of PKG in the penis include potassium sensitization, suppression of the calcium sensitizing RhoA-Rho Kinase pathway, and depletion of intracellular calcium by sequestration in the sarcoplasmic reticulum and expulsion through membrane-bound calcium channels. The net effect of all these pathways is to oppose the activation of the actin–myosin cross-bridge formation in smooth muscle cells of penile arteries and corporal erectile tissue, leading to muscular relaxation and subsequent vasodilation. With vasodilation, penile blood flow is increased and the corporal bodies become engorged with blood.

With the cessation of sexual arousal, production of NO declines. Production of cGMP declines in turn and the processes that mediate corporal vasodilation cease. cGMP is broken down by the action of phosphodiesterases. The most clinically relevant isoform of phosphodiesterase in the penis is type 5 (PDE5). Selective inhibitors of PDE5 (PDE5i) are potent erectogenic agents that work by prolonging the vasodilatory effects of cGMP in the penis. These highly efficacious agents have been the mainstay of ED therapy for over 2 decades; their unique mechanism of action explains the important observation that these drugs are primarily useful for maintaining rather than attaining erection. Reliance on initial NO activity for efficacy also makes clear how these agents are less effective in men with neurogenic etiologies for ED (eg, postpelvic surgery, severe diabetes).[9]

While the NO/cGMP/PDE5 pathway is arguably the most fundamental and clinically important molecular pathway mediating erection, a number of other vascular mechanisms are also at play and may be manipulated pharmacologically to induce erections. Sympathetic tone is dominant in the penis at baseline and limits the inflow of blood. Therefore, erections are mediated by parasympathetic neural input from the sacral (S2–S4) spinal cord.[10] Cessation of sympathetic tone to the penis via cortical inhibition of sympathetic projections from the thoracic spinal cord is an important mechanism of psychogenic arousal contributing to penile erection. Sympatholytic drugs administered to the penis may also have erectogenic effects. Protein Kinase A (PKA) works in a fashion similar to PKG and can have similar vasodilatory effects mediated by many of the same mechanisms. PKA may be produced by the action of various other drugs known to be associated with the induction of erections, specifically prostaglandin E1.[7]

ORAL PHARMACOTHERAPY FOR ERECTILE DYSFUNCTION

Dr. Louis Ignarro, Dr. Jacob Rajfer, and colleagues at the University of California, Los Angeles reported that nitric oxide (NO) was the chemical mediator of penile erections in 1992.[5] Dr. Ignarro would later be awarded the Nobel prize for his discovery of the role of NO in vasodilation. Subsequent elucidation of the presence of PDE5I in the penis and discovery of drugs that were selective inhibitors of this enzyme lead to the use of PDE5i as a mainstay of ED treatment, a development that persists to this day.[5,6,11] The creation of an effective and safe oral therapy for ED had profound effects on culture and society that were out of proportion to its medical utility. The advent of PDE5 put sex and sexuality at the forefront of public consciousness and altered the way the world views and discusses sex.

The PDE5 gene is localized to chromosome 4q26.[12,13] It encodes the PDE5 enzyme, which is a homodimer that is about 200 kDa large.[13] PDE5 selectively hydrolyzes only cGMP, in contrast to other PDE isoforms which may catalyze both cAMP and cGMP or just cAMP.[14,15] There are 3 main components to PDE5: the N-terminal fold, the linker region, and the L-terminal helix.[16,17] The N-terminal serves to regulate the catalytic domain and is activated by cGMP binding and phosphorylation. Though there are 3 unique isoforms of PDE5, the catalytic domain is conserved across isoforms. The catalytic domain of PDE5 consists of a core pocket, a lid region, a hydrophobic pocket, and a metal-binding site. The core pocket consists of 3 components: the saddle, which in PDE5I is specific to cGMP, and

2 deep pockets which serve as hydrophilic clamps that "sandwich" cGMP or PDE5i and help potentiate the activity of PDE5i.[18]

PDE5i are currently used on-label in the treatment of both ED and pulmonary hypertension. All currently approved oral pharmacotherapies for ED are of the PDE5i class (**Table 2**). These agents have revolutionized the care of men with ED and improved the quality of life for many men and their partners. All of these drugs have proven efficacy. Limited published data, typically industry-sponsored, tout the advantages or patient preferences of one drug over the others but ultimately it is not clear that anyone is superior across the board for all patients. Selection of PDE5i ultimately comes down to issues of individual patient preferences and (often) access in terms of insurance coverage and costs.

PDE5i have accrued a very favorable safety profile over the past 22+ years they have been available.[19] The only class-specific medical contraindication is the use of concomitant daily dose nitrate therapy as the combination of a nitrate drug and PDE5i may lead to a precipitous drop in blood pressure.[20] PDE5i may be offered to patients who have been prescribed short-acting nitrate medications (eg sublingual nitroglycerin) but it must be made clear to such patients that they should not use these drugs within 24 hours of one another (and possibly 36 in the case of long-acting PDE5i such as tadalafil). Alpha-blocker therapy is a relative contraindication due to the potential for the exacerbation of orthostatic hypotension; this effect is typically mild and can be mitigated by providing an interval between dosing.[21]

Common adverse reactions associated with PDE5i include headaches (12%–15%), flushing (4%–14%), indigestion (<1–10%), stuffy nose/congestion (4%–10%), vision disturbances (0%–5%), and myalgias (rare-4%). Serious side effects include angina, sudden decrease or loss of vision, serious skin reactions, and seizures.[22] The mechanism of these adverse events and whether they

Table 2
Pharmacokinetics of PDE5is available in the United States

Generic Name	Dosage (mg)	Half-Life (hours)	Volume of Distribution (L)	Onset of Action (minutes)
Sildenafil	25–100	3–5	105	60
Vardenafil	5–20	4–6	208	30
Tadalafil	5–20	17.5	60–70	60–120
Avanafil	50–100	6	47–83	30

are truly related to the use of the medication is somewhat unclear; the absolute incidence of these events appears to be quite rare given the long clinical history of PDE5i and the numerous prescriptions dispensed as they became commercially available.

The incidence of priapism with the use of PDE5i, while frequently mentioned in advertising, seems to be lower than for some other common medications that are not explicitly given with the intention of inducing erections (eg trazodone, second-generation antipsychotics).[23] Patients should be counseled on this potential but may be reassured that the likelihood of prolonged erection is low.

A number of clinical syndromes have been reported in association with PDE5i, including Non-Arteric Ischemic Optic Neuropathy (NAION, a source of sudden unilateral vision loss), sensorineural hearing loss, major adverse cardiac events, and melanoma.[23] Evidence in support of these syndromes being clearly linked to PDE5i as an independent risk factor is generally scant with the possible exception of NAION. However, NAION is a rare clinical entity with an estimated annual incidence of about 1 case per 10,000 person years.[24] Given very low baseline probability, even a statistically significant increase in incidence with PDE5i use translates into a very low absolute risk for this condition in PDE5i users.

Sildenafil

Sildenafil was the first PDE5i and was originally synthesized in Sandwich, UK. In 1991, the drug underwent a phase 1 clinical trial for angina. Although the drug did not have efficacy for angina, it was speculated that it may help with erectile problems. In 1992, a multi-dose phase 1 trial in healthy volunteers was conducted in Wales, and erections were noted to be a side effect. The efficacy of the medication was further demonstrated in 1993 during a pilot cross-over study of 16 men, in which "clear differences between sildenafil and placebo" were noted. Phase 2 and Phase 3 clinical trials were conducted between 1994 and 1997. Importantly, the drug demonstrated excellent tolerability, with main adverse effects of headache, flushing, dyspepsia, and congestion. No significant differences were noted in the rate of MI, CVA, or serious cardiac events.[25] In 1998, Viagra was approved as the first oral agent for the treatment of ED.[6]

Sildenafil consists of a pyrazolopyrimidine group (which binds to the core pocket of the catalytic domain of PDE5), an ethoxyphenyl group (which binds to the hydrophobic pocket), and methylpiperazine (which lies in the lid region). This drug has no interaction with the metal-binding site.[26] Inhibition of PDE5 in this fashion leads to the diminished breakdown of cGMP.

Typical dosages of sildenafil are 25 to 100 mg taken on demand. This medication is also sold under the trade name Revatio, administered at 20 mg three times daily for the management of pulmonary hypertension.[27] Sildenafil has a half-life of 3 to 5 hours and a mean apparent steady-state volume of distribution of approximately 105 L.[28] This substantially exceeds the body's total volume of water, which is approximately 42 L. The onset of action typically occurs within 60 minutes. Sildenafil is metabolized by the hepatic P450 enzymes CYP3A4 and CYP2C9. Patients using strong inhibitors of these cytochromes (eg ritonavir, erythromycin, ketoconazole) and those patients with liver failure or severe renal failure experience increased exposure to the drug at a given dose[29]; low starting doses should be considered in these patients. Of note, absorption of sildenafil is slowed by intake of dietary lipids. Thus, this medication should not be taken after a meal, and it is often recommended that this medication be taken preprandially.

Vardenafil

Vardenafil, approved by the FDA in 2003, has similar pharmacokinetics to those of sildenafil. The pyrazolopyrimidine structure of this drug is very similar to sildenafil. Trade names for this medication are Levitra and Staxyn. Typical dosages of vardenafil are 5 to 20 mg. Vardenafil has a half-life of 4 to 6 hours and a mean apparent steady-state volume of distribution of 208 L.[28] Fifty percent of users report getting an erection within 30 minutes of oral dosing. Vardenafil is also available in a sublingually administered 10 mg formulation. Side effects are similar to those listed above.

Vardenafil is predominantly metabolized in the liver via CYP3A4 and like sildenafil the dosing should be adjusted to lower concentrations in patients taking inhibitors of this cytochrome. Similar to sildenafil, absorption of vardenafil is slowed by dietary lipid intake, and it is recommended that vardenafil not be taken after a meal and instead be taken preprandially. Vardenafil is also contraindicated in patients with congenital QT syndrome and also patients using Type IA or III antiarrhythmics.[30] The FDA also recommends against the use of vardenafil in patients on hemodialysis or with severe hepatic failure.[31]

Tadalafil

Tadalafil was initially approved by the FDA in November 2003 and is sold under the brand name Cialis. Its chemical composition creates a rigid structure, which improves the drug's selectivity and at least hypothetically may reduce the likelihood of adverse reactions related to the cross-binding of this drug to other PDE isoforms in other parts of the body. Typical dosages of this medication for ED are 5 to 20 mg on-demand or 2.5 to 5 mg daily dose. Tadalafil has a half-life of 17.5 hours and a mean apparent steady-state volume of distribution of 60 to 70 L.[28] Unlike sildenafil and vardenafil, the absorption of tadalafil is not affected by food intake. Tadalafil is predominantly metabolized by hepatic enzyme CYP3A. Unique features of Tadalafil's structure are that there is a hydrogen bond to the saddle, that methylenedioxyphenyl binds to the Q2 pocket, and that there is extensive interaction with the hydrogen pocket which leads to a rigid structure and decreased entropy with binding. Its patent protection expired from 2017 to 2020.

Of note, tadalafil is the only PDE5i that is approved to be taken daily (the other PDE5i medications are approved for on-demand use). Daily tadalafil has also been shown to be effective for treating benign prostatic hyperplasia that causes lower urinary tract symptoms.[32]

Avanafil

Avanafil was approved by the FDA in 2012 after meeting primary efficacy and safety endpoints and is commercially available as Stendra. The side effect profile is consistent with other existing PDE5is and includes congestion, headache, flushing, and rhinorrhea. Typical dosages are 50 to 200 mg dosed on-demand. Of note, avanafil is purported to have a more rapid onset of action compared with other FDA-approved PDE5i; direct comparison data on the onset of action are limited. The half-life of avanafil is approximately 6 hours and a steady-state volume of distribution of 47 to 83L.[22]

Avanafil is unique structurally in that it contains a chloromethoxy benxylamino group, pyrimidine carboxyamide, and a pyrimidinylmethyl group. Additionally, the catalytic site binding is irrespective of the molecule's orientation.[33] The FDA recommends against the use of avanafil in patients with severe renal or hepatic impairment.[34] At the time of this writing, there is no generic form of this medication available.

Other phosphodiesterase type V inhibitors

Numerous PDE5I have been developed and approved outside of the United States. Examples include mirodenafil, udenafil, and lodenafil. These agents differ in terms of absorption and half-life but estimates of overall efficacy seem similar to what is observed in studies of agents available in the United States. Mirodenafil is sold under the trade name Mvix and has a Tmax of 1.125 hours and a half-life of 2.5 hours. The typical dose is 5 to 100 mg. Udenafil is sold under the trade name Zydena. Its Tmax is 1 to 1.5 hours and its half-life is 11 to 13 hours. Typical dosages are 100 to 200 mg. Lodenafil, sold under the brand name Helleva, has a Tmax of 1.2 hours and a half-life of approximately 2 hours. Its typical dosages are 40 to 80 mg.[22]

INJECTION PHARMACOTHERAPY FOR ERECTILE DYSFUNCTION

Prostaglandin E1 (PgE1, also known as Alprostadil) is the only agent that has been approved by the US FDA as an intracavernosal injection for the management of ED. PgE1 acts to stimulate the production of cAMP and works to induce vasodilation, smooth muscle relaxation, and inhibits platelet aggregation.[35] In studies, intracavernous Alprostadil was either significantly more efficacious or comparable to comparative medications.

Although not formally approved as treatments for ED, a number of other vasodilatory agents have been widely used with good efficacy and safety for the management of ED. The alpha-antagonist phentolamine opposes sympathetic tone to the penis; when administered as an injection this drug has the effect of "removing the brakes" of sympathetic induced vasoconstriction and inducing erection response. The nonspecific PDE inhibitor papaverine is also widely used as an injectable medication for ED; inhibition of PDE in the penis has the net effect of helping to maintain the presence of cGMP and cAMP in the corporal bodies, leading to the preservation of vasodilation by mechanisms addressed in the above section on selective PDE5i. These injectable medications are most commonly used as compounded mixtures combining 2 or 3 agents (known as bimix and trimix, respectively). The cholinergic drug atropine is sometimes added to produce so-called "quadmix." The clinical utility of atropine for the potentiation of penile erection is ambiguous and has not been supported in clinical trials.[36]

To determine the pharmacodynamic profile of intracavernous prostaglandin E1, one study randomized patients to 1 of 5 dose groups (placebo, 2.5 μg, 5 μg, 10 μg, or 20 μg).[37] Interestingly, no significant differences were identified among the various formulations and there was little or no intrapatient variation in dose response. To determine whether "slow" versus "bolus" injection is superior, an open clinical study of 52 patients was performed using the same dosage.[38] This study found that 28 of the 52 patients reported improved penile rigidity with bolus injection rather than slow injection, while 24 patients reported no difference. There seems to be no particular utility to slow administration although the authors of this article did not clarify the functional parameters of a "slow" versus bolus injection.

One study measuring the local intracavernous and peripheral venous concentration curves of papaverine and prostaglandin E1 found that papaverine slowly drains into the systemic circulation and shows a slightly higher level in the peripheral blood approximately 30 to 60 minutes after injection.[39] Prostaglandin E1 shows a much more rapid decrease in the local concentration with no measurable increase in the peripheral concentration, which is presumably due to the short half-time of the drug after it passes the lungs.

Corporal fibrosis/Peyronie's Disease and priapism are the 2 most common serious adverse effects that have been reported in the context of intracavernous injections for ED.

Fibrosis is thought to occur after multiple intracavernosal injections and led to plaques similar to those seen in Peyronie's disease, which may lead to penile curvature and/or worsening ED. One study of 92 patients found that fibrosis occurred in 12% of men after a mean of 10 months of use. Interestingly, this study did not find that fibrosis incidence was associated with the number of injections, but rather, that it is associated with inadequate compression of injection sites after intracavernosal injections.[40] Onset of fibrosis has also been reported after relatively low numbers of injections, in particular when there are complications of injection technique such as subcutaneous injections or hematoma formation.[41] For these reasons it is deemed essential to instruct patients to hold pressure on the injection site as a routine recommendation. Interpretation of the incidence of penile fibrosis/Peyronie's Disease in the context of penile injections is complicated in that many men who use injections have not had a full/rigid penile erection for years before the treatment. For this reason, clinically occult scars/fibrosis may become clinically apparent only after the injection is administered, in which case the injection itself may be falsely implicated as the cause.

Priapism is the most serious common adverse reaction clearly linkable to penile injection therapy. This form of priapism is generally amenable to the irrigation/aspiration of the corporal bodies. It is common practice to also include intracorporal injection of the sympathomimetic agent, preferably phenylephrine due to its selective binding to alpha-1-receptors.[42,43] The efficacy of this therapy for the resolution of priapism declines with the duration of erection so patients should be advised to not delay presentation for therapy in the context of injection-induced priapism. Prevention of priapism in the first place is preferred; for this reason, it is typical to start injection therapy for ED at a very low dose under the direct supervision of a clinician. Dose escalation may be considered under the guidance of the prescribing physician.[1]

INTRAURETHRAL PHARMACOTHERAPY FOR ERECTILE DYSFUNCTION

The mucosal lining of the urethra is permeable to prostaglandin. This property permitted the development of a urethral suppository that delivers concentrated prostaglandin to facilitate erection. The cleverly named Medicated Urethral Suppository for Erections (MUSE) is available in concentrations of 125, 250, 500, and 1000 mcg. The half-life is approximately 5 to 10 minutes, with the onset of action within 30 to 60 minutes.[44]

The most common side effects are urethral burning and pain, reported in 12% of patients. Less common side effects include urethral bleeding (5%), and even less frequently, blurred vision, confusion, dizziness, sweating, and fatigue. Rarely, this medication can cause fainting. MUSE is contraindicated in patients with PGE1 hypersensitivity, and it is recommended to use only with caution in patients with a known urethral stricture, balanitis, severe hypospadias, and curvature, and in patients with acute or chronic urethritis. MUSE should not be used if the man is engaging in vaginal intercourse with a pregnant partner unless a condom is used to mitigate the possible transfer of prostaglandin and subsequent induction of labor.

COMBINATION THERAPY

Combination therapy (most commonly an oral PDE5i and an intracavernosal injection agent) has been suggested as a potential treatment modality for some men who do not have success with a single therapy. This approach is associated with an increased risk of adverse events, in particular priapism. Combination therapy is currently considered off-label use and should be conducted with caution and careful patient selection.

One study of 34 men postradical prostatectomy demonstrated that two-thirds had increased response after combining ICI with a PGE1 with maximum dose PDE5i.[45] This was also demonstrated in a larger study of 93 men, though this study also demonstrated a higher side effect rate when compared with PDE5i use alone.[46] MUSE combined with PDE5i has also been demonstrated to result in improved erections. In a study of 23 men who had undergone prostatectomy and had failed maximum dose sildenafil, 83% reported enhanced erections using combination therapy and reported that approximately 80% of the time they were able to achieve an erection that was sufficient for penetrative intercourse.[22]

FUTURE DIRECTIONS

The efficacy and safety of PDE5i for ED has dampened enthusiasm for the investment required to develop truly novel pharmacotherapies for ED. That said, a number of compounds have been developed to modulate other molecular pathways and/or steps in the NO-cGMP pathway.

Tissue and receptor selectivity is a major roadblock in the development of novel ED pharmacotherapies. The predominance of a specific PDE isoform (PDE5) in the penis makes targeting with a selective inhibitor feasible. Other molecular messengers are more widely expressed in the body, increasing the odds of undesirable side effects, particularly for medications that are dosed orally and subsequently have the potential to be distributed to other body regions.

Soluble guanylate cyclase activators are a promising class of agents for ED that work to stimulate the production of cGMP without reliance on nitric oxide. The promise of these agents largely revolves around use in men who have neurogenic ED (eg related to pelvic surgery or diabetic neuropathy) and hence the absence of the nNOS required for initiating erectile processes. These agents may be beneficial as monotherapy or as an adjunct to PDE5i. Both soluble and insoluble forms are under investigation. Preliminary evidence has been promising.[47] However, none of these agents have at this time achieved approval by a regulatory body and the potential clinical utility of such agents remains ambiguous based on the absence of recent peer-reviewed published data.[48]

The RhoA/Rho Kinase pathway has been of considerable interest as a management strategy for ED for some time. Rho Kinase enhances calcium activity/sensitivity in corporal smooth muscle, leading to increased muscle tone and vasoconstriction.[7,8] Animal studies have suggested a beneficial effect of Rho Kinase Inhibitors (RKI) in the induction of penile erection.[49] *In vitro* studies of human corporal tissues have demonstrated that a specific RKI can induce smooth muscle relaxation, and effect that is potentiated by the addition of a PDE55i.[50] Whether these encouraging findings can be translated into clinical application remains uncertain.

At the time of this writing, there is no pharmacotherapy approved specifically for the management of hypoactive sexual desire disorder in men. Testosterone supplementation is an approved treatment of testosterone deficiency syndrome (TDS) with improvements in a libido a commonly sought beneficial effect of therapy.[51] A discussion of testosterone merits much more consideration than can be incorporated into a review of this nature.

Flibanserin is a novel multifunctional serotonin agonist and antagonist that has been approved as an oral formulation for the management of HSDD in women. This medication acts as a full agonist at postsynaptic 5HT1A receptors and as an antagonist at postsynaptic 5HT2A receptors.[52,53] This medication acts selectively on pyramidal neurons to release dopamine and norepinephrine and to reduce serotonin. Bremelanotide is a melanocortin analog that has been approved as a dopamine receptor agonist for the management of the same condition. A limited body of evidence support the use of these agents for men with HSDD but neither has been submitted for FDA approval in men.[54]

SUMMARY

A wide variety of pharmacotherapies are available for men with ED. The appropriate treatment of a given man depends on the severity of his ED, his comorbid risk factors, and his tolerance for treatment-related adverse events.

DISCLOSURE

F. Nik-Ahd has no financial conflicts of interest. A.W. Shindel has had no commercial conflicts of interest since August 2017.

REFERENCES

1. Burnett AL, Nehra A, Breau RH, et al. Erectile Dysfunction: AUA Guideline. J Urol 2018;200(3): 633–41.
2. Nair R, Sellaturay S, Sriprasad S. The history of ginseng in the management of erectile dysfunction in ancient China (3500-2600 BCE). Indian J Urol 2012;28(1):15–20.
3. Borrelli F, Colalto C, Delfino DV, et al. Herbal Dietary Supplements for Erectile Dysfunction: A Systematic Review and Meta-Analysis. Drugs 2018;78(6): 643–73.
4. Klotz L. How (not) to communicate new scientific information: a memoir of the famous Brindley lecture. BJU Int 2005;96(7):956–7.
5. Rajfer J, Aronson WJ, Bush PA, et al. Nitric oxide as a mediator of relaxation of the corpus cavernosum in

response to nonadrenergic, noncholinergic neurotransmission. N Engl J Med 1992;326(2):90–4.

6. Goldstein I, Lue TF, Padma-Nathan H, et al. Oral sildenafil in the treatment of erectile dysfunction. Sildenafil Study Group. N Engl J Med 1998;338(20):1397–404.

7. Dean RC, Lue TF. Physiology of penile erection and pathophysiology of erectile dysfunction. Urol Clin North Am 2005;32(4):379–95, v.

8. MacDonald SM, Burnett AL. Physiology of Erection and Pathophysiology of Erectile Dysfunction. Urol Clin North Am 2021;48(4):513–25.

9. Aversa A, Francomano D, Lenzi A. Does testosterone supplementation increase PDE5-inhibitor responses in difficult-to-treat erectile dysfunction patients? Expert Opin Pharmacother 2015;16(5):625–8.

10. Steers WD. Pharmacologic treatment of erectile dysfunction. Rev Urol 2002;4(Suppl 3):S17–25.

11. Rajfer J. Discovery of NO in the penis. Int J Impot Res 2008;20(5):431–6.

12. Loughney K, Hill TR, Florio VA, et al. Isolation and characterization of cDNAs encoding PDE5A, a human cGMP-binding, cGMP-specific 3',5'-cyclic nucleotide phosphodiesterase. Gene 1998;216(1):139–47.

13. Yanaka N, Kotera J, Ohtsuka A, et al. Expression, structure and chromosomal localization of the human cGMP-binding cGMP-specific phosphodiesterase PDE5A gene. Eur J Biochem 1998;255(2):391–9.

14. Zhang M, Kass DA. Phosphodiesterases and cardiac cGMP: evolving roles and controversies. Trends Pharmacol Sci 2011;32(6):360–5.

15. Lugnier C. Cyclic nucleotide phosphodiesterase (PDE) superfamily: a new target for the development of specific therapeutic agents. Pharmacol Ther 2006;109(3):366–98.

16. Omori K, Kotera J. Overview of PDEs and their regulation. Circ Res 2007;100(3):309–27.

17. Blount MA, Zoraghi R, Ke H, et al. A 46-amino acid segment in phosphodiesterase-5 GAF-B domain provides for high vardenafil potency over sildenafil and tadalafil and is involved in phosphodiesterase-5 dimerization. Mol Pharmacol 2006;70(5):1822–31.

18. Ahmed WS, Geethakumari AM, Biswas KH. Phosphodiesterase 5 (PDE5): Structure-function regulation and therapeutic applications of inhibitors. Biomed Pharmacother 2021;134:111128.

19. Yafi FA, Sharlip ID, Becher EF. Update on the Safety of Phosphodiesterase Type 5 Inhibitors for the Treatment of Erectile Dysfunction. Sex Med Rev 2018;6(2):242–52.

20. Schwartz BG, Kloner RA. Drug interactions with phosphodiesterase-5 inhibitors used for the treatment of erectile dysfunction or pulmonary hypertension. Circulation 2010;122(1):88–95.

21. Kallidonis P, Adamou C, Kotsiris D, et al. Combination Therapy with Alpha-blocker and Phosphodiesterase-5 Inhibitor for Improving Lower Urinary Tract Symptoms and Erectile Dysfunction in Comparison with Monotherapy: A Systematic Review and Meta-analysis. Eur Urol Focus 2020;6(3):537–58.

22. Charles Welliver WH. Erectile Dysfunction: Medical Treatment. AUA Core Curriculum. 2021. Available at: https://university.auanet.org/core/sexual-medicine-andrology/erectile-dysfunction-medical-treatment/index.cfm. Accessed May 1 2021.

23. Rezaee ME, Gross MS. Are We Overstating the Risk of Priapism With Oral Phosphodiesterase Type 5 Inhibitors? J Sex Med 2020;17(8):1579–82.

24. Hattenhauer MG, Leavitt JA, Hodge DO, et al. Incidence of nonarteritic anterior ischemic optic neuropathy. Am J Ophthalmol 1997;123(1):103–7.

25. Katzenstein LGEB. Viagra (sildenafil citrate) : the remarkable story of the discovery and launch. New York: Medical Information Press; 2001.

26. Jeon YH, Heo YS, Kim CM, et al. Phosphodiesterase: overview of protein structures, potential therapeutic applications and recent progress in drug development. Cell Mol Life Sci CMLS 2005;62(11):1198–220.

27. Michelakis ED, Tymchak W, Noga M, et al. Long-term treatment with oral sildenafil is safe and improves functional capacity and hemodynamics in patients with pulmonary arterial hypertension. Circulation 2003;108(17):2066–9.

28. Mehrotra N, Gupta M, Kovar A, et al. The role of pharmacokinetics and pharmacodynamics in phosphodiesterase-5 inhibitor therapy. Int J Impot Res 2007;19(3):253–64.

29. Highlights of prescribing information. 2014. Available at: https://www.accessdata.fda.gov/drugsatfda_docs/label/2014/20895s039s042lbl.pdf.

30. Corona G, Razzoli E, Forti G, et al. The use of phosphodiesterase 5 inhibitors with concomitant medications. J Endocrinol Invest 2008;31(9):799–808.

31. Langtry HD, Markham A. Sildenafil: a review of its use in erectile dysfunction. Drugs 1999;57(6):967–89.

32. Roehrborn CG, McVary KT, Elion-Mboussa A, et al. Tadalafil Administered Once Daily for Lower Urinary Tract Symptoms Secondary to Benign Prostatic Hyperplasia: A Dose Finding Study. J Urol 2008;180(4):1228–34.

33. Bell AS, Palmer MJ. Novel phosphodiesterase type 5 modulators: a patent survey (2008 - 2010). Expert Opin Ther Pat 2011;21(10):1631–41.

34. Vivus. HIGHLIGHTS OF PRESCRIBING INFORMATION. 2012. Available at: https://www.accessdata.fda.gov/drugsatfda_docs/label/2012/202276s000lbl.pdf.

35. Heidrich H, Breddin HK, Rudofsky G, et al. Cardiopulmonary effects and safety of prostaglandin E1: A review. Int J Angiology 1994;3(1):160–8.

36. Sogari PR, Telöken C, Souto CA. Atropine role in the pharmacological erection test: study of 228 patients. J Urol 1997;158(5):1760–3.

37. Defining the Therapeutic Ratio for Intracavernosal Administration of Prostaglandin E1 (Alprostadil). In: Key clinical trials in erectile dysfunction. London: Springer London; 2007. p. 20–3.

38. de Meyer JM, Oosterlinck W. Influence of the method of intracavernous injection on penile rigidity: a possible pharmacokinetic explanation. Urology 1997;49(2):248–52.

39. van Ahlen H, Peskar BA, Sticht G, et al. Pharmacokinetics of vasoactive substances administered into the human corpus cavernosum. J Urol 1994; 151(5):1227–30.

40. Montorsi F, Guazzoni G, Rigatti P, et al. Pharmacological management of erectile dysfunction. Drugs 1995;50(3):465–79.

41. Chen J, Godschalk M, Katz PG, et al. Peyronie's-like plaque after penile injection of prostaglandin E1. J Urol 1994;152(3):961–2.

42. Bivalacqua TJ, Allen BK, Brock G, et al. Acute Ischemic priapism: an AUA/SMSNA Guideline. J Urol; 2021. 101097ju0000000000002236.

43. Corporation BH. Phenylephrine hydrochloride-phenylephrine hydrochloride injection. 2015. Available at: https://dailymed.nlm.nih.gov/dailymed/lookup.cfm?setid=72348406-e74f-46c5-b93d-34d07cffe1fd.

44. Gesundheit N, Peterson C, Cowley C, et al. The pharmacokinetics of transurethral alprostadil (Prostaglandin E1) in men with erectile dysfunction. J Urol 1997;157(259):A1013.

45. Mydlo JH, Viterbo R, Crispen P. Use of combined intracorporal injection and a phosphodiesterase-5 inhibitor therapy for men with a suboptimal response to sildenafil and/or vardenafil monotherapy after radical retropubic prostatectomy. BJU Int 2005; 95(6):843–6.

46. McMahon CG, Samali R, Johnson H. Treatment of intracorporeal injection nonresponse with sildenafil alone or in combination with triple agent intracorporeal injection therapy. J Urol 1999;162(6):1992–7.

47. Lasker GF, Pankey EA, Kadowitz PJ. Modulation of soluble guanylate cyclase for the treatment of erectile dysfunction. Physiology (Bethesda) 2013;28(4): 262–9.

48. Mónica FZ, Antunes E. Stimulators and activators of soluble guanylate cyclase for urogenital disorders. Nat Rev Urol 2018;15(1):42–54.

49. Hannan JL, Albersen M, Kutlu O, et al. Inhibition of Rho-kinase improves erectile function, increases nitric oxide signaling and decreases penile apoptosis in a rat model of cavernous nerve injury. J Urol 2013; 189(3):1155–61.

50. Uvin P, Albersen M, Bollen I, et al. Additive effects of the Rho kinase inhibitor Y-27632 and vardenafil on relaxation of the corpus cavernosum tissue of patients with erectile dysfunction and clinical phosphodiesterase type 5 inhibitor failure. BJU Int 2017; 119(2):325–32.

51. Mulhall JP, Trost LW, Brannigan RE, et al. Evaluation and Management of Testosterone Deficiency: AUA Guideline. J Urol 2018;200(2):423–32.

52. Stahl SM. Mechanism of action of flibanserin, a multifunctional serotonin agonist and antagonist (MSAA), in hypoactive sexual desire disorder. CNS Spectr 2015;20(1):1–6.

53. Stahl SM, Sommer B, Allers KA. Multifunctional pharmacology of flibanserin: possible mechanism of therapeutic action in hypoactive sexual desire disorder. J Sex Med 2011;8(1):15–27.

54. Diamond LE, Earle DC, Garcia WD, et al. Co-administration of low doses of intranasal PT-141, a melanocortin receptor agonist, and sildenafil to men with erectile dysfunction results in an enhanced erectile response. Urology 2005;65(4):755–9.

Medical Treatment of Disorders of Ejaculation

Tony Chen, MD*, Evan A. Mulloy, MD, Michael L. Eisenberg, MD

KEYWORDS

- Premature ejaculation • Delayed ejaculation • Retrograde ejaculation • Delayed orgasm
- Postorgasmic illness syndrome • Pharmacology

KEY POINTS

- Ejaculation and orgasm are under complex neurohormonal control pathways.
- Studies investigating the effects of pharmacologic therapies for disorders of ejaculation are limited by small sample sizes and inconsistent methodologies including varied definitions of the disease and/or outcome.
- The vast majority of pharmacologic therapies for disordered ejaculation are only available as an off-label treatment.

INTRODUCTION

During the male sexual response cycle, peak arousal culminates in ejaculation and orgasm, 2 distinct and typically simultaneous phenomena. While men normally have a degree of conscious control over the timing of ejaculation during penetrative intercourse, a loss of this control can result in significant distress or embarrassment to the subject or his partner. Ejaculatory dysfunction (EjD) is a range of disorders defined by when ejaculation occurs, if at all, and whether there are any sequelae such as pain. EjD disorders include premature ejaculation (PE), delayed ejaculation (DE), retrograde ejaculation, anejaculation, painful ejaculation, and postorgasmic illness syndrome (POIS). EjD is not rare conditions but are less understood and less studied compared with sexual conditions such as erectile dysfunction (ED). The biochemical, myological, and neurohormonal pathways involved in ejaculation and orgasm have yet to be fully elucidated, and as a result, pharmacotherapy options remain limited and mostly lacking in approval from the United States Food and Drug Administration (FDA). Standard treatment by specialists for the pharmacologic treatment of these conditions is currently prescribed in an off-label fashion. This article will review the physiology of ejaculation, before reviewing currently prescribed pharmacologic treatments for EjD with a particular focus on the 2 most prevalent disorders, PE and DE.

PHYSIOLOGY OF ORGASM AND EJACULATION

The 4 stages of the sexual response cycle progress linearly in men from desire, arousal, climax, and resolution. Normally, the climax that results from a progressive accumulation of sexual arousal and stimulation comprises ejaculation and orgasm, which are 2 separate phenomena.

Ejaculation is made up of two phases: emission and expulsion. Emission is a coordinated process mediated by the sympathetic nervous system via the hypogastric nerve and pelvic plexus during which the bladder neck closes, and seminal fluid from the prostate and seminal vesicles, and sperm via the epididymis and vas deferens are deposited in the posterior urethra.[1] Expulsion, sometimes referred to as ejection, is the second phase when somatic nervous system-mediated rhythmic contractions of the ischiocavernosus muscle and bulbospongiosus muscle lead to antegrade forceful

Stanford University School of Medicine, Center for Academic Medicine, Urology -5656, 453 Quarry Road, Palo Alto, CA 94304, USA
* Corresponding author.
E-mail address: chentony@stanford.edu

Urol Clin N Am 49 (2022) 219–230
https://doi.org/10.1016/j.ucl.2021.12.001
0094-0143/22/© 2021 Elsevier Inc. All rights reserved.

expulsion of seminal fluid from the urethra.[1] A small group of neurons located in the ventral horns of the S2–S4 sacral spinal cord, sometimes referred to as Onuf's nucleus, innervate the striated muscles of the pelvic floor and are involved in coordinating expulsion.[2] Gabaninergic neurons within the spinal cord sometimes referred to as the "spinal ejaculation generator" also play a significant role in coordinating and integrating stimuli from cerebral and central origins to trigger the ejaculatory reflex.[3]

Orgasm is one of the most pleasurable sensations known to man and is mediated by cerebral processing of peripheral sensory nerve signaling that occurs with the contraction of accessory sexual organs and the release of distal urethral pressure that typically accompanies ejaculation.[4] However, the fact that men often report normal orgasm after radical prostatectomy suggests our understanding of the triggers remains incomplete.[5]

Neurotransmitter and hormonal control of ejaculation and orgasm are complex due to the existence of multiple receptor types and sites of action, and much of what is known is derived from animal studies. Generally speaking, oxytocin and dopamine stimulate ejaculation and orgasm. Serotonin (5-HT), nitric oxide (NO) and gamma-aminobutyric acid (GABA), and opioid-receptor agonist signaling inhibit ejaculation and orgasm[6–8] Hyperthyroidism has been associated with PE, whereas hypothyroidism has been associated with DE. Testosterone plays a central role in modulating the sexual response, and in ejaculation specifically, high levels have been associated with PE and low levels with DE.[9]

PREMATURE EJACULATION

There are 2 types of PE: lifelong and acquired. Lifelong PE is defined in the American Urologic Association (AUA)/Sexual Medicine Society of North America (SMSNA) 2021 clinical guideline as "poor ejaculatory control, associated bother, and ejaculation within about 2 minutes of initiation of penetrative sex that has been present as sexual debut," whereas acquired PE is "consistently poor ejaculatory control, associated bother, and ejaculation latency that is markedly reduced from prior sexual experience during penetrative sex.[10] Estimates of PE prevalence vary widely depending on research methodology and definition of PE, and range from less than 5% in carefully selected symptomatic men with evidence of distress, to as high as 50%.[11,12] PE treatments are typically aimed at increasing the intravaginal ejaculation latency time (IELT), the time between the beginning of vaginal penetration and the start of intravaginal ejaculation during penetrative sex.[13] Several pharmacologic therapies have been used in the treatment of PE, including the use of topical anesthetic agents, selective serotonin reuptake inhibitors (SSRIs), tricyclic antidepressants (TCAs), tramadol, and alpha-adrenergic blockers.

Topical Anesthetics

The first known pharmacologic treatments of PE used topical anesthetics such as benzocaine, prilocaine, or lidocaine to reduce sensory input from the glans penis.[14] Reducing sensitivity in the glans penis potentially minimizes afferent stimuli which in turn inhibit the spinal reflex arc involved in ejaculation.[15] Topical agents are today considered among first-line treatment options for PE. These agents may come in ointment, gel, spray, or topical wipe forms. Benefits of this modality include "on-demand" usage and avoidance of adverse effects (AEs) on ejaculatory or orgasmic sensation.[16]

Topical anesthetics (AUA guideline first-line therapy) are often used in a eutectic formulation, which mixes medications in an emulsion which results in a lower melting point than its individual components, which allows for a higher concentration of absorbable medication and penetration of intact skin.[15] Eutectic mixture of local anesthetics (EMLA) cream is a 1:1 mixture of prilocaine 2.5% and lidocaine 2.5% in cream base. A placebo-controlled study of 40 patients applying cream 20 to 45 minutes before intercourse found significant improvement of IELT in subjects of almost 9 minutes over baselines by applying EMLA cream compared with placebo, and importantly, that the optimal time of application was 20 minutes before sex in the intervention arm.[17] One of the largest double-blind trials of 42 men studying EMLA Cream usage reported a 5.6-fold increase in IELT compared with no improvement with placebo.[18] EMLA cream is available by prescription in the United States and has approval from the Food and Drug Administration (FDA) for use on normal intact skin for local analgesia, but not specifically for PE.[19]

The first topical therapy explicitly approved for use in PE treatment is FortacinTM, A metered-dose spray containing a eutectic mixture of prilocaine 50 mg/mL and lidocaine 150 mg/mL that earned regulatory approval in the European Union and sold in the United Kingdom in 2016.[20] During clinical development, Fortacin was also known by the names PSD502 and Topical Eutectic Mixture for Premature Ejaculation (TEMPE). Two double-blind, placebo-controlled phase III studies of PSD502 applied 5 minutes before intercourse demonstrated 4.6- to 6.3-fold increases in IELT as well as significant improvements in survey-based measures of ejaculatory control and sexual satisfaction compared with placebo.[21,22] There were no systemic side-effects of this topical anesthetic delivery system and local adverse reactions were typically mild. 4.5% of patients reported genital hypoesthesia, and 4.4% reported ED, and 3.9% of female partners reported vulvovaginal burning, but discontinuation rates due to these side effects were rare in the 0.2% to 0.5% range.[20] As of this writing, Fortacin is not available in the United States.

Several over the counter treatment options are available in the United States in local and online pharmacies. K-Y© Duration Spray for Him, Promescent©, Stud-100©, and Hims© Delay Spray are examples of lidocaine-based sprays with a strength of 10 mg of lidocaine per spray and an instruction to apply 3 to 10 sprays in intervals of 5 to 15 minutes before intercourse. A single-blind placebo-controlled trial of 150 lifelong patients with PE using a lidocaine 5% spray containing 5 to 10 mg of lidocaine over 8 weeks reported an improvement of IELT from 0.61 minutes on average to 6.26 minutes.[23] Mild local AEs such as penile numbness, local burning sensation, and genital erythema were reported in less than 5% of subjects, and no systemic effects or transference to partner were seen. Roman© Swipes and Preboost are medicated benzocaine 4% wipes, which patients apply to the penis 5 minutes before sex to allow the solution to dry. Preboost has been shown in a placebo-controlled trial of 21 men using the product for 8 weeks, to lead to an improvement of IELT from an average of 1.25 minutes to 5.5 minutes. No transference of benzocaine to the receiving partner was observed and only local AEs of mild skin irritation was reported.[24]

Finally, medicated condoms are also available in the United States for the topical treatment of PE. No controlled trials are available to evaluate the efficacy and safety of these products. Examples include Durex Mutual Climax, Durex Extended Pleasure, and Trojan Extended Pleasure, which all use Benzocaine ranging from 4% to 5% concentrations. Potential side effects disclosed on product inserts include possible rash, irritation, burning itching, or ED.[15]

Selective Serotonin Reuptake Inhibitors and Tricyclic Antidepressants

Oral medication first-line treatments for PE include the class of drugs called SSRIs and TCAs. These classes of medications inhibit axonal reabsorption and clearance of 5-HT in the synaptic cleft of central serotonergic neurons which increases extracellular levels of 5-HT and enhances postsynaptic membrane 5-HT receptor activity.[25]

Off-label use of SSRIs (sertraline 50–200 mg, fluoxetine 20–40 mg, citalopram 20–40 mg, paroxetine 10–40 mg), and TCAs (clomipramine 12.5–50 mg) that are available by prescription in the United States have been studied for their potential effects in the setting of PE treatment. A 2004 meta-analysis of 79 studies published between 1943 and 2003 concluded that the abovementioned pharmacologic interventions significantly improved IELT, averaging an increase of 1 to 5 minutes. The improvements were comparable among clomipramine, fluoxetine, citalopram, and sertraline, but paroxetine resulted in the most significant ejaculation delay, increasing IELT 8.8-fold over baseline.[26]

Administration of these drugs can be conducted on a continual or on-demand basis. With daily dosing, IELT improvement can occur within 5 to 10 days of treatment initiation, but maximal therapeutic effect is not typically seen until 2 to 3 weeks.[27] On-demand dosing, on the other hand, is given 3 to 6 hours before intercourse and shown to be moderately efficacious but offers less substantial IELT improvement than daily dosing.[28] On-demand dosing can be initiated on its own after a trial of daily dosing, or in addition to a low-dose daily regimen.[29] On-demand dosing may be more suitable for men who engage in sexual intercourse less frequently, whereas daily dosing may offer men in regularly sexually active relationships more convenience.

Importantly, AEs of SSRIs used in PE treatment occur approximately in 1 in 3 individuals.[27] Common AEs can include fatigue, headache, nausea, diarrhea, increased perspiration.[30] Significant mood changes including increased agitation have been reported in small numbers of patients as well. Decreased libido and ED, while reported in SSRI safety studies in the treatment of clinical depression, are less frequently seen in nondepressed men receiving SSRI treatment of PE.[31] TCAs are less selective in the inhibition of reuptake and have additional anticholinergic, histaminergic, and adrenergic side effects including dry mouth, dizziness, blurred vision, tachycardia, and orthostatic hypotension.[32] Off-label SSRI use is thus typically favored over TCA clomipramine use due to these differences in AEs.

More dangerous but less common AE's from SSRI therapy include upper-gastrointestinal bleeding especially when used with nonsteroidal inflammatory drugs,[33] priapism,[34] and serotonin syndrome, which is a potentially life-threatening condition characterized by clonus, agitation, fever, seizure, and rhabdomyolysis requiring immediate cessation of serotonergic medications and immediate medical attention.[35]

In patients who have taken SSRIs continuously for a month, sudden reduction or cessation of therapy may precipitate withdrawal symptoms that may include flu-like symptoms, nausea, vertigo, sensory disturbances, or mood disturbances.[36] Thus, patients should be counseled that changes in SSRI therapy should be made with their prescribing physician's guidance.

SSRI treatment of PE should be avoided in men with a history of bipolar depressive disorder due to the risk of triggering mania.[37] SSRIs should also be avoided in adolescent men under the age of 18 due to an increased risk of suicide attempt and suicidal ideation.[38] Men with depression over the age of 18 were not found to have a higher risk of suicidality when treated with antidepressants compared with placebo, but the AUA recommends exercising caution nonetheless in prescribing SSRIs to men with PE and comorbid depression.[10] Suicidal ideation has not been reported in trials of SSRIs to treat PE in men without depression.

Caution should also be taken when considering prescribing SSRIs to treat PE in men who are actively trying to conceive. Chronic SSRI use has been linked to elevated DNA fragmentation levels and impairments in sperm concentration, motility, and morphology. desire fertility.[39,40] While semen parameters seem to recover within 1 to 2 months of medication discontinuation, appropriate counseling of patients regarding the potential for fertility-related AEs at the time of therapy initiation is recommended.[41]

Dapoxetine is a short half-life SSRI that is rapidly acting and has received regulatory approval for the treatment of PE in over 50 countries, but is not yet available in the United States, which limits its clinical utility at this time. Data from randomized placebo-controlled trials from over 6000 men with lifelong or acquired PE in over 25 countries demonstrated that 30 mg or 60 mg doses taken on-demand 1 to 3 hours before penetrative intercourse resulted in 2.5- to 3-fold increases in IELT.[42] Common AEs included headache, nausea, diarrhea, dizziness. Notably, there were no reported changes in mood, suicidality, anxiety, or withdrawal symptoms.

Tramadol

Men who have failed first-line therapies may be considered for on-demand, off-label tramadol hydrochloride for the treatment of PE. Tramadol is a centrally acting μ-opioid agonist that also has peripheral inhibition of 5-HT and norepinephrine reuptake.[43] Because of tramadol's rapid absorption when taken orally, and short half-life of 6 hours,

it has the appropriate pharmacokinetic characteristics of an on-demand treatment of PE.[44]

The majority of studies investigating Tramadol's effects on IELT outcomes are open-label studies that report heterogeneous efficacy rates. A 2013 study of 300 men with lifelong PE from Egypt taking doses of either 25 mg, 50 mg, or 100 mg of on-demand Tramadol after a 4 week washout period demonstrated a dose-dependent 10- to 20-fold increase in IELT.[45] A well-designed European phase 3 randomized double-blind placebo-controlled multi-site trial of 62 mg and 89 mg tramadol on-demand doses demonstrated a moderate improvement in IELT compared with placebo of 2.4- and 2.5-fold, respectively.[46] An open-label crossover study of 35 men with lifelong PE comparing long-term daily paroxetine 20 mg therapy with on-demand tramadol 50 mg showed that IELT increased by 7-fold in the tramadol arm and 11-fold in the paroxetine arm before crossover. After crossover, IELT increase in the Tramadol arm decreased to 5-fold above baseline, whereas the IELT increase in the daily paroxetine arm continued to increase to a maximum of 22-fold.[47] Two meta-analyses from 2015 concluded that on-demand Tramadol is effective in treating PE compared with placebo, and well-tolerated, particularly in the 25 and 50 mg dosing.[48,49]

Tramadol is generally well-tolerated with few AEs that occur in a dose-dependent fashion. At lower doses, AEs commonly include somnolence, dry mouth, and gastrointestinal symptoms such as nausea and vomiting. Rare cases of tramadol causing serotonin syndrome have also been reported.[50]

While not studied specifically in doses used for PE treatment, Tramadol's potential for addiction, abuse, and dependency are considered low.[51] Abuse rates of tramadol mirror those of nonsteroidal antiinflammatory drugs and tend to be much lower than opioid medications such as hydrocodone, benzodiazepines, and oxycodone.[52,53] Among patients taking higher doses of Tramadol than typically used for PE, withdrawal symptoms have been reported following only 3 to 4 days of drug therapy.[54] Despite these reassurances, clinicians are recommended to exercise caution and vigilance when considering prescribing tramadol for the management of PE.

Alpha-Blockers

Alpha-1 adrenergic receptor antagonists (also known as alpha-blockers) are another off-label option for men who have failed first-line therapies for PE. This drug class is commonly used to treat lower urinary tract symptoms (LUTS) in men with or without benign prostatic hyperplasia (BPH). A well-known side effect of alpha-blocker therapy is a decrease in ejaculatory volume due to decreased seminal emission by the direct inhibitory action of the drug on alpha-1 subtype-A adrenergic receptors in the seminal vesicles.[55] Several studies investigating various alpha-blockers have shown benefit in the treatment of PE, but have inherent limitations in methodologies including small sample sizes, broad inclusion criteria, variable PE definitions, and variable outcomes.

A small study of 8 patients by Sato and colleagues given on-demand silodosin 4 mg 2 hours before sexual intercourse demonstrated an improvement of IELT from a baseline of 3.4 to 10.1 minutes. Unfortunately, 75% of the patients had concomitant ED, and were instructed to use the silodosin with or without phosphodiesterase type-5 inhibitors (PDE5is), making it difficult to discern the specific impact of silodosin alone.[56] Akin and colleagues studied 5 different types of alpha-blockers among 108 men with PE and showed that with tamsulosin hydrochloride 0.4 mg, alfuzosin 10 mg, silodosin 4 mg, terazosin 5 mg, and doxazosin mesylate 4 mg, IELT improved significantly from a baseline ranging from 18.8 to 23.6 seconds to a posttreatment range of 80 to 151 seconds with improvement in quality of life survey responses as well.[57] The largest improvement was seen in the Silodosin treatment group. In a separate placebo-controlled study of 64 patients with PE who were dissatisfied with on-demand dapoxetine 30 mg, silodosin 4 mg given 3-h before intercourse was shown to significantly improve IELT over placebo from 0.55 minutes to 4.5 minutes.[58]

Alpha-blockers are generally safe but can have systemic side effects such as orthostatic hypotension, dizziness, rhinitis, and diminished ejaculation or anejaculation. Ejaculatory side effects are more commonly seen in alpha-1 subtype-A-selective blockers such as tamsulosin and silodosin with rates as high as 30%, compared with rates lower than 1.5% for nonselective alpha-blockers such as terazosin, doxazosin, or alfuzosin.[59]

Phosphodiesterase Type-5 Inhibitors

PDE5is such as sildenafil, tadalafil, and vardenafil are well-known effective treatments for ED. These drugs have also been investigated as off-label treatments for PE either alone or in combination with other drugs. PDE5is modulate the NO/cyclic guanosine monophosphate (cGMP) pathway which enhances central and peripheral inhibitory signaling in the urogenital tract and may, in turn, inhibit seminal vesicle secretory activity and smooth muscle contraction.[60,61] Data on efficacy are mixed and limited by inadequately designed studies. A double-blind, placebo-controlled trial of sildenafil in men with PE did not show any difference in IELT, but did show improved confidence levels and perceived ejaculatory control.[62] A separate placebo-controlled study looking at vardenafil reported significant improvements in IELT from a baseline of 0.6 to 4.5 minutes in the treatment group versus 0.7 to 0.9 in the placebo group.[63] A 2017 systematic review of 15 randomized controlled trials concluded that on-demand PDE5is are more effective than placebo, and that PDE5is combined with SSRIs are more effective than SSRIs alone.[64] However, concerns over the methodological flaws and significant outcome heterogeneity of these studies limit the ability to recommend PDE5is as monotherapy for patients with PE alone without comorbid ED.[65]

Future Directions

While there are many effective treatments for PE, side effects may lead to discontinuation, which continues to generate interest in investigations of novel therapeutics.

Modafinil is a wake-promoting drug used to alleviate daytime sleepiness and acts on the central nervous system through poorly understood pathways involving dopamine, serotonin, and GABA signaling.[66] Animal studies have supported modafinil as a possible treatment of PE and 1 uncontrolled proof-of-concept study of on-demand 100 mg modafinil in 55 patients with lifelong PE showed a modest improvement of ILET from approximately 25 seconds to 50 seconds.[67]

Oxytocin antagonists are another class of drug being investigated as a potential treatment of PE. Oxytocin is a peptide hormone that is released by the posterior pituitary at the time of orgasm and mediates contractility through action on oxytocin receptors present in the human epididymis.[68] Two separate Phase II randomized controlled trials of cligosiban, a small-molecule oxytocin receptor antagonist capable of crossing the blood–brain barrier, had mixed results. One study reported an increase of IELT by 61 seconds in the treatment group versus 16.4 seconds in the placebo group, and the other trial with no differences was observed. The medication was well-tolerated without significant AEs. Differences in study design may explain the discrepancy.

Summary

PE is a common disorder of ejaculation that can present either as a lifelong or acquired condition. First-line therapies currently include topical anesthetics, and on-demand or daily SSRIs or clo-mipramine. Second-line therapies include tramadol hydrochloride, or alpha-1 adrenergic antagonists. There are no FDA-approved treatments for PE in the United States as of publication, and medicines are prescribed in an off-label fashion.

DELAYED EJACULATION

DE is a condition in which there is difficulty in obtaining ejaculation/orgasm. This can happen for numerous reasons, inherently making the precise definition of the condition difficult. The International Consultation on Sexual Dysfunctions (ICSD) defines DE as an IELT beyond 20 to 25 minutes of sexually associated with negative personal feelings such as bother or distress.[69] Other classifications of the disorder, such as in Diagnostic and Statistical Manual of Mental Disorders, do not require an objective minimum latency time, but rather require the disorder be present in a majority of sexual encounters and occur persistently over several months.[70] In 2015, the ICSD further recognized 2 types of DE: lifelong and acquired. Lifelong DE is DE occurring in all or almost all (75%–100%) of sexual experiences and acquired DE occurs in at least 50% of sexual experiences after the period of normal ejaculatory function. All definitions require associated symptoms of bothering to the patient to meet criteria and that there are no other comorbid or concomitant diagnoses present that could better explain the disorder.

The prevalence of DE is estimated at 2% to 4% in the general population of sexually active men though the prevalence may increase with age.[71,72] In the European Male Aging Study, 6% of men aged 40 to 79 experienced severe orgasmic/ejaculatory impairment.[73]

DE is associated with other medical conditions including ED, LUTS, chronic/prostatitis/chronic pelvic pain syndrome, depression, testosterone deficiency, and aging.[74–76] Commonly prescribed medications associated with DE include antidepressants, opioid medicines, and alpha-blockers (**Table 1**).[77–79] The mechanism by which delayed orgasm occurs is variable and may be due to inadequate sexual stimulation which may occur in men with penile neuropathy or suppression of central nervous system arousal response. Common causes of the latter include alcohol, antipsychotics, and opioids. Some urologic procedures such as transurethral resection of the prostate or radical prostatectomy may contribute to DE as well. In addition to biological variables, there are also psychosocial factors such as relationship stress that may affect the male sexual response and disrupt climax.[79]

DE is a clinical diagnosis. The initial evaluation of the male with DE should include a medical, relationship, and sexual history and a focused physical examination. If DE is suspected, then a clinician should attempt to determine if it is lifelong or acquired and if it is situational or generalized. The examination should include an assessment for physical signs of metabolic disarray or hypogonadism including a male genital exam assessing penile morphology, testicular size, and genital skin condition.[10] A serum testosterone is an adjunct test if a man is suspected to be hypogonadal. Over 25% of men with DE have hypogonadism.[76] Routine imaging of men with DE is likely unnecessary. However, one study obtained functional MRIs and identified abnormal brain activity and increased neuron activation (in both the right occipital lobe and hippocampus) in men with DE and found, areas that may be areas of future pharmacologic therapy for DE.[80]

Psychogenic Treatments

Management of men with DE can be multi-factorial and may involve psychologically and physiologically based treatments. A mental health professional specializing in sexual health play an integral role in treating these patients. There are multiple psychogenic approaches available for men and are dependent on identifying any psychosexual irregularities that may be present, such as comparing ejaculatory patterns between masturbation and partnered experiences. In men whereby there is a discrepancy between penile and psychological stimulation between masturbation and sexual activity with their partner, penile vibratory therapy may help may restore ejaculation and orgasm. Mulhall and colleagues noted the restoration of ejaculation and orgasm in 72% of anejaculatory men within 6 months of initiating penile vibratory stimulation during intercourse.[81] The routine clinical implication of this practice is unclear given the lack of other robust evidence but may be of benefit for some men. If there is a discrepancy between masturbatory fantasy and reality of sexual intercourse with the partner, adapting masturbatory habits to what is reflective of partnered sex may help in restoring ejaculation.[82] Behavioral modifications are low risk. These include elements such as using different positions during intercourse or alternative sex practices (such as oral sex) and are implemented to improve psychosexual arousal and pleasure. Psychological conflicts such as fear of impregnation or hurting or defiling one's partner with sex and ejaculation may be addressed and mediated to help normalize ejaculatory habits.[82,83] Regardless of the

Table 1
Common medications and substances associated with delayed ejaculation

Medication class	Examples
Alcohol	Ethanol
Alpha-Blockers	Alfuzosin, Doxazosin, Silodosin, Tamsulosin, Terazosin
Anti-Hypertensives	Labetalol, Methyldopa, Prazosin, Phenoxybenzamine,
Anti-inflammatories	Naproxen
Antiepileptics	Carbamazepine, Pregabalin
Antipsychotics	Chlorpromazine, Haloperidol,
Anxiolytic Medicine	Alprazolam, Chlordiazepoxide
Cannabis	
Diuretics	Thiazides
GABA Transaminase Inhibitors	Aminocaproic acid
Monoamine Oxidase Inhibitors	Isocarboxazid, Pargyline, Phenelzine, Tranylcypromine
Muscle Relaxers	Baclofen
Neuroleptics	Mesoridazine
Opiates	Methadone, Tramadol, Oxycodone, Hydrocodone
Selective Norepinephrine-Serotonin Inhibitors	Duloxetine, Venlafaxine,
Selective Serotonin Reuptake Inhibitors	Citalopram, Escitalopram, Fluoxetine, Paroxetine, Sertraline
Tricyclic Anti-Depressants	Amitriptyline, Amoxapine, Clomipramine, Desipramine, Imipramine, Nortriptyline, Mirtazapine

approach used, it is imperative that men maintain open communication between their partners about sexual needs and desires to facilitate improvement in ejaculatory patterns and sexual dysfunction.

Medical Therapy

There are no FDA-approved pharmacologic therapies to lower the ejaculatory threshold and decrease latency time. However, there are a number of medications associated with DE and cessation of these may be considered. However, it is important to consider the risks and benefits of medication cessation before doing so with the physical and psychological well-being of the patient being the top priority. Consultation with other treating providers is also helpful. In men whereby cessation may not be possible, adjusting or offering adjunct therapy may be of benefit. For example, in men treated with SSRIs or TCA for depression, dose adjustments may be made after shared decision making discussion. In addition, augmenting therapy with agents such as buspirone, bupropion, cyproheptadine bethanechol either as an adjunct or alternative has been shown to improve orgasmic dysfunction in these men.[84–87]

While there are no FDA-approved medications for DE, there are several medicines that have been described for the treatment of DE including bupropion, oxytocin, pseudoephedrine, ephedrine, midodrine, bethanechol, yohimbine, cabergoline, and imipramine. Cabergoline (dopamine agonist) and bupropion (norepinephrine-dopamine reuptake inhibitor) are more commonly used.[88] One randomized trial comparing bupropion 150 mg or 300 mg a day to placebo in nondepressed men and women showed significant improvement in orgasm delay and up to 70% of subjects reported improvement in sexual function overall.[89] Lipshultz and colleagues note that 0.5 mg cabergoline twice weekly resulted in subjective orgasm improvement in 87/131(66.4%) of men.[90] The evidence from all of the studies involving the pharmacologic therapies for DE are limited and less robust compared with those for PE. In fact, the American Urologic Association panel that developed recent guidelines for ejaculatory disorders rendered "insufficient evidence to assess risk-benefit ratio" on oral medical therapies for DE though can be offered to appropriately selected patients through shared decision making that is in line with the patient's own personal principles.[10]

Nonmedical Therapy

There have been other therapies suggested for DE including pudendal nerve release, platelet-rich plasma, and intracavernosal injection. As with other therapies; robust, published, peer-reviewed data supporting these modalities do not exist. As such, these therapies are not recommended outside the context of a clinical trial.

Testosterone Supplementation

25% of men with DE have testosterone deficiency; however, it is unclear if testosterone supplementation helps restore ejaculatory function. One randomized control trial failed to find any improvement in ejaculatory function in men treated with 2% testosterone solution compared with placebo.[91] There are limitations to this trial in that few of the men in the treatment group achieved normal testosterone levels. Men with DE and normal testosterone levels should not be offered testosterone replacement therapy. Testosterone replacement may be offered to men with DE and other symptoms of hypogonadism such as fatigue, low energy, and low libido. In men who are treated with testosterone, the goal therapeutic range is within the 50th percentile and therapy in men who do not have subjective symptomatic improvement within 90 days should be discontinued. As with other treatments for DE, initiating testosterone therapy should be conducted through a shared decision-making model with adherence to society testosterone therapy guidelines.[92]

Summary

DE is a disorder that can cause significant physical and emotional distress for sexually active men and their partners. The etiology of this disorder is multifactorial involving both physiologic and psychological variables. Much like PE, treatment of this disorder ranges from psychosocial interventions to pharmacologic therapy. Further research is needed to discern the etiologies of DE to allow the development of novel, rational therapies.

OTHER EJACULATORY DISORDERS

Retrograde ejaculation is a condition in which semen flows into the bladder instead of antegrade through the urethra during ejaculation. This occurs when the bladder neck does not close properly during the emission phase of ejaculation and may be secondary to bladder neck surgery, a side effect of pharmacologic treatment, or nerve injury from insults such as diabetic neuropathy or retroperitoneal surgery.[93] First-line medical treatments comprise of off-label sympathomimetic (synephrine, pseudoephedrine hydrochloride, ephedrine sulfate, phenylpropanolamine, midodrine) or anticholinergic (imipramine hydrochloride, brompheniramine maleate) drugs that enhance bladder outlet resistance and encourage antegrade propulsion of semen. Studies are unfortunately limited by small sample sizes and case reports. A systematic review of available studies reported rates of antegrade ejaculation are higher in patients receiving a combination of sympathomimetics (39%) and anticholinergics compared with either drug class alone (28% and 22%, respectively).

POIS is a rare cluster of postejaculatory flu-like symptoms that typically last between 2 and 7 days.[94] Hypotheses on the pathophysiology of POIS have postulated an allergic or autoimmune etiology that causes a malreaction to a man's own seminal fluid, as evidenced by positive skin-prick tests on patients with POIS.[95] Others have postulated that the symptoms mimic an opioid-withdrawal-like state possibly resulting from the depletion of a patient's reserve of endogenous opioid with orgasm.[96] Due to the condition being underdiagnosed and underreported, there are no standard pharmacologic treatments. Studies of potential treatments are limited to small case series and case reports, and have included antihistamines, SSRIs, benzodiazepines, and NSAID therapy.

Dysejaculation, ejaculodynia, or painful ejaculation is a condition that is not well understood, but is thought to have both psychogenic and organic components. Conditions such as chronic prostatitis, urogenital tract infection, cancer, postsurgical complications may lead to dysejaculation.[93] Management depends on treating suspected underlying causes, and no specific pharmacotherapy exists.

SUMMARY

Ejaculation and orgasm are physiologic sequelae of sexual arousal that are under complex neuronal and hormonal control. The most common disorders are PE and DE, of which effective but off-label medical treatments are available. Additional research to obtain a deeper understanding of the involved pathways are needed and may potentially lead to novel therapies.

CLINICS CARE POINTS

- Men with ejaculatory disorders such as premature ejaculation and delayed ejaculation should be considered for referral to a mental health professional specializing in sexual health counseling and therapy.

- First-line medical therapies for premature ejaculation include selective serotonin reuptake inhibitors (SSRIs), certain tricyclic antidepressants (TCAs), and topical anesthetics.
- Men with delayed ejaculation and concomitant testosterone deficiency may be offered treatment to normalize testosterone levels.

DISCLOSURE

M.L. Eisenberg advises the following companies: Dadi, Ro, Sandstone Diagnostics, Underdog Fertility, and Hannah Life Technologies. T. Chen and E. Mulloy have nothing to disclose.

REFERENCES

1. Giuliano F, Clément P. Physiology of ejaculation: emphasis on Serotonergic control. Eur Urol 2005; 48(3):408–17.
2. Schellino R, Boido M, Vercelli A. The Dual nature of Onuf's Nucleus: Neuroanatomical Features and Peculiarities, in Health and Disease. Front Neuroanat 2020; 14. https://doi.org/10.3389/fnana.2020.572013.
3. Chéhensse C, Facchinetti P, Bahrami S, et al. Human spinal ejaculation generator. Ann Neurol 2017; 81(1):35–45.
4. El-Hamd M, Saleh R, Majzoub A. Premature ejaculation: an update on definition and pathophysiology. Asian J Androl 2019;21(5):425.
5. Koeman M, van Driel MF, Weijmar Schultz WCM, et al. Orgasm after radical prostatectomy. BJU Int 1996;77(6):861–4.
6. Hull EM, Lumley LA, Matuszewich L, et al. The roles of nitric oxide in sexual function of male rats. Neuropharmacology 1994;33(11):1499–504.
7. Clement P, Giuliano F. Physiology and Pharmacology of ejaculation. Basic Clin Pharmacol Toxicol 2016;119:18–25.
8. Alwaal A, Breyer BN, Lue TF. Normal male sexual function: emphasis on orgasm and ejaculation. Fertil Steril 2015;104(5):1051–60.
9. Corona G, Jannini EA, Vignozzi L, et al. The hormonal control of ejaculation. Nat Rev Urol 2012;9(9):508–19.
10. AW. Shindel, SE Althof, SCarrier, et al, Disorders of ejaculation: an AUA/SMSNA Guieline. https://doi.org/10.1097/JU.0000000000002392.
11. Althof SE, McMahon CG, Waldinger MD, et al. An update of the International Society of sexual Medicine's Guidelines for the Diagnosis and treatment of premature ejaculation (PE). Sex Med 2014;2(2): 60–90. https://doi.org/10.1002/sm2.28.
12. Shindel AW, Nelson CJ, Naughton CK, et al. Premature ejaculation in infertile couples: prevalence and correlates. J Sex Med 2008;5(2):485–91.
13. Waldinger MD, Quinn P, Dilleen M, et al. A multinational population survey of intravaginal ejaculation latency time. J Sex Med 2005;2(4):492–7.
14. Schapiro B. Premature ejaculation: a review of 1130 Cases. J Urol 1943;50(3):374–9.
15. Butcher MJ, Zubert T, Christiansen K, et al. Topical Agents for premature ejaculation: a review. Sex Med Rev 2020;8(1):92–9.
16. Morales A, Barada J, Wyllie MG. A review of the current status of topical treatments for premature ejaculation. BJU Int 2007;100(3):493–501.
17. Atikeler MK, Gecit I, Senol FA. Optimum usage of prilocaine-lidocaine cream in premature ejaculation. Andrologia 2002;34(6):356–9.
18. Busato W, Galindo CC. Topical anaesthetic use for treating premature ejaculation: a double-blind, randomized, placebo-controlled study. BJU Int 2004; 93(7):1018–21.
19. EMLA® CREAM - U.S. Food and drug administration. Available at: https://www.accessdata.fda.gov/drugsatfda_docs/label/2000/19941s11lbl.pdf. Accessed September 10, 2021.
20. Porst H, Burri A. Fortacin™ spray for the treatment of premature ejaculation. Urol J 2017;84(2_suppl): 1–10.
21. Carson C, Wyllie M. Improved ejaculatory latency, control and sexual satisfaction when PSD502 is applied topically in men with premature ejaculation: results of a phase III, double-blind, placebo-controlled study. J Sex Med 2010;7(9):3179–89.
22. Dinsmore WW, Wyllie MG. PSD502 improves ejaculatory latency, control and sexual satisfaction when applied topically 5 min before intercourse in men with premature ejaculation: results of a phase III, multicentre, double-blind, placebo-controlled study. BJU Int 2009;103(7):940–9.
23. Abu El-Hamd M. Effectiveness and tolerability of lidocaine 5% spray in the treatment of lifelong premature ejaculation patients: a randomized single-blind placebo-controlled clinical trial. Int J Impot Res 2021;33(1):96–101.
24. Shabsigh R, Perelman MA, Getzenberg RH, et al. Randomized, placebo-controlled study to evaluate the efficacy, Safety, and tolerability of Benzocaine Wipes in Subjects with premature ejaculation. J Mens Health 2019;15(3):80.
25. Artigas F, Nutt DJ, Shelton R. Mechanism of action of antidepressants. Psychopharmacol Bull 2002; 36(Suppl 2):123–32.
26. Waldinger MD, Zwinderman AH, Schweitzer DH, et al. Relevance of methodological design for the interpretation of efficacy of drug treatment of premature ejaculation: a systematic review and meta-analysis. Int J Impot Res 2004;16(4):369–81.
27. McMahon CG. Long term results of treatment of premature ejaculation with selective serotonin re-uptake inhibitors. Int J Impot Res 2002;14(Suppl 3):S19.

28. McMahon CG. Current and Emerging treatments for premature ejaculation. Sex Med Rev 2015;3(3): 183–202.

29. McMahon CG, Touma K. Treatment of premature ejaculation with paroxetine hydrochloride as needed: 2 single-blind placebo controlled crossover studies. J Urol 1999;161(6):1826–30. McMahon CG, Touma K. Treatment of premature ejacula-tion with paroxetine hydrochloride as needed: 2 single-blind-placebo controlled crossover studies. J Urol 1999; 161:1826–30.

30. McMahon C. Premature ejaculation. Indian J Urol 2007;23(2):97.

31. Sun Y, Yang L, Bao Y, et al. Efficacy of PDE5Is and SSRIs in men with premature ejaculation: a new systematic review and five meta-analyses. World J Urol 2017;35(12):1817–31.

32. Ferguson JM. SSRI antidepressant Medications. Prim Care Companion J Clin Psychiatry 2001; 03(01):22–7.

33. Anglin R, Yuan Y, Moayyedi P, et al. Risk of Upper Gastrointestinal Bleeding with selective serotonin re-uptake inhibitors with or without Concurrent NonSte-roidal Anti-Inflammatory Use: a systematic review and meta-analysis. Am J Gastroenterol 2014; 109(6):811–9.

34. Dent LA, Brown WC, Murney JD. Citalopram-Induced Priapism. Pharmacotherapy 2002;22(4): 538–41.

35. Wang RZ, Vashistha V, Kaur S, et al. Serotonin syndrome: Preventing, recognizing, and treating it. Cleve Clin J Med 2016;83(11):810–6.

36. Gabriel M, Sharma V. Antidepressant discontinua-tion syndrome. Can Med Assoc J 2017;189(21): E747.

37. McInerney SJ, Kennedy SH. Review of Evidence for Use of antidepressants in Bipolar Depression. Prim Care Companion CNS Disord 2014. https://doi.org/ 10.4088/PCC.14r01653.

38. Sharma T, Guski LS, Freund N, et al. Suicidality and aggression during antidepressant treatment: sys-tematic review and meta-analyses based on clinical study reports. BMJ Published Online January 2016; 27:i65.

39. Tanrikut C, Feldman AS, Altemus M, et al. Adverse effect of paroxetine on sperm. Fertil Steril 2010; 94(3):1021–6.

40. Koyuncu H, Serefoglu EC, Ozdemir AT, et al. Delete-rious effects of selective serotonin reuptake inhibitor treatment on semen parameters in patients with life-long premature ejaculation. Int J Impot Res 2012; 24(5):171–3.

41. Tanrikut C, Schlegel PN. Antidepressant-Associated Changes in semen parameters. Urology 2007;69(1): 185.e5-e7.

42. McMahon CG, Althof SE, Kaufman JM, et al. Efficacy and Safety of Dapoxetine for the treatment of premature ejaculation: Integrated analysis of results from five phase 3 Trials. J Sex Med 2011;8(2): 524–39.

43. Sansone RA, Sansone LA. Tramadol: seizures, sero-tonin syndrome, and coadministered antidepres-sants. Psychiatry (Edgmont) 2009;6(4):17–21.

44. Grond S, Sablotzki A. Clinical Pharmacology of tra-madol. Clin Pharmacokinet 2004;43(13):879–923.

45. Eassa BI, El-Shazly MA. Safety and efficacy of tra-madol hydrochloride on treatment of premature ejaculation. Asian J Androl 2013;15(1):138–42.

46. Bar-Or D, Salottolo KM, Orlando A, et al. A random-ized double-blind, placebo-controlled Multicenter study to evaluate the efficacy and Safety of Two Doses of the tramadol orally Disintegrating Tablet for the treatment of premature ejaculation within Less than 2 Minutes. Eur Urol 2012;61(4):736–43.

47. Alghobary M, El-Bayoumy Y, Mostafa Y, et al. Evalu-ation of tramadol on demand Vs. Daily paroxetine as a Long-term treatment of lifelong premature ejacula-tion. J Sex Med 2010;7(8):2860–7.

48. Kirby EW, Carson CC, Coward RM. Tramadol for the management of premature ejaculation: a timely sys-tematic review. Int J Impot Res 2015;27(4):121–7.

49. Martyn-St James M, Cooper K, Kaltenthaler E, et al. Tramadol for premature ejaculation: a systematic re-view and meta-analysis. BMC Urol 2015;15(1):6.

50. Takeshita J, Litzinger MH. Serotonin syndrome asso-ciated with tramadol. Prim Care Companion J Clin Psychiatry 2009;11(5):273.

51. McDiarmid T, Mackler L, Schneider DM. Clinical in-quiries. What is the addiction risk associated with tramadol? J Fam Pract 2005;54(1):72–3.

52. Adams EH, Breiner S, Cicero TJ, et al. A Compari-son of the Abuse Liability of tramadol, NSAIDs, and Hydrocodone in patients with Chronic Pain. J Pain Symptom Manage 2006;31(5):465–76.

53. Inciardi JA, Cicero TJ, Muñoz A, et al. The Diversion of Ultram®, Ultracet®, and Generic tramadol HCl. J Addict Dis 2006;25(2):53–8.

54. Senay EC, Adams EH, Geller A, et al. Physical dependence on Ultram® (tramadol hydrochloride): both opioid-like and atypical withdrawal symptoms occur. Drug Alcohol Depend 2003;69(3):233–41.

55. HISASUE S-I, FURUYA R, ITOH N, et al. Ejaculatory disorder caused by alpha-1 adrenoceptor antago-nists is not retrograde ejaculation but a loss of sem-inal emission. Int J Urol 2006;13(10):1311–6.

56. Sato Y, Tanda H, Nakajima H, et al. Silodosin and its potential for treating premature ejaculation: a prelim-inary report. Int J Urol 2012;19(3):268–72.

57. Akin Y, Gulmez H, Ates M, et al. Comparison of alpha Blockers in treatment of premature ejacula-tion: a Pilot clinical trial. Iran Red Crescent Med J 2013;15(10). https://doi.org/10.5812/ircmj.13805.

58. Khera M, Bhattacharya RK, Blick G, et al. Changes in Prostate Specific Antigen in Hypogonadal men

after 12 Months of Testosterone Replacement therapy: Support for the Prostate Saturation theory. J Urol 2011;186(3):1005–11.

59. Kaplan SA. Side effects of alpha-Blocker Use: retrograde ejaculation. Rev Urol 2009;11(Suppl 1): S14–8.

60. Mamas MA, Reynard JM, Brading AF. Nitric oxide and the lower urinary tract: current concepts, future prospects. Urology 2003;61(6):1079–85.

61. Machtens S, Ckert S, Stief CG, et al. Effects of various nitric oxide-donating drugs on adrenergic tension of human seminal vesicles in vitro. Urology 2003;61(2):479–83.

62. McMahon CG, Stuckey BGA, Andersen M, et al. Efficacy of Sildenafil Citrate (Viagra) in men with premature ejaculation. J Sex Med 2005;2(3):368–75.

63. Aversa A, Pili M, Francomano D, et al. Effects of vardenafil administration on intravaginal ejaculatory latency time in men with lifelong premature ejaculation. Int J Impot Res 2009;21(4):221–7.

64. Martyn-St James M, Cooper K, Ren S, et al. Phosphodiesterase type 5 inhibitors for premature ejaculation: a systematic review and meta-analysis. Eur Urol Focus 2017;3(1):119–29.

65. McMahon CG, McMahon CN, Leow LJ, et al. Efficacy of type-5 phosphodiesterase inhibitors in the drug treatment of premature ejaculation: a systematic review. BJU Int 2006;98(2):259–72.

66. Ballon JS, Feifel D. A systematic review of Modafinil. J Clin Psychiatry 2006;67(04):554–66.

67. Tuken M, Kiremit MC, Serefoglu EC. On-demand Modafinil improves ejaculation time and patient-reported Outcomes in men with lifelong premature ejaculation. Urology 2016;94:139–42.

68. Filippi S, Vignozzi L, Vannelli GB, et al. Role of oxytocin in the ejaculatory process. J Endocrinol Invest 2003;26(3 Suppl):82–6.

69. Rowland D, McMahon CG, Abdo C, et al. Disorders of orgasm and ejaculation in men. J Sex Med 2010; 7(4):1668–86.

70. American Psychiatric Association. Diagnostic and Statistical Manual of Mental Disorders. American Psychiatric Association; 2013. https://doi.org/10.1176/appi.books.9780890425596.

71. Di Sante S, Mollaioli D, Gravina GL, et al. Epidemiology of delayed ejaculation. Transl Androl Urol 2016;5(4):541–8.

72. Laumann EO, Nicolosi A, Glasser DB, et al. Sexual problems among women and men aged 40–80 y: prevalence and correlates identified in the Global Study of Sexual Attitudes and Behaviors. Int J Impot Res 2005;17(1):39–57.

73. Corona G, Lee DM, Forti G, et al. Age-related Changes in General and sexual Health in Middle-aged and Older men: results from the European male Ageing study (EMAS). J Sex Med 2010;7(4): 1362–80.

74. Rosen R, Altwein J, Boyle P, et al. Lower urinary tract symptoms and male sexual dysfunction: the multinational survey of the Aging male (MSAM-7). Eur Urol 2003;44(6):637–49.

75. Seyam R. A systematic review of the correlates and management of nonpremature ejaculatory dysfunction in heterosexual men. Ther Adv Urol 2013;5(5): 254–97.

76. Corona G, Jannini EA, Mannucci E, et al. Different Testosterone Levels Are associated with ejaculatory dysfunction. J Sex Med 2008;5(8):1991–8.

77. Corona G. Psychobiological correlates of delayed ejaculation in male patients with sexual Dysfunctions. J Androl 2006;27(3):453–8.

78. Vallejo-Medina P, Sierra JC. Effect of drug Use and Influence of Abstinence on sexual Functioning in a Spanish male drug-Dependent Sample: a Multisite study. J Sex Med 2013;10(2):333–41.

79. Abdel-Hamid IA, Ali OI. Delayed ejaculation: pathophysiology, Diagnosis, and treatment. World J Mens Health 2018;36(1):22.

80. Flannigan R, Heier L, Voss H, et al. Functional Magnetic Resonance Imaging Detects Between-Group Differences in Neural Activation among men with delayed orgasm Compared with Normal Controls: preliminary report. J Sex Med 2019;16(8):1246–54.

81. Nelson CJ, Ahmed A, Valenzuela R, et al. Assessment of Penile Vibratory Stimulation as a management Strategy in men with Secondary Retarded orgasm. Urology 2007;69(3):552–5.

82. Perelman MA. Psychosexual therapy for delayed ejaculation based on the Sexual Tipping Point model. Transl Androl Urol 2016;5(4):563–75.

83. Althof SE. Psychological interventions for delayed ejaculation/orgasm. Int J Impot Res 2012;24(4): 131–6.

84. Abdel-Hamid IA, Saleh E-S. Primary lifelong delayed ejaculation: Characteristics and Response to Bupropion. J Sex Med 2011;8(6):1772–9.

85. Landen M, Eriksson E, Agren H, et al. Effect of Buspirone on sexual dysfunction in Depressed patients treated with selective serotonin reuptake inhibitors. J Clin Psychopharmacol 1999;19(3):268–71.

86. Arnott S, Nutt D. Successful treatment of Fluvoxamine-induced Anorgasmia by Cyproheptadine. Br J Psychiatry 1994;164(6):838–9.

87. Bernik M, Vieira AHG, Nunes PV. Bethanecol chloride for treatment of clomipramine-induced orgasmic dysfunction in males. Rev Hosp Clin Fac Med Sao Paulo 2004;59(6):357–60.

88. Sadowski DJ, Butcher MJ, Köhler TS. A review of pathophysiology and management Options for delayed ejaculation. Sex Med Rev 2016;4(2):167–76.

89. Modell G, May RS, Charles J. Effect of Bupropion-SR on orgasmic dysfunction in Nondepressed Subjects: a Pilot study. J Sex Marital Ther 2000;26(3): 231–40.

90. Hollander AB, Pastuszak AW, Hsieh T-C, et al. Cabergoline in the treatment of male orgasmic disorder—a Retrospective Pilot analysis. Sex Med 2016; 4(1):e28–33.

91. Paduch DA, Polzer PK, Ni X, et al. Testosterone Replacement in Androgen-Deficient men with ejaculatory dysfunction: a randomized controlled trial. J Clin Endocrinol Metab 2015;100(8):2956–62.

92. Mulhall JP, Trost LW, Brannigan RE, et al. Evaluation and management of Testosterone Deficiency: AUA Guideline. J Urol 2018;200(2):423–32.

93. Parnham A, Serefoglu EC. Retrograde ejaculation, painful ejaculation and hematospermia. Transl Androl Urol 2016;5(4):592–601.

94. Nguyen HMT, Bala A, Gabrielson AT, et al. Post-Orgasmic Illness syndrome: a review. Sex Med Rev 2018;6(1):11–5.

95. Waldinger MD, Meinardi MMHM, Zwinderman AH, et al. Postorgasmic Illness syndrome (POIS) in 45 Dutch Caucasian males: clinical Characteristics and Evidence for an Immunogenic Pathogenesis (Part 1). J Sex Med 2011;8(4):1164–70.

96. Jiang N, Xi G, Li H, et al. Postorgasmic Illness syndrome (POIS) in a Chinese man: No Proof for IgE-Mediated Allergy to semen. J Sex Med 2015;12(3): 840–5.

Medical Treatment of Benign Prostatic Hyperplasia

Alexander Plochocki, MD, MPH, Benjamin King, MD*

KEYWORDS

- BPH • LUTS • BOO • Alpha-1 antagonist • Male • Urinary retention

KEY POINTS

- Selective alpha-1 antagonists (eg, Tamsulosin) are safe, effective, and fast-acting first-line BPH treatment that targets voiding and storage LUTS
- 5-alpha reductase inhibitors (eg, finasteride, dutasteride) are effective mono- or combination for men with large prostates and/or urinary retention
- Anticholinergics (eg, oxybutynin, tolterodine, solifenacin) combined with alpha-1 antagonists can target storage-LUTS with low rates of causing urinary retention
- Men with erectile dysfunction and/or desire to preserve sexual function can start tadalafil monotherapy for BPH/LUTS

INTRODUCTION

Benign prostatic hyperplasia (BPH) and its associated is one of the most common diagnoses seen by the urologist, with previous studies estimating greater than half of the men having at least one symptom of lower urinary tract symptoms (LUTS),[1] with the prevalence increasing as our population ages with the majority of men older than 70 having BPH/LUTS.[2] Over the last 2 decades, we have seen a decrease in surgical management and an increase in medical BPH management across the United States, especially with increasing patient age at the time of diagnosis.[3]

An enlarged prostate by itself is not an indication for treatment, but it is rather the symptoms and impact on the quality of life (QoL) that bring patients to the urologist. While many of these symptoms may be mild, by the time a man presents to the urologist, they have generally crossed the threshold into bothersome. While the primary issue of BPH was first believed to be solely from bladder outlet obstruction (BOO), we know now that LUTS is more complex and a combination of both voiding and storage issues. The gold standard to assess LUTS is with the international prostate symptom score (IPSS; **Table 1**), which has been validated extensively and features both voiding and storage symptoms (ie, overactive bladder). While symptom relief and patient perception of treatment efficacy is inherently subjective, a score improvement of 4 points is often considered a significant improvement in most men.[4]

ALPHA-ADRENERGIC ANTAGONISM

The prostate contains a large amount of smooth muscle which responds to alpha-adrenergic stimulation by increasing the prostatic urethral resistance, by blocking this stimulation we can induce relaxation to lessen bladder outlet resistance. The bladder and prostate contain mostly alpha-1 receptors which led to the development of our arsenal of selective blockers. While most alpha-1 blockers in use today are well-tolerated, their side effect profile stems from the alpha blockade both in the prostate and systemically. Generally,

Department of Urology, University of Vermont Medical Center, 111 Colchester Avenue, Burlington, VT 05401, USA
* Corresponding author.
E-mail address: Benjamin.King@uvmhealth.org

Urol Clin N Am 49 (2022) 231–238
https://doi.org/10.1016/j.ucl.2021.12.003
0094-0143/22/© 2021 Elsevier Inc. All rights reserved.

Table 1
International prostate symptom score (IPSS) symptoms. LUTS: Lower urinary tract symptoms

Symptom	Nature of LUTS
Incomplete Emptying	Voiding
Urinary Frequency	Storing
Intermittency	Voiding
Urgency	Storing
Weak Stream	Voiding
Straining	Voiding
Nocturia	Storing
Impact on Quality of Life	N/A

patients may experience retrograde ejaculation, rhinitis, and orthostatic hypotension. As the bladder contains alpha receptors, which can explain why overactive bladder (OAB) symptoms can be lessened. The exact physiology of this is unclear, but is theorized to involve an increase in detrusor blood flow stimulated by alpha blockade.[5]

The first selective alpha-1 blocker was tested as *prazosin*, which demonstrated effectiveness, but required twice-daily dosing.[6] Prazosin is no longer used for LUTS, but has interestingly found use in the treatment of posttraumatic stress disorder. *Doxazosin* and *terazosin* are selective alpha-1 blockers that are dosed daily, in general, they require a titration period to get to a full therapeutic dose and are not often first-line agents.[7,8]

Tamsulosin is arguably the most well-known alpha-1 blocker, it is not just alpha-1 selective, but uro-selective which allows it to maintain good symptom control with minimal side effects. Generally, you can expect symptom relief within a few days to a week of starting therapy. Tamsulosin has been studied extensively, and has been shown to decrease IPSS by about 9.5 points.[9] Tamsulosin is generally prescribed at a dose of 0.4 mg, ideally taken 30 minutes after the same meal every day. The dose can be increased to 0.8 mg daily for patients with breakthrough symptoms.

Alfuzosin and *silodosin* are additional uro-selective agents that are able to be dosed daily and have been additionally shown to be effective. Silodosin may be associated with worse sexual side effects, but less chance of orthostatic hypotension.[10,11]

Doxazosin has a gastrointestinal therapeutic system (*Doxazosin GITS*) formulation of doxazosin mesylatethat provides a more sustained release of the drug, which allows patients to start the drug at a therapeutic dose and forego titration. Interestingly, this GITS formation has been shown in some studies to provide better symptom relief for patients with a similar side-effect profile.[12] In a similar way to tamsulosin, you can start doxazosin GITS at 4 mg daily and titrate up to 8 mg daily for breakthrough symptoms.

As alpha-1 antagonists as a class will demonstrate effect within a few days, patients who were started on these drugs for acute urinary retention requiring catheterization should be continued on these medications for a few days before a trial without a catheter. The AUA guidelines suggest at least 3 days of treatment.[13]

Patients should be counseled that, any time after starting alpha-1 blockers, they are at an increased risk of developing floppy iris syndrome during cataract surgery. This has been noted even years after stopping alpha-1 blockade therapy, so any patient who has been on alpha-1 blockers for any period of time may be at risk.[14]

5-ALPHA REDUCTASE INHIBITION

BPH is hormonally mediated almost exclusively by prostatic levels of dihydrotestosterone (DHT) and suppression of DHT leads to decreased prostate volume and therefore less prostatic urethral compression. Testosterone is converted to DHT by steroid 5-alpha reductase; there are 2 isozymes expressed in the body: Type 1 steroid 5-alpha reductase (predominately expressed in extraprostatic tissues) and type 2 steroid 5-alpha reductase (predominately expressed in prostatic tissues).

Finasteride (selective type 2 steroid 5-alpha reductase) and *dutasteride* (nonselective inhibitor of both isozymes) are the two 5-alpha reductase inhibitors (5ARIs) available. Given that these medications work on hormonal expression in the prostate, there is a significant lag time until symptom relief, patient's should expect to wait 6 months to see results. Additionally, generally patients with larger prostates will see better results.[15] The AUA guidelines suggest using a 30 cc prostate as the lower cut-off for starting 5ARI therapy.[13] Prostate size can be estimated with cross-sectional imaging, or estimated with digital rectal examination.

Finasteride and dutasteride have been extensively studied independently and head-to-head and found to decrease IPSS scores and decrease prostate volume by about 30%.[16,17] There is no difference in outcomes or side effects with either medications. Side effects are usually well-tolerated and include erectile dysfunction (8.1%), decreased libido (6.4%), ejaculatory dysfunction (0.8%) gynecomastia (0.5%), all of which seem within the first year of treatment. Studies have shown that the incidence of side effects do not increase with longer treatment periods, with the exception of ejaculatory dysfunction, which did worsen with longer treatment.[18] Interestingly, there is an increased reported incidence of "post-finasteride syndrome" which is characterized by sexual side effects and mood depression that persists despite drug cessation irrespective of the length of treatment, the pathophysiology of this is unclear, and it is an area of current research.[19]

The MTOPS trial demonstrated the safety and efficacy of 5ARI and alpha-1 antagonist combination therapy with men having less symptom progression on combination therapy compared with monotherapy. Men on finasteride alone or on combination therapy exhibited a decrease in rates of acute urinary retention and need for surgical intervention compared with doxazosin monotherapy.[17] It is hypothesized that as men continue to age, their prostatic growth continues to cause increased urethral pressure that outpaces the effect of the 5ARI and the reduced smooth muscle relaxation of the alpha-1 antagonist;[17] however, it should always be noted that as men age they may develop more medical comorbidities that may make them more susceptible to urinary retention independent of their BPH.

Controversial use of 5ARIs is in reducing prostatic bleeding associated with BPH either for gross hematuria with clot retention or given preoperatively before transurethral resection of the prostate (TURP). While there is significant anecdotal evidence for this use, there is a paucity of evidence-based data,[20] but some studies suggest even short-term courses, on the order of 4 to 6 weeks, of 5ARIs may have clinical significance.[21] Anecdotally, some urologists would continue patients on 5ARIs until a few weeks postop from a TURP and start it empirically on someone presenting with gross hematuria and LUTS.

ANTICHOLINERGICS

The detrusor muscle of the bladder is innervated by parasympathetic fibers and mediated through muscarinic receptors, which in turn mediates bladder capacity and involuntary detrusor contractions which can contribute to storage-associated LUTS. By inhibiting these with muscarinic receptor antagonists (anticholinergics), we can decrease involuntary detrusor contractions, which in turn lead to better urine storage capacity. As we are inhibiting detrusor contractions, there is a risk of urinary retention, especially in patients with voiding LUTS.[22]

Oxybutynin, solifenacin, and *tolterodine* are 3 of the most commonly prescribed anticholinergics. While they do serve a role for patients with only overactive bladder symptoms, patients with BPH often have a combination of voiding and storage LUTS. Therefore, anticholinergics are often not used as monotherapy, as studies have shown that this can be far less effective than combination therapy.[23] However, patients on tolterodine ER monotherapy were noted to have decreased urinary urgency incontinence without an increase in rates or urinary retention.

While acute urinary retention (AUR) is the oft-cited side effect of anticholinergics, the actual rates AUR have been quite low across the literature, likely on the magnitude of 0.3%.[24] Generally, a cut-off PVR off 200 cc has been used as a soft contraindication to starting anticholinergic therapy, which should obviously be stopped if a patient develops AUR. If a patient does develop AUR, we would not routinely trial a different anticholinergic. The most common side effects are dry mouth, constipation, and blurry vision. It should be noted that CNS side effects, such as confusion and delirium are more common in older men and men with preexisting neurologic conditions, and should be used with caution. There has been data to suggest that CNS side effects vary based on drug, with one study demonstrating oxybutynin having worse CNS adverse events in comparison to darifenicin.[25]

Combination therapy for anticholinergics and alpha-1 antagonists has been proven to be successful with many different combinations of drugs. Tamsulosin and tolterodine ER were studied each as monotherapy, combined therapy, and compared with placebo; combination therapy was found to provide the most significant reduction in symptoms, with a larger reduction in storage symptoms, with no effect on urinary retention rates.[23] This is further supported by a meta-analysis of multiple studies of different combinations of anticholinergic + alpha-1 antagonist combination therapy that support that patients with storage-LUTS experience a significant decrease in symptoms without an increase in urinary retention rates, suggesting that over 100 patients would need to be treated with combination therapy to induce an additional case of urinary retention.[26]

PHOSPHODIESTERASE TYPE 5 INHIBITION

Phosphodiesterase type 5 inhibitors (PDE5i) are most widely known as a treatment of erectile dysfunction (ED), through their vasodilator effect by blocking cGMP breakdown and promoting nitrous oxide production. Patients taking PDE5i have been noted to have a decrease in LUTS. While the overall mechanism for this is unclear, possible theories include increased oxygenation of the bladder and prostate as well as possible bladder neck and prostatic smooth muscle relaxation.[27,28] ED and LUTS are often coexistent in the aging male as well, so a drug that can target both would be ideal across this population.

Sildenafil was the first PDE5i studied[29] and further research demonstrated that among men with a baseline IPSS greater than 10, taking sildenafil a mean of 2 times a week was associated with a statistically significant decrease in IPSS by 4.6 points.[30] Given sildenafil's on-demand dosing, this can create a difficult treatment regimen for men to take, further exacerbated by sildenafil's poor absorption, requiring it to be taken on an empty stomach. So while the decrease in LUTS could be viewed as a potential added benefit, a more stable drug would be preferred for primary treatment of LUTS.

This is whereby tadalafil has an advantage, as it has a much longer half-life in the body and can be taken daily. After tadalafil was proven to be effective in reducing LUTS,[31] a randomized controlled dose-finding trial-tested tadalafil 2.5, 5, 10, and 20 mg daily over a 12 week period. All men demonstrated decreases in IPSS, but a 5 mg daily dose was found to have the most favorable risk-benefit profile.[32] Currently, tadalafil dosed at 5 mg daily is the only PDE5i with FDA approval for treatment of BPH/LUTS. It is recommended to take it at the same time every day and can be taken with or without food. While 5 mg is the most common dose, it can be titrated for men with refractory ED or LUTS, we generally do not titrate past 10 mg daily. Side effects of tadalafil are generally well-tolerated by most men and include headache, flushing dyspepsia, and nasal congestion, myalgias, and back pain. The adverse effect rate is similar to sildenafil; however, myalgias and back pain may be more prevalent with taldalifil.[33] As tadalafil does not have the ejaculatory dysfunction side effects of alpha-blockers, this may make it a more attractive first-line therapy in younger men who prioritize sexual function.

While tadalafil is not as well studied with combination treatment as drugs in other classes, a recent meta-analysis[34] of tamsulosin and tadalafil combination therapy demonstrated overall very positive results, that combination therapy results in an improvement in IPSS (mostly with improvement in voiding symptoms), increase in Qmax, as well as has an ameliorating effect on the ejaculatory dysfunction of tamsulosin monotherapy when on combination therapy. The study did note that there were more patients that had to stop treatment due to adverse events in the combination therapy cohorts. Overall, tadalafil and tamsulosin can be recommended to patients, but a discussion on the possibility of worsening side effects and possibly a contingency plan to return to monotherapy.

BETA-3 ADRENERGIC AGONISM

Beta-3 adrenergic receptors are present on the bladder and their activation leads to smooth muscle relaxation in the detrusor, by activating these receptors we can induce bladder relaxation, inhibit microcontractions of the bladder, which leads to increased storage and a decrease in storage LUTS.[35] Animal-based studies suggest that beta-3 agonists also induce relaxation of the urethra[36] providing possible physiology for relief of voiding-LUTS. Given that beta-3 agonists use a completely different pathway than their anticholinergic counterparts, it allows us to treat storage LUTS with a different side effect profile.

Mirabegron is the primary beta-3 agonist available, and while initially studied in men and women with OAB, there has been data specifically looking at this drug in men with BPH and storage symptoms. Mirabegron has been studied against solifenacin and found to provide similar relief of urgency, frequency, and incontinence.[37] Mirabegron doses of 50 mg and 100 mg demonstrated no change from placebo in worsening BOO, as patients' detrusor pressures and max flow rate were unaffected from placebo. Patients demonstrated decreased frequency and urgency on mirabegron.[38] Mirabegron is started at a dose of 25 mg daily and is increased to 50 mg after 4 to 8 weeks, while some studies tested doses up to 100 mg, most patients are only titrated up to 50 mg.

While mirabegron is well-tolerated, previous studies have shown that an increase in systolic blood pressure with mirabegron, it should be avoided in patients with difficult to control hypertension. Additionally, the patient's blood pressures should be monitored while starting and up-titrating. Anecdotally, it has been difficult to get insurance approval for mirabegron without demonstrating prior failure or intolerance of anticholinergics, and it is for this reason that we recommend against starting mirabegron on inpatients with the plan to continue through discharge.

Vibegron received FDA approval for use in OAB in 2020 and has shown promising results and safety, with the EMPOWUR clinical trial studying vibegron against tolterodine ER was

Table 2
BPH medications with dosing and mechanism of action

Drug	Dosing	Drug Class/Notes
Tamsulosin	Start 0.4 mg daily with dinner up to 0.8 mg daily	*Uro-selective alpha-1 antagonist*
Alfuzosin	7.5–10 mg daily with same meal	*Uro-selective alpha-1 antagonist*
Silodosin	4-8 mg daily	*Uro-selective alpha-1 antagonist,* potentially more sexual side effects, less hypotension
Terazosin	1 mg at bedtime x 3 d, 2 mg × 3 d, then 5 mg therapeutic dose, up to 10 mg	*Alpha-1 selective alpha-1 antagonist,* hypotension can happen whenever uptitrating. Up titrate more slowly if patient symptomatic.
Doxazosin IR	2 mg at bedtime x 3 d, titrate to 4 or 8 mg	*Alpha-1 selective alpha-1 antagonist*
Doxazosin GITS	4 mg after breakfast, up to 8 mg	*Alpha-1 selective alpha-1 antagonist,* may provide superior symptom relief
Finasteride	5 mg daily	*5-alpha reductase inhibitor,* selective for type 2
Dutasteride	0.5 mg daily	*5-alpha reductase inhibitor,* non-selective
Tolterodine ER	4 mg daily	*Anticholinergic*
Oxybutynin	5mg BID up to 5 mg TID	*Anticholinergic*
Oxybutynin ER	5–30 mg daily	*Anticholinergic*
Solifenacin	3–9 mg daily	*Anticholinergic*
Mirabegron	Start 25 mg daily and increase to 50 mg after 4–8 wk, can increase to 100 mg daily	*Beta-3 agonist,* monitor for hypertension
Tadalafil	5–20 mg daily	*Phosphodiesterase type 5 inhibitor,* 5 mg ideal dose for LUTS

Abbreviations: ER, Extended release; GITS, Gastrointestinal therapeutic system; IR, Immediate release; LUTS, Lower urinary tract symptoms

demonstrating a better reduction in urge incontinence and a comparable decrease in urgency.[39] The study was extended to 40 weeks and demonstrated continued safety and efficacy.[40] Vibegron is currently being studied for use in BPH with storage LUTS.

PHYTOTHERAPY

There are a plethora of naturally-obtained compounds marketed for LUTS; studying and comparing these drugs are difficult, especially as controlling for drug contents and formulations is difficult between studies, disrupting the reproducibility and generalizability of results. The most commonly seen treatment of BPH is arrangements of saw palmetto (*Serenoa repens*). Multiple meta-analyses have demonstrated that, while well-tolerated, saw palmetto does not afford any change in LUTS.[41] Side effects are usually stomach/abdominal upset, diarrhea, nausea, headache, rhinitis, decreased libido, and there are no published drug-herb interactions.[42] *Pygeum* (*Pygeum africanum*), the bark of an African tree, is purported to also decrease LUTS, but—again—there is a lot of inter-study variability. Pygeum is well-tolerated through many of their studies without any major side effects documented.[42] *Nettle* (*Urtica dioica*) are the roots of an herbaceous wild plant found worldwide that has a paucity of data supporting its use, but is generally well-tolerated without serious side

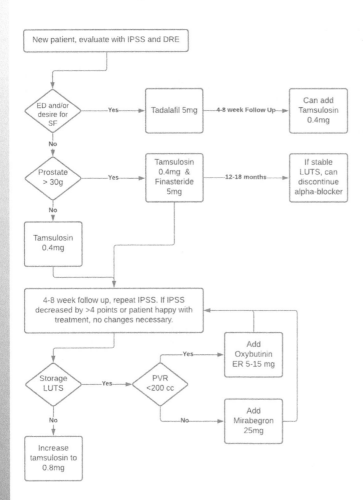

Fig. 1. *Suggested BPH Medical Management Pathway.* Drug choice is derived from our institution's practice pattern, clinicians may substitute for other drugs within the same class based on their comfort level. ED, Erectile Dysfunction; IPSS, International Prostate Symptom Score; LUTS, Lower urinary tract symptoms; PVR, Post-void residual; SF, Sexual Function.

effects.[42] *Rye grass pollen* (*Secale cereale*) is microbially digested pollen that is then extracted, with the active ingredients not entirely known, some clinical trials suggest it may help with LUTS, with side-effects mostly of gastrointestinal upset and skin rash. *Pumpkin seed* (*Cucurbita pepo*) has not been well studied as a BPH treatment, but has no documented side effects.[42] The complete list of phytotherapy options would be quite extensive, but most of these treatments have little clinical evidence of their efficacy, but are usually well-tolerated; clinicians should advise their patients accordingly.

SUMMARY AND SUGGESTIONS

Given the vast spectrum of medication classes and drugs in each category, there is variation in treatment across urologists. For BPH/LUTS, we start our work up with a digital rectal examination, urinalysis, and history to rule out other non-BPH causes of LUTS, such as urethral stricture. If

patients have symptoms of urinary retention, we will get a postvoid residual in our office as well. Additionally, we discuss possible lifestyle management options such as caffeine cessation for storage-LUTS and limiting evening fluid intake for nocturia. For most men, our treatment starts with 0.4 mg of tamsulosin taken with dinner or nightly, which they can increase to 0.8 mg daily if they are getting a partial response and otherwise tolerating the medication well. Even if patients have predominately storage LUTS, we will often still start an alpha-1 antagonist before starting an anticholinergic. If the patient has very severe LUTS and a large prostate volume (>30 cc), we also discuss starting finasteride concomitantly, with the tentative plan to withdraw tamsulosin at 12 to 18 months. For patients presenting with urinary retention due to BPH, we will also start finasteride and tamsulosin. The commonly prescribed drugs and their dosages can be found in **Table 2** and we present our general work flow for the medical management of BPH in **Fig. 1**.

CLINICS CARE POINTS

- LUTS can be quantified with an IPSS, allowing more objective tracking of symptomatology throughout treatments.

- Uro-selective alpha-1 antagonists (tamsulosin, alfuzosin, silodosin) are well-tolerated and effective first-line treatments for LUTS.

- 5-alpha reductase inhibitors are slow-onset medications indicated for men with large (>30 cc) prostates and have been shown to decrease rates of urinary retention.

- Anticholinergics are ideal for combination therapy for patients with refractory storage LUTS, with generally low risk of developing acute urinary retention in men with baseline low PVRS less than 200 cc.

- Patients presenting with LUTS and erectile dysfunction can be started on a course of daily tadalafil.

- Patients should be aware that as they age they may "outgrow" their current therapy and may need to progress to combination therapies or consider surgical intervention.

DISCLOSURE

The authors have nothing to disclose.

REFERENCES

1. Irwin DE, Milsom I, Hunskaar S, et al. Population based survey of urinary incontinence, overactive bladder, and other lower urinary tract symptoms in five countries: results of the EPIC study. Eur Urol 2006;50(6):1306–14.

2. Egan KB. The Epidemiology of Benign Prostatic Hyperplasia Associated with Lower Urinary Tract Symptoms: Prevalence and Incident Rates. Urol Clin North Am 2016;43(3):289–97.

3. Welliver C, Feinstein L, Ward JB, et al. Trends in Lower Urinary Tract Symptoms Associated with Benign Prostatic Hyperplasia, 2004 to 2013: the Urologic Diseases in America Project. J Urol 2020; 203(1):171–8.

4. Barry MJ, Williford WO, Chang Y, et al. Benign prostatic hyperplasia specific health status measures in clinical research: how much change in the American Urological Association symptom index and the benign prostatic hyperplasia impact index is perceptible to patients? J Urol 1995;154(5):1770–4.

5. Andersson K-E, Boedtkjer DB, Forman A. The link between vascular dysfunction, bladder ischemia, and aging bladder dysfunction. Ther Adv Urol 2017;9(1):11–27.

6. Chapple CR, Christmas TJ, Milroy EJ. A twelve-week placebo-controlled study of prazosin in the treatment of prostatic obstruction. Urol Int 1990; 45(Suppl 1):47–55.

7. Wilt TJ, MacDonald R. Doxazosin in the treatment of benign prostatic hypertrophy: an update. Clin Interv Aging 2006;1(4):389–401.

8. Lepor H, Auerbach S, Puras-Baez A, et al. A Randomized, Placebo-Controlled Multicenter Study of the Efficacy and Safety of Terazosin in the Treatment of Benign Prostatic Hyperplasia. J Urol 1992;148(5 Part 1):1467–74.

9. Narayan P, Tunuguntla HSGR. Long-Term Efficacy and Safety of Tamsulosin for Benign Prostatic Hyperplasia. Rev Urol 2005;7(Suppl 4):S42–8.

10. MacDonald R, Wilt TJ. Alfuzosin for treatment of lower urinary tract symptoms compatible with benign prostatic hyperplasia: a systematic review of efficacy and adverse effects. Urology 2005; 66(4):780–8.

11. Jung JH, Kim J, MacDonald R, et al. Silodosin for the treatment of lower urinary tract symptoms in men with benign prostatic hyperplasia. Cochrane Database Syst Rev 2017;2017(11):CD012615.

12. Guo J, Tang R. Efficacy and tolerability of doxazosin gastro-intestinal therapeutic system versus tamsulosin in patients with lower urinary tract symptoms associated with benign prostatic hyperplasia. Medicine (Baltimore) 2021;100(33):e26955.

13. Lerner LB, McVary KT, Barry MJ, et al. Management of Lower Urinary Tract Symptoms Attributed to Benign Prostatic Hyperplasia: AUA GUIDELINE PART I, Initial Work-up and Medical Management. J Urol 2021. https://doi.org/10.1097/JU. 0000000000002183.

14. Christou CD, Tsinopoulos I, Ziakas N, et al. Intraoperative Floppy Iris Syndrome: Updated Perspectives. Clin Ophthalmol Auckl NZ 2020;14:463–71.

15. Tacklind J, Fink HA, Macdonald R, et al. Finasteride for benign prostatic hyperplasia. Cochrane Database Syst Rev 2010;10:CD006015.

16. Nickel JC, Gilling P, Tammela TL, et al. Comparison of dutasteride and finasteride for treating benign prostatic hyperplasia: the Enlarged Prostate International Comparator Study (EPICS). BJU Int 2011; 108(3):388–94.

17. McConnell JD, Roehrborn CG, Bautista OM, et al. The long-term effect of doxazosin, finasteride, and combination therapy on the clinical progression of benign prostatic hyperplasia. N Engl J Med 2003; 349(25):2387–98.

18. Fwu C-W, Eggers PW, Kirkali Z, et al. Change in sexual function in men with lower urinary tract

symptoms/benign prostatic hyperplasia associated with long-term treatment with doxazosin, finasteride and combined therapy. J Urol 2014;191(6):1828–34.

19. Diviccaro S, Melcangi RC, Giatti S. Post-finasteride syndrome: An emerging clinical problem. Neurobiol Stress 2019;12:100209.

20. Bruha M, Welliver C. Is There a Role for Preoperative 5 Alpha Reductase Inhibitors in Reducing Prostate Vascularity and Blood Loss? Curr Urol Rep 2017; 18(10):75.

21. Bansal A, Arora A. Transurethral Resection of Prostate and Bleeding: A Prospective, Randomized, Double-Blind Placebo-Controlled Trial to See the Efficacy of Short-Term Use of Finasteride and Dutasteride on Operative Blood Loss and Prostatic Microvessel Density. J Endourol 2017;31(9):910–7.

22. Chapple CR, Yamanishi T, Chess-Williams R. Muscarinic receptor subtypes and management of the overactive bladder. Urology 2002;60(5 Suppl 1):82–8.

23. Kaplan SA, Roehrborn CG, Rovner ES, et al. Tolterodine and Tamsulosin for Treatment of Men With Lower Urinary Tract Symptoms and Overactive BladderA Randomized Controlled Trial. JAMA 2006; 296(19):2319–28.

24. Blake-James BT, Rashidian A, Ikeda Y, et al. The role of anticholinergics in men with lower urinary tract symptoms suggestive of benign prostatic hyperplasia: a systematic review and meta-analysis. BJU Int 2007;99(1):85–96.

25. Kay GG, Ebinger U. Preserving cognitive function for patients with overactive bladder: evidence for a differential effect with darifenacin. Int J Clin Pract 2008;62(11):1792–800.

26. Filson CP, Hollingsworth JM, Clemens JQ, et al. The Efficacy and Safety of Combined Therapy with α-Blockers and Anticholinergics for Men with Benign Prostatic Hyperplasia: A Meta-Analysis. J Urol 2013;190(6). https://doi.org/10.1016/j.juro.2013.05.058.

27. Gacci M, Eardley I, Giuliano F, et al. Critical analysis of the relationship between sexual dysfunctions and lower urinary tract symptoms due to benign prostatic hyperplasia. Eur Urol 2011;60(4):809–25.

28. Angulo J, Cuevas P, Fernández A, et al. Tadalafil enhances the inhibitory effects of tamsulosin on neurogenic contractions of human prostate and bladder neck. J Sex Med 2012;9(9):2293–306.

29. Sairam K, Kulinskaya E, McNicholas TA, et al. Sildenafil influences lower urinary tract symptoms. BJU Int 2002;90(9):836–9.

30. Mulhall JP, Guhring P, Parker M, et al. Assessment of the impact of sildenafil citrate on lower urinary tract symptoms in men with erectile dysfunction. J Sex Med 2006;3(4):662–7.

31. McVary KT, Roehrborn CG, Kaminetsky JC, et al. Tadalafil relieves lower urinary tract symptoms secondary to benign prostatic hyperplasia. J Urol 2007; 177(4):1401–7.

32. Roehrborn CG, McVary KT, Elion-Mboussa A, et al. Tadalafil administered once daily for lower urinary tract symptoms secondary to benign prostatic hyperplasia: a dose finding study. J Urol 2008; 180(4):1228–34.

33. Gong B, Ma M, Xie W, et al. Direct comparison of tadalafil with sildenafil for the treatment of erectile dysfunction: a systematic review and meta-analysis. Int Urol Nephrol 2017;49(10):1731–40.

34. Zhou Z, Zheng X, Wu J, et al. Meta-Analysis of Efficacy and Safety of Tadalafil Plus Tamsulosin Compared with Tadalafil Alone in Treating Men with Benign Prostatic Hyperplasia and Erectile Dysfunction. Am J Mens Health 2019;13(5). 1557988319882597.

35. Aizawa N, Homma Y, Igawa Y. Effects of mirabegron, a novel β3-adrenoceptor agonist, on primary bladder afferent activity and bladder microcontractions in rats compared with the effects of oxybutynin. Eur Urol 2012;62(6):1165–73.

36. Alexandre EC, Kiguti LR, Calmasini FB, et al. Mirabegron relaxes urethral smooth muscle by a dual mechanism involving β3 -adrenoceptor activation and α1 -adrenoceptor blockade. Br J Pharmacol 2016;173(3):415–28.

37. Tubaro A, Batista JE, Nitti VW, et al. Efficacy and safety of daily mirabegron 50 mg in male patients with overactive bladder: a critical analysis of five phase III studies. Ther Adv Urol 2017;9(6):137–54.

38. Nitti VW, Rosenberg S, Mitcheson DH, et al. Urodynamics and safety of the β3-adrenoceptor agonist mirabegron in males with lower urinary tract symptoms and bladder outlet obstruction. J Urol 2013; 190(4):1320–7.

39. Staskin D, Frankel J, Varano S, et al. International Phase III, Randomized, Double-Blind, Placebo and Active Controlled Study to Evaluate the Safety and Efficacy of Vibegron in Patients with Symptoms of Overactive Bladder: EMPOWUR. J Urol 2020; 204(2):316–24.

40. Staskin D, Frankel J, Varano S, et al. Once-Daily Vibegron 75 mg for Overactive Bladder: Long-Term Safety and Efficacy from a Double-Blind Extension Study of the International Phase 3 Trial (EMPOWUR). J Urol 2021;205(5):1421–9.

41. Tacklind J, MacDonald R, Rutks I, et al. Serenoa repens for benign prostatic hyperplasia. Cochrane Database Syst Rev 2012;2012(12):CD001423.

42. Pagano E, Laudato M, Griffo M, et al. Phytotherapy of Benign Prostatic Hyperplasia. A Minireview Phytother Res 2014;28(7):949–55.

Nutraceuticals and Phytotherapy in Men's Health: Antioxidants, Pro-oxidants, and a Novel Opportunity for Lifestyle Changes

Mark A. Moyad, MD, MPH

KEYWORDS

- Dietary supplements • BPH • Erectile dysfunction • Male infertility • Prostate cancer • Anthelmintic
- Testosterone replacement • Lifestyle changes

KEY POINTS

- Patients interested or currently using nutraceuticals represent a diverse patient population with a keen potential interest and adherence to heart-healthy lifestyle changes, and behavioral changes should be a primary prevention and initial treatment option along with conventional therapy when needed for numerous men's health conditions.
- BPH nutraceuticals, including saw palmetto were as safe, but not more effective than placebo in the STEP and CAMUS methodologically rigorous clinical trials, and another product known as Permixon continues to accumulate positive data, but should be tested in phase 3 trial against or even with an oral conventional treatment option and/or a high-quality placebo.
- ED supplements, including Panax ginseng, and the more prominent nitric oxide (NO) enhancing amino acids arginine and citrulline have positive preliminary efficacy data with and without PDE-5 inhibitors, but safety signals with some of these agents in specific patient populations need to be resolved.
- "Less is more" supplementation should be the current mantra in the prostate cancer milieu, and recent efficacy and/or safety concerns with some male infertility antioxidants used in the FAZST and MOXI trials also need more research, and whether some antioxidants are exhibiting prooxidant activity in some clinical settings.
- DHEA and other DHEA and testosterone enhancing mimicking products have multiple concerns from HDL reductions to questionable utilization in some patients with BPH or prostate cancer.

INTRODUCTION

Dietary supplements, or "nutraceuticals," could arguably be considered an area of medicine in need of its own appreciated or accepted specialty for multiple reasons such as past and increasing current utilization by many patients in most medical disciplines, notable number of publications (positive, neutral or negative), and ongoing clinical trials being conducted.[1,2]

For example, within COVID-19 there are approximately 200 clinical trials being initiated, recruiting, ongoing, or completed using a dietary supplement.[2] Whether consumer, patient, or health care professional the impact of dietary supplements seems more palpable than ever, as is the necessity for updated objective knowledge. Furthermore, complementary and alternative medicine (CAM) is already an accepted vernacular expression within

University of Michigan Medical Center, Department of Urology, Ann Arbor, MI 48109, USA
E-mail address: moyad@med.umich.edu

Urol Clin N Am 49 (2022) 239–248
https://doi.org/10.1016/j.ucl.2021.12.006
0094-0143/22/© 2021 Elsevier Inc. All rights reserved.

medical specialties, but in reality, CAM is an umbrella term of a multitude of options, but dietary supplements occupy the largest part of the spectrum in terms of expenditure and prevalence.[1] This should place dietary supplement education at the forefront of CAM awareness. Emphasis should also be placed on quality control (QC) issues within dietary supplements, and ideally, a third-party verification process for any supplement would be a partial solution to this issue. Numerous QC companies exist today (NSF, UL, USP, etc.), and recently one national pharmacy company decided to only sell nutraceutical products on their shelves that contain some type of reputable or accepted QC verification seal,[3] which is an admirable decision, and will hopefully be mirrored 1 day by other supplement retailers.

NUTRACEUTICALS AND THE GREATER PERSPECTIVE

Patients interested or using dietary supplements, in general, are often more open and accepting of lifestyle changes to improve personal health.[4,5] In other words, supplement discussions are a potential bridge to healthier lifestyle dialogues and adherence, which for this author has been one of the most attractive unsung features of this area of medicine. Interestingly, even among male physicians, it seems supplement utilization has been associated with an increased commitment toward multiple healthy behaviors.[6]

Heart-healthy lifestyle changes continue to garner evidence as a salubrious overall method to reduce the risk of being diagnosed with severe benign prostatic hyperplasia (BPH), aggressive prostate cancer, prostatitis, sexual dysfunction, low testosterone, and even infertility.[1,7–10] Thus, these lifestyle changes should be discussed and emphasized initially with patients. For example, exercise, healthy weight/waist, blood pressure, cholesterol, glucose, diet, smoking cessation, minimizing alcohol exposure, stress, improving sleep hygiene, etc. should receive as much attention as any over-the-counter (OTC) pill. It is of interest that seemingly separate medical conditions within men's health share such similar risk factors, which provides impressive and ample educational opportunities. An additional emphasis on the impact of lifestyle changes on proven medical interventions should also be reviewed. This includes synergistic benefits with medications when heart healthy behaviors are accomplished, but when heart unhealthy behaviors occur then detrimental impacts on these same interventions could also occur.[11,12] Research continues to suggest it is never too late in life to impact urologic outcomes with healthy lifestyle changes.[13]

BPH AND HERBAL CONUNDRUMS

Beta-sitosterol enjoyed several positive preliminary BPH publications over 2 decades ago including a prominent meta-analysis.[14] However, it has not been part of a rigorous phase 3 trial compared with a prescription and/or placebo since this time, which is unfortunate as it is such a commonly used ingredient in many BPH supplements. Additionally, multiple other BPH herbal and multi-ingredient products also have beta-sitosterol as a component including numerous saw palmetto options. One could argue beta-sitosterol has become of the most essential compounds whereby products are allowed to make some form of structure and function claims ("prostate healthy").

On a related subject, higher intakes of dietary plant sterols (1300 mg or more), such as beta-sitosterol, could significantly reduce cholesterol, which is a part of an FDA approved heart healthy claim,[15] and theoretically one potential mechanism of action to improve heart and prostate health.[16] However, the FDA approved claim for plant sterols from food sources applies to products in appreciable excess of what was used in several successful BPH pill-based studies of the same compound (60–195 mg/d). Interestingly, the FDA health claim was also permitted when plant sterols were used in addition to a diet low in saturated fat and cholesterol. In other words, the FDA claim was allowed for some "food" sources if other dietary changes were also advertised on the label. This needs to be explained to patients interested in plant sterols.

The authors of the previous prominent beta-sitosterol BPH meta-analysis also emphasized the lack of long-term efficacy and safety data,[14] which is arguably still an issue. Although one specific unresolved safety signal needs further clarification when dealing with any large source of plant sterols, and this is the updated potential impact of an inherited metabolic condition known as "sitosterolemia."[17–20] Paradoxically, in some patients with this "rare" autosomal recessive disease rather than blocking the absorption of cholesterol or even minimally absorbing plant sterols these patients seem to experience increased uptake and/or an inability to adequately eliminate these compounds from the body, which could lead to significant increases in LDL cholesterol and a higher risk of premature cardiovascular events. This condition is specifically caused by a biallelic (homozygous/compound heterozygous) loss-of-function (LOF) genetic mutations in ATP-binding cassette (ABC) subfamily ABCG5 or ABCG8, which both normally function to eliminate sterols from the liver and intestines. Interestingly, some recent estimates suggest loss of function

(LOF) mutation in either gene could be more common than previous estimates, which would question the past accepted "rare" label placed on this condition. For example, it is plausible some patients diagnosed with familial hypercholesterolemia (FH) in the past were misdiagnosed sitosterolemia cases. Regardless, the issue of sitosterolemia does not seem to garner sufficient awareness within cardiology or urology.

Another popular BPH supplement is known as "Pygeum africanum" has a somewhat similar unresolved clinical story to beta-sitosterol in terms of a positive past meta-analysis,[21] but a lack of recent or updated phase 3 research to better construe advantages and disadvantages of this herbal nutraceutical. Although, there was an admirable but unsuccessful attempt to use Pygeum in a phase 3 U.S. trial known as "CAMUS,"[22] which ultimately became a dose-escalation study of saw palmetto.[23] Pygeum bark products also potentially contain beta-sitosterol as one of its active potential ingredients,[24] but a different concern over using these products needs better resolution. Pygeum bark appears on some endangered lists and there is a concern over the ongoing utilization of these trees for BPH and other medical conditions.[25–27] The relative supply, or environmental impact of removing wild Pygeum bark needs more attention and discussion, as does alternative and more sustainable farming sources of these trees.

Other herbal BPH products including pumpkin seed extract and saw palmetto have multiple potential beneficial compounds, and again beta-sitosterol is a compound often found in both products,[28] which has also been associated with a dampening in proinflammatory cytokines.[29] A phase 3 trial is needed for pumpkin seed extract, but there are some preliminary clinical studies demonstrating safety and potential efficacy,[30] but again plant sterol issues (if any) need further elucidation. However, saw palmetto seems to have reached a perplexing clinical scenario. Two methodologically robust phase-3 type clinical trials have been conducted with saw palmetto including the CAMUS and STEP studies.[23,31] Neither trial demonstrated a benefit compared with placebo even when dose-escalation was used in CAMUS, and no changes in PSA occurred compared with placebo.[32] These findings call into question the precise mechanism of action attributed to saw palmetto, quality of the placebo from past studies, placebo response rates, or even ideal form of saw palmetto and standardization needed to demonstrate clinical success. The ongoing perplexity centers around other uniquely derived or proprietary isolation methods of saw palmetto with a history of pharmacologic QC demonstrating consistent clinical benefits in numerous BPH studies, especially the product known as "Permixon" (Pierre Fabre Medicament, Castres, France), which is a hexane lipidosterolic extract of saw palmetto.[33,34] Regardless of the reasons, Permixon was not used in either phase 3 type U.S. studies (CAMUS or STEP). In the STEP trial, a carbon dioxide extract was used and in the CAMUS study, a lipidic ethanolic derived product was chosen. Whether it is a higher quantitative and/or qualitative fatty acid content found in Permixon, the additional potential contribution of some plant sterols,[35] or simply the need to be in a more updated rigorous head-to-head clinical trial against placebo and medications used in clinical guidelines for BPH, the debate will continue as to why this form of saw palmetto continues to demonstrate positive outcomes over other notable sources. Regardless of the opinion of any clinician on supplement utilization for BPH or another condition, it must be reiterated that the interest or even utilization of nutraceuticals by many consumers represents one potential opportunity for health care professionals to engage in a dialogue with a diverse patient population more open and in some cases more likely to derive some benefit from lifestyle changes.[5,36]

ERECTILE DYSFUNCTION (ED) AND NITRIC OXIDE OPTIONS AND LIMITATIONS

Panax ginseng (Asian ginseng, Korean red ginseng) has been thoroughly reviewed and seems to have multiple proposed mechanisms of action from prolactin reduction to increasing nitric oxide (NO) levels.[37–39] The overall safety and short-term efficacy record of this herbal product has been adequate, but more research on the long-term objective effectiveness beyond placebo and the optimal dosage and ginsenoside content (standardized ingredients) for efficacy is needed (phase 3 trial). The subjective improvement from randomized trials has been consistent, which would suggest it could be an option for some patients with ED. Arguably, the future issue for ginseng is not a dearth of preliminary clinical data, but a reliable source, or proven QC verification method for these unique phytotherapies, and this is true of the entire herbal product category within urology.[37–39] Known standardized active ingredient concentrations, specific compounds extracted from specific sources (roots, seeds, stems, leaves), heavy metal and other contaminant levels, potential drug interactions, and even similarity or differences from past products used in phase 3 trials should become the minimal threshold for herbal supplement acceptance.

Perhaps the compound with the largest amount of attention or publications as a single ingredient is L-arginine with and without PDE-5 inhibitors.[40–42] Mechanistically, the conversion of this amino acid to NO and reasonable pricing, in general, equates to a logical choice among many clinicians with mild-to-moderate ED of several different etiologies, but coverage of the disadvantages of this approach needs more attention. L-arginine requires large oral dosages for potential efficacy in part because of extensive first-pass metabolism, deactivating enzymes (arginases), and microbiome strains along the intestinal tract, which ultimately discourage systemic exposure.[43,44] One solution would be the utilization of oral L-citrulline, which does not seem to harbor many of these pharmacologic limitations, and although L-citrulline has some positive preliminary data it is in urgent need of long-term efficacy, safety and even compliance studies.[45,46] If one capsule of either NO precursor equates to approximately 500 mg then even 2 to 3 g/d would still be tantamount to 4 to 6 pills daily, which makes long-term utilization of L-arginine or even L-citrulline at lower dosages more challenging. Other formulations, more diluted delivery systems, and the lowest concentration for efficacy especially in terms of L-citrulline utilization are needed.

Another related issue with L-arginine has been the surprise adverse effects, or lack of an effect observed in some notable past cardiovascular disease trials of at least 6 months duration, which has not received adequate attention in urology.[47–49] Whether these concerns are relevant today in some patients with a history of certain forms of cardiovascular disease (myocardial infarction, peripheral artery disease, and so forth.) simply needs more research.[50] Also, whether these cardiovascular concerns also could apply to L-citrulline has not been determined. Ironically, it is of interest L-arginine and L-citrulline have blood pressure lowering properties,[50–52] which have been consistent in short-term trials, and this could be perceived as an advantage or disadvantage based on the clinical scenario, but again it does reflect the importance of testing the lowest potential dosage of safety and efficacy.

Another issue is the best form or version of these ingredients. Many nutraceutical products use one, or the other amino acid, and often with additional ingredient(s), but solving this complexity was not the purpose of this review. Still, an issue of free form or combined/complexed arginine or citrulline needs to be addressed in terms of efficacy and safety. For example, the free form of L-citrulline seems to have been used in some preliminary ED studies with some efficacy,[45] but the citrulline malate combination has been generally used within exercise enhancement studies,[53,54] and whether there are clinical efficacy differences between them need

further study. Still, the generally encouraging news has to be the recent acknowledgment in some clinical guidelines of specific supplements and their potential future role in ED management if more safety and efficacy research is completed.[55]

Even more interesting from this author's standpoint is the plethora of positive data and endorsement of lifestyle changes to prevent ED, the progression of ED, or to synergistically assist with conventional treatment.[56–59] One accepted method for encouraging healthy NO availability or production is regular physical activity. Exercise seems to also reduce one of the most well recognized competitive inhibitors of NO synthesis known as "asymmetrical dimethylarginine" (ADMA), which is upregulated in a variety of diverse disease states.[60,61]

MALE INFERTILITY: ANTI-VERSUS PRO-OXIDANTS

The enthusiasm for a nutraceutical to reduce oxidative stress and improve some parameters of male fertility and ideally improve pregnancy and live-birth rates has received a considerable number of positive past publications.[62,63] Still, there has been adequate caution from many of these publications as to the quality of the evidence, the need for more randomized trials, and specific subgroups of infertile men qualifying for a nutraceutical intervention. Recently, 2 methodologically impressive clinical trials were published to address some of these past issues. The Folic Acid and Zinc Supplementation Trial (FAZST) used an intervention of 5 mg/d folic acid and 30 mg elemental zinc daily versus placebo in 2370 men receiving infertility treatment in the U.S. and found no significant effects on semen parameters over 6-month, or live birth rates over 9-months .[64] A statistically significant increase in DNA fragmentation was observed with this intervention, and a higher incidence of gastrointestinal symptoms and erythema were also noted.

Another separate multi-site trial was The Males, Antioxidants, and Infertility (MOXI) study, which used a diverse daily combination antioxidant intervention (500 mg vitamin C, 400 mg vitamin E, 0.20 mg selenium, 1000 mg L-carnitine, 20 mg zinc, 1 mg folic acid, 10 mg lycopene, and 2000 IU vitamin D) in 174 men with male factor infertility.[65] Overall, no differences in semen characteristics, DNA integrity, pregnancy, or live birth rates occurred in favor of the intervention except a statistically significant difference in sperm concentration ($P = .03$), total sperm count ($P = .02$), and total motile sperm count ($P = .04$) in favor of placebo after 3-months of treatment. No difference in overall and serious adverse events between the antioxidant and placebo groups was found.

Is it plausible higher concentrations of some antioxidants could function as a pro-oxidant or encourage oxidative stress in some men with infertility?[66] What is plausible is the antithesis of what was expected in some clinical urologic situations could become the actual observed outcome as witnessed for example, from the phase 3 SELECT trial of prostate cancer prevention.[67] Also, the added impact of increasing fortification in some food supplies, such as the U.S., also questions the true definition and prevalence of "nutrient deficiency" in many situations and what constitutes over exposure. However, it is too early to argue the benefits and limitations of antioxidant treatment, and which subgroups of infertile men would benefit or not from nutraceuticals. More high-quality trials such as FAZST or MOXI will help urology and patients arrive at this answer, but the antioxidant versus pro-oxidant debate abounds in urology.

FAZST and MOXI may provide another indirect lesson in terms of male infertility, which is an appreciation of the challenging and changing landscape of the average patient in need of assistance. In FAZST the mean male participant was 32 years of age, obese, and with an elevated blood pressure at baseline while female partners were overweight and in the proximity of being obese.[64] In the MOXI trial men on average were overweight and a mean age of 34.[65] Thus, it is possible the solution to infertility in some men, and couples, has become more challenging with the increasing prevalence and severity of unhealthy health parameters found in younger and older age groups over the past decade.[68] Are the expectations simply too great for any nutraceutical to solve under some of these conditions? Are these unhealthy baseline parameters increasing inflammation as well as pro-oxidation? Perhaps, a more positive angle is the increasing relevance of behavioral changes within this current milieu. Weight loss, exercise, smoking cessation, and other lifestyle changes are included in some recent male infertility clinical guidelines, which bring further awareness to these issues.[69] Healthier parameters and lifestyles need to be recognized as a more lucid path toward mitigating inflammation or oxidation.

PROSTATE CANCER: LESS IS MORE

Few conditions in all of the medicine are more symbolic of the potential consequences of over exposure to some nutrients in some specific clinical conditions other than prostate cancer prevention. SELECT was a methodologically robust phase 3 clinical trial and vitamin E at a dosage well above the recommended dietary allowance (RDA) was found to significantly increase the risk of prostate cancer.[67] Additional ancillary and further concerning findings from this trial suggested men replete with selenium or with higher alpha-tocopherol levels at baseline, and then exposed to the selenium supplement in this trial seemed to have an increased risk of being diagnosed with high-grade prostate cancer.[70,71] Other observational and clinical studies echo some of these concerns, including after being diagnosed with prostate cancer and the potential for accelerated PSA kinetics in some men with higher baseline selenium status,[72] or even a higher risk of progression associated with ingesting supplemental selenium.[73] Again, is this another case of a common antioxidant engaging in pro-oxidant activity when excessive exposure or supra-physiologic blood levels are attained? Interestingly, no other individual supplemental antioxidant has emerged as a consensus candidate to prevent prostate cancer despite such a strong emphasis in locating such a nutrient over the last 25 years.[74]

Observing other urologic cancers, but with higher recurrence levels after treatment, such as nonmuscle invasive bladder cancer (NMIBC), suggests other common nutrients in excessive dosages, such as folic acid, could increase the risk of relapse.[75] Higher folate or folic acid exposure has also been implicated in potentially increasing the risk and progression of prostate cancer.[76,77] Men on active surveillance (AS) have been preliminarily tested with a folate reduced protocol with promising initial results,[78] which should lead to more research using this unique "less is more approach." In summary, the current state of several nutraceutical compounds in prostate cancer prevention or treatment suggests excessive exposure seems to offer minimal benefits and could increase the risk of progression.

ANTIPARASITIC ALTERNATIVE PRODUCTS FOR PROSTATE CANCER?

This article would be remiss in objectively educating practitioners on the current landscape of OTC products without mentioning the ongoing controversies with accessing and using off-label, often veterinary-based, antiparasitic compounds in cancer and other conditions. Although not officially "nutraceuticals" from this author's standpoint, some of these agents are accessible OTC, which deserves some commentary. For example, ivermectin procurement occurred during the COVID-19 pandemic as patients seemed to seek out alternative products, but ordering, prescribing, or even distributing this compound to prevent or treat COVID-19 has been discouraged based on a current lack of high-quality evidence and safety concerns.[79] However, before the ivermectin controversy evolved there has been interest in using other primarily intestinal anthelmintic products as potential repurposed medications against various cancers including prostate cancer with a focus on mebendazole over albendazole due to the potential for microtubule disruption as one possible mechanistic pathway along with a suggestion of a better safety profile (less neutropenia).[80] Still, the current clinical support for using these anthelmintics outside of a clinical trial is questionable. Mebendazole recently demonstrated no notable clinical efficacy in 10 patients with advanced gastrointestinal cancer,[81] and in combination with temozolomide in patients with recently diagnosed high-grade gliomas from a phase 1 trial (n = 24) there was no statistically significant impact on survival, but the authors observed an appropriate safety profile (reversible liver enzyme increases) and "encouraging" activity in this adjuvant setting.[82] Clinicians should continue to observe the data with these anthelmintic compounds to provide the most objective assessment for patients inquiring about their use from the internet or other sources. Multiple other mebendazole trials are expected to be completed in the future against a variety of cancers. Regardless, another anthelmintic known as "fenbendazole" used in some animals and with minimal human safety and clinical trial data seems to have gained interest by some patients with prostate and other cancers.[83] Perhaps this is due to the attention it was given within some social media circles, its relation to mebendazole, or because it can be procured OTC. A recent case-study in a patient with non-small cell lung cancer using fenbendazole via social media sources demonstrated enhanced hepatotoxicity requiring hospitalization, no observed cancer treatment effects, and resolution of toxicity on the discontinuation of the drug and the reutilization of pembrolizumab, which had demonstrated previous efficacy.[84] This case exemplifies a serious concern when using some unproven OTC therapies, which could delay proven and effective treatments and enhance toxicity in some cases. Numerous previous preliminary studies have suggested for some time the potential for liver toxicity with fenbendazole.[85,86] Another concern with these specific broad-spectrum anthelmintic compounds is the minimal absorption capabilities of these drugs after ingestion, which is part of the reasoning for primarily using them in the treatment of intestinal parasites. If these agents do not demonstrate efficacy for intestinal cancers, then is it plausible to expect some efficacy for other nongastrointestinal disease states? Again, the ongoing and numerous cancer clinical trials using mebendazole should soon provide more lucid advantages and disadvantages of this specific drug class against a variety of cancers, but currently, the clinical concerns seem to outweigh the early preliminary promise. Yet, this author humbly recognizes that a plethora of ongoing clinical trials await publication. Regardless, the potential efficacy for lifestyle changes to improve some prognostic outcomes or to reduce toxicity from conventional therapy in prostate and other cancers continues to gain momentum from recent clinical research.[87–89] It would seem prudent to consider using and further intrinsically investing in some of these lifestyle changes while waiting for the data to mature from these other more controversial extrinsic interventions.

TESTOSTERONE REPLACEMENT RISKS: PILLS VERSUS RX VERSUS LIFESTYLE

Minimal attention can be placed on testosterone replacement (TRT) nutraceuticals at this time because of the limited space remaining within this article for such a formidable and extensive subject. However, it should be reiterated that the parent nutraceutical compound for testosterone enhancement, DHEA, continues to have multiple ongoing concerns including: an unreliable ability to increase male hormone levels, significant HDL reductions, potential for BPH and cancer progression, and simply whether a statistically significant numerical increase in testosterone, if it even occurs in some patients, is tantamount to any appreciable objective and subjective clinically relevant parameter changes.[90–95] Thus, when some nutraceuticals have the potential to enhance DHEA production, but need more rigorous data,[96,97] then it would seem logical to express somewhat similar concerns until proven otherwise. Prescription testosterone products have reliable QC data and perhaps more clinical research. However, the cost and short- and long-term safety issues with these products, in some patients, should also not be dismissed, and more objective open communication of the advantages and disadvantages should always be encouraged.[98]

What does seem to receive a lack of sufficient attention is the impact of diet on a total testosterone blood test in potentially misdiagnosing hypogonadism,[99] and the increasing impact on weight loss and other healthy lifestyle changes to increase testosterone in many patients without the added costs and safety issues.[100] And, if heart-healthy lifestyle alterations cannot intrinsically change these metabolic parameters and/or tangibly impact some of the more notable male hypogonadal symptoms, then it would seem more appropriate to address and potentially entertain the extrinsic treatment options, but not vice versa.

SUMMARY

Consumer, patient, and healthcare professional interest or the utilization of nutraceuticals are associated with an increased interest and compliance with heart-healthy lifestyle changes. Thus, opportunity abounds in these unique situations to improve the overall personal health of patients, and this is a critical take-home message of this article. Men's health is replete with nutraceutical options and simply and objectively communicating the advantage and disadvantages of each option based on the specific medical condition are needed. It seems easier to generalize the impact, or lack of impact, of dietary supplements, but this is an antiquated method of dealing with the subject as the plethora of publications now available, including phase 3 trials, should encourage a constructive conversation on any specific men's health subject.

CLINICS CARE POINTS

- Supplement QC verification, especially with herbal products, should be the rule and not the exception.
- Men's health supplements, in general, need more comprehensive and regularly updated safety & efficacy information.
- Lifestyle changes have an ability to enhance conventional treatment efficacy and outcomes.

DISCLOSURE

Quality control consultant to Max International on cosmetic products.

REFERENCES

1. Moyad MA. Integrative medicine and urology: bladder and prostate cancer, supplements and lifestyle changes. AUA Update Ser 2020;39. lesson 10.
2. U.S. National Library of Medicine. Available at: https://clinicaltrials.gov. October 1, 2021.
3. CVS pharmacy tested to be trusted. Available at: https://www.cvs.com/content/tested-trusted. October 1, 2021.
4. Kao TC, Kazman JB, Cheng Y-H, et al. Healthy lifestyles among military active duty service members, and associations with body-building and weight-loss supplement use. Ann Epidemiol 2021;53: 27–33.
5. Tank M, Franz K, Cereda E, et al. Dietary supplement use in ambulatory cancer patients: a survey on prevalence, motivation and attitudes. J Cancer Res Clin Oncol 2021;147:1917–25.
6. Rautiainen S, Wang L, Gaziano JM, et al. Who use multivitamins? A cross-sectional study in the Physicians' Health Study. Eur J Nutr 2014; 53:1065–7.
7. Moyad MA. Integrative medicine and urology: lifestyle changes, supplements and acupuncture-noncancerous conditions. AUA Update Ser 2021; 40. lesson 33.
8. Giubilei G, Mondaini N, Minervini A, et al. Physical activity of men with chronic prostatitis/chronic pelvic pain syndrome not satisfied with conventional treatments-could it represent a valid option? The physical activity and male pelvic pain trial: a double-blind, randomized study. J Urol 2007;177: 159–65.
9. Terentes-Printzios D, Loakeimidis N, Rokkas K, et al. Interactions between erectile dysfunction, cardiovascular disease and cardiovascular drugs. Nat Rev Cardiol 2021. https://doi.org/10.1038/s41569-021-00593-6.
10. Agarwal A, Baskaran S, Parekh, et al. Male infertility. Lancet 2021;397:319–33.
11. Maio G, Saraeb S, Marchiori A. Physical activity and PDE5 inhibitors in the treatment of sexual dysfunction: results of a randomized controlled study. J Sex Med 2010;7:2201–8.
12. Muller RL, Gerber L, Moreira DM, et al. Obesity is associated with increased prostate growth and attenuated prostate volume reduction by dutasteride. Eur Urol 2013;63:1115–21.
13. Khan S, Wolin KY, Pakpahan R, et al. Body size throughout the life-course and incident benign prostatic hyperplasia-related outcomes and nocturia. BMC Urol 2021. https://doi.org/10.1186/s12894-021-00816-5.
14. Wilt T, Ishani A, MacDonald R, et al. Beta-sitosterols for benign prostatic hyperplasia. Cochrane Database Syst Rev 2000;(2):CD001043.
15. FDA. Part 101-Food labeling. Subpart E-specific requirements for health claims. Sec. 101.83 Health Claims: plant sterol and stanol esters and risk of coronary heart disease (CHD). Available at: https://www.accessdata.fda.gov/scripts/cdrh/cfdocs/cfcfr/CFRSearch.cfm?fr=101.83. June 1, 2020.
16. Semczuk-Kaczmarek K, Platek AE, Szymanski FM. Co-treatment of lower urinary tract symptoms and cardiovascular disease-where do we stand? Cent Eur J Urol 2020;73:42–5.
17. Yamada Y, Sugi K, Gatate Y, et al. Premature acute myocardial infarction in a young patient with sitosterolemia. CJC Open 2021;3:1085–8.

18. Yoo EG. Sitosterolemia: a review and update of pathophysiology, clinical spectrum, diagnosis, and management. Ann Pediatr Endocrinol Metab 2016;21:7–14.

19. Tada H, Nohara A, Ogura M, et al. Diagnosis and management of sitosterolemia 2021. J Atheroscler Thromb 2021;28:791–801.

20. Lek M, Karczewski KJ, Minikel EV, et al. Analysis of protein-coding genetic variation in 60,706 humans. Nature 2016;536:285–91.

21. Wilt T, Ishani A, Mac Donald R, et al. Pygeum africanum for benign prostatic hyperplasia. Cochrane Database Syst Rev 2002;1:CD001044.

22. Lee J, Andriole G, Avins A. Redesigning a large-scale clinical trial in response to negative external trial results: the CAMUS study of phytotherapy for benign prostatic hyperplasia. Clin Trials 2009;6:628–36.

23. Barry MJ, Meleth S, Lee JY, et al. Effect of increasing doses of saw palmetto extract on lower urinary tract symptoms: a randomized trial. JAMA 2011;306:1344–51.

24. Thompson RQ, Katz D, Sheehan B. Chemical comparison of Prunus africana bark and pygeum products marketed for prostate health. J Pharm Biomed Anal 2019;163:162–9.

25. Cunningham A, Anoncho VF, Sunderland T. Power, policy and the Prunus Africana bark trade, 1972-2015. J Ethnopharmacol 2016;178:323–33.

26. Bodeker G, van 't Klooster C, Weisbord E. Prunus Africana (Hook.f.) Kalkman: the overexploitation of a medicinal plant species and its legal context. J Altern Complement Med 2014;20:810–22.

27. Stewart KM. The African cherry (Prunus Africana): can lessons be learned from an over-exploited medicinal tree? J Ethnopharmacol 2003;89:3–13.

28. Patel S, Rauf A. Edible seeds from Cucurbitaceae family as potential functional foods: immense promises. Few concerns. Biomed Pharmacother 2017;91: 330–7.

29. Kwon Y. Use of saw palmetto (Serenoa repens) extract for benign prostatic hyperplasia. Food Sci Biotechnol 2019;28:1599–606.

30. Vahlensieck W, Theurer C, Pfitzer E, et al. Effects of pumpkin seed in men with lower urinary tract symptoms due to benign prostatic hyperplasia in the one-year, randomized, placebo-controlled GRANU study. Urol Int 2015;94:286–95.

31. Bent S, Kane C, Shinohara K, et al. Saw palmetto for benign prostatic hyperplasia. N Engl J Med 2006;354:557–66.

32. Andriole GL, McCullum-Hill C, Sandhu GS, et al. The effect of increasing doses of saw palmetto fruit extract on serum prostate specific antigen: analysis of the CAMUS randomized trial. J Urol 2013; 189:486–92.

33. Vela-Navarrete R, Alcaraz A, Rodriguez-Antolin A, et al. Efficacy and safety of a hexanic extract of Serenoa repens (Permixon) for the treatment of lower urinary tract symptoms associated with benign prostatic hyperplasia (LUTS/BPH): systematic review and meta-analysis of randomized controlled trials and observational studies. BJU Int 2018;122:1049–65.

34. Novara G, Giannarini G, Alcaraz A, et al. Efficacy and safety of hexanic lipidosterolic extract of Serenoa repens (Permixon) in the treatment of lower urinary tract symptoms due to benign prostatic hyperplasia: systematic review and meta-analysis of randomized controlled trials. Eur Urol Focus 2016;2:553–61.

35. Keehn A, Taylor J, Lowe FC. Phytotherapy for benign prostatic hyperplasia. Curr Urol Rep 2016; 17:53.

36. Lee JY, Foster HE, McVary KT, et al. Recruitment of participants to a clinical trial of botanical therapy for benign prostatic hyperplasia. J Alt Comp Med 2011;17:469–72.

37. Lee HW, Lee MS, Kim TH, et al. Ginseng for erectile dysfunction: a Cochrane systematic review. World J Mens Health 2021. https://doi.org/10.5534/wjmh. 210071.

38. Leisegang K, Finelli R. Alternative medicine and herbal remedies in the treatment of erectile dysfunction: a systematic review. Arab J Urol 2021;19:323–39.

39. Sin VJ-E, Anand GS, Koh H-L. Botanical medicine and natural products used for erectile dysfunction. Sex Med Rev 2021;9:568–92.

40. Rhim HC, Kim MS, Park Y-J, et al. The potential role of arginine supplements on erectile dysfunction: a systemic review and meta-analysis. J Sex Med 2019;16:223–34.

41. Xu Z, Liu C, Liu S, et al. Comparison of efficacy and safety of daily oral L-arginine and PDE5Is alone or in combination in treating erectile dysfunction: a systematic review and meta-analysis of randomized controlled trials. Andrologia 2021. https://doi. org/10.1111/and.14007.

42. Gallo L, Pecoraro S, Sarnacchiaro P, et al. The daily therapy with L-arginine 2500 mg and tadalafil 5 mg in combination for the treatment of erectile dysfunction: a prospective, randomized multicentre study. Sex Med 2020;8:178–85.

43. Morris SM Jr. Enzymes of arginine metabolism. J Nutr 2004;134:2743S–7S.

44. Schwedhelm E, Maas R, Freese R, et al. Pharmacokinetic and pharmacodynamic properties of oral L-citrulline and L-arginine: impact on nitric oxide metabolism. Br J Clin Pharmacol 2008;65: 51–9.

45. Cormio L, De Siati M, Lorusso F, et al. Oral L-citrulline supplementation improves erection hardness in men with mild erectile dysfunction. Urology 2011;77:119–22.

46. Osadchiy V, Eleswarpu SV, Mills SA, et al. Efficacy of preprostatectomy multi-modal penile rehabilitation regimen on recovery of postoperative erectile function. Int J Impot Res 2020;32:323–8.

47. Schulman SP, Becker LC, Kass DA, et al. L-arginine therapy in acute myocardial infarction: the vascular interaction with age in myocardial infarction (VINTAGE MI) randomized clinical trial. JAMA 2006;295:58–64.

48. Wilson AM, Harada R, Nair N, et al. L-arginine supplementation in peripheral arterial disease: no benefit and possible harm. Circulation 2007;116:188–95.

49. Rodriguez-Krause J, Krause M, da Rocha IMG, et al. Association of L-arginine supplementation with markers of endothelial function in patients with cardiovascular or metabolic disorders: a systematic review and meta-analysis. Nutrients 2018. https://doi.org/10.3390/nu11010015.

50. Boger RH. L-arginine therapy in cardiovascular pathologies: beneficial or dangerous? Curr Opin Clin Nutr Metab Care 2008;11:55–61.

51. Dong J-Y, Qin L-Q, Zhang Z, et al. Effect of oral L-arginine supplementation on blood pressure: a meta-analysis of randomized, double-blind, placebo-controlled trials. Am Heart J 2011;162:959–65.

52. Khalaf D, Kruger M, Wehland M, et al. The effects of oral l-arginine and l-citrulline supplementation on blood pressure. Nutrients 2019. https://doi.org/10.3390/nu11071679.

53. Trexler ET, Persky AM, Ryan ED, et al. Acute effects of citrulline supplementation on high-intensity strength and power performance: a systematic review and meta-analysis. Sports Med 2019;49:707–18.

54. Varvik FT, Bjornsen T, Gonzalez AM. Effect of citrulline malate on repetition performance during strength training: a systematic review and meta-analysis. Int J Sport Nutr Exerc Metab 2021;31:350–8.

55. Domes T, Najafabadi BT, Roberts M, et al. Canadian Urological Association guideline: erectile dysfunction. Can Urol Assoc J 2021;15:310–22.

56. Esposito K, Giugliano F, Di Palo C, et al. Effect of lifestyle changes on erectile dysfunction in obese men: a randomized controlled trial. JAMA 2004; 291:2978–84.

57. Kratzik CW, Lackner JE, Mark I, et al. How much physical activity is needed to maintain erectile function? Results of the Androx Vienna Municipality Study. Eur Urol 2009;55:509–17.

58. Palm P, Zwisler A-DO, Svendsen JH, et al. Sexual rehabilitation for cardiac patients with erectile dysfunction: a randomised clinical trial. Heart 2019;105:775–82.

59. Gerbild H, Larsen CM, Graugaard C, et al. Physical activity to improve erectile function: a systematic review of intervention studies. Sex Med 2018;6:75–89.

60. Goto C, Nishioka K, Umemura T, et al. Acute moderate-intensity exercise induces vasodilation through an increase in nitric oxide bioavailability in humans. Am J Hypertens 2007;20:825–30.

61. Riccioni G, Scotti L, Guagnano MT, et al. Physical exercise reduces synthesis of ADMA, SDMA, and L-arg. Front Biosci (Elite Ed) 2015;7:417–22.

62. Smits RM, Mackenzie-Proctor R, Yazdani A, et al. Antioxidants for male subfertility. Cochrane Database Syst Rev 2019;3:CD007411.

63. Agarwal A, Leisegang K, Majzoub A, et al. Utility of antioxidants in the treatment of male infertility: clinical guidelines based on systematic review and analysis of the evidence. World J Mens Health 2021;39:233–90.

64. Schisterman EF, Sjaarda LA, Clemons T, et al. Effect of folic acid and zinc supplementation in men on semen quality and live birth among couples undergoing infertility treatment: a randomized clinical trial. JAMA 2020;323:35–48.

65. Steiner AZ, Hansen KR, Barnhart KT, et al, for the Reproductive Medicine Network. The effects of antioxidants on male factor infertility: the Males, Antioxidants, and Infertility (MOXI) randomized clinical trial. Fertil Steril 2020;113:552–60.

66. Henkel R, Sandhu IS, Agarwal A. The excessive use of antioxidant therapy: a possible cause of male infertility? Andrologia 2019;51:e13162. https://doi.org/10.1111/and.13162.

67. Klein EA, Thompson IM Jr, Tangen CM, et al. Vitamin E and the risk of prostate cancer: the selenium and vitamin E Cancer prevention trial. (SELECT). JAMA 2011;306:1549–56.

68. Obesity and overweight. Center for Disease Control and Prevention (CDC). Available at: https://www.cdc.gov/nchs/fastats/obesity-overweight.htm. June 15, 2020.

69. Minhas S, Bettocchi C, Boeri L, et al. European association of urology guidelines on male sexual and reproductive health: 2021 update on male infertility. Eur Urol 2021. https://doi.org/10.1016/j.eururo.2021.08.014.

70. Kristal AR, Darke AK, Morris JS, et al. Baseline selenium status and effects of selenium and vitamin e supplementation on prostate cancer risk. J Natl Cancer Inst 2014. https://doi.org/10.1093/jnci/djt456.

71. Albanes D, Till C, Klein EA, et al. Plasma tocopherols and risk of prostate cancer in the selenium and vitamin E cancer prevention trial (SELECT). Cancer Prev Res 2014;7:886–95.

72. Stratton MS, Algota AM, Ranger-Moore J, et al. Oral selenium supplementation has no effect on prostate-specific antigen velocity in men undergoing active surveillance for localized prostate cancer. Cancer Prev Res (Phila) 2010;3:1035–41.

73. Kenfield SA, Van Biarigan EL, DuPre N, et al. Selenium supplementation and prostate cancer mortality. J Natl Cancer Inst 2014. https://doi.org/10.1093/jnci/dju360.

74. Moyad MA. Preventing lethal prostate cancer with diet, supplements, and Rx: heart healthy continues to be prostate healthy and "first do no harm" part II. Curr Urol Rep 2020. https://doi.org/10.1007/s11934-020-0967-4.

75. Tu H, Dinney CP, Ye Y, et al. Is folic acid safe for non-muscle-invasive bladder cancer patients? An evidence-based cohort study. Am J Clin Nutr 2018; 107:208–16.

76. Bo Y, Zhu Y, Tao Y, et al. Association between folate and health outcomes: an umbrella review of meta-analyses. Front Public Health 2020. https://doi.org/10.3389/fpubh.2020.550753.

77. Liss MA, Ashcraft K, Satsangi A, et al. Rise in serum folate after androgen deprivation associated with worse prostate cancer-specific survival. Urol Oncol 2020;682:e21–7.

78. Ullevig SL, Bacich DJ, Gutierrez JM, et al. Feasibility of dietary folic acid reduction intervention for men on active surveillance for prostate cancer. Clin Nutr ESPEN 2021;44:270–5.

79. FDA Consumer Health. Why you should not use ivermectin to treat or prevent COVID-19. Available at: https://www.fda.gov/consumers/consumer-updates/why-you-should-not-use-ivermectin-treat-or-prevent-covid-19. October 1, 2021.

80. Chai J-Y, Jung B-K, Hong S-J. Albendazole and mebendazole as anti-parasitic and anti-cancer agents: an update. Korean J Parasitol 2021;59:189–225.

81. Mansoori S, Fryknas M, Alvfors C, et al. A phase 2a clinical study on the safety and efficacy of individualized dosed mebendazole in patients with advanced gastrointestinal cancer. Sci Rep 2021. https://doi.org/10.1038/s41598-021-88433-y.

82. Gallia GL, Holdhoff M, Brem H, et al. Mebendazole and temozolomide in patients with newly diagnosed high-grade gliomas: results of a phase 1 clinical trial. Neurooncol Adv 2021;3. https://doi.org/10.1093/noajnl/vdaa154.

83. Heo DS. Anthelmintics as potential anti-cancer drugs? J Korean Med Sci 2020;35:e75.

84. Yamaguchi T, Shimizu J, Oya Y, et al. Drug-induced liver injury in a patient with nonsmall cell lung cancer after the self-administration of febendazole based on social media information. Case Rep Oncol 2021;14:886–91.

85. Shoda T, Onodera H, Takeda M, et al. Liver tumor promoting effects of fenbendazole in rats. Toxicol Pathol 1999;27:553–62.

86. Gardner CR, Mishin V, Laskin JD, et al. Exacerbation of acetaminophen hepatotoxicity by the antihelmentic drug febendazole. Toxicol Sci 2012;125:607–12.

87. Kang D-W, Fairey AS, Boule NG, et al. Effects of exercise on cardiorespiratory fitness and biochemical progression in men with localized prostate cancer under active surveillance: the ERASE randomized clinical trial. JAMA Oncol 2021. https://doi.org/10.1001/jamaoncol.2021.3067.

88. Orgel E, Framson C, Buxton R, et al. Caloric and nutrient restriction to augment chemotherapy efficacy for acute lymphoblastic leukemia: the IDEAL trial. Blood Adv 2021;5:1853–61.

89. de Groot S, Lugtenberg RT, Cohen D, et al. Fasting mimicking diet as an adjunct to neoadjuvant chemotherapy for breast cancer in the multicentre randomized phase 2 DIRECT trial. Nat Commun 2020. https://doi.org/10.1038/s41467-020-16138-3.

90. Acacio BD, Stanczyk FZ, Mullin P, et al. Pharmacokinetics of dehydroepiandrosterone metabolites after long-term daily oral administration to healthy young men. Fertil Steril 2004;81:595–604.

91. Arnold JT, Gray NE, Jacobowitz K, et al. Human prostate stromal cells stimulate increased PSA cell production in DHEA-treated prostate cancer epithelial cells. J Steroid Biochem Mol Biol 2008;111:240–6.

92. Jones JA, Nguyen A, Straub M, et al. Use of DHEA in a patient with advanced prostate cancer: a case report and a review. Urology 1997;50:784–8.

93. Poretsky L, Brillon DJ, Ferrando S, et al. Endocrine effects of oral dehydroepiandrosterone in men with HIV infection: a prospective, randomized, double-blind, placebo-controlled trial. Metabolism 2006; 55:858–70.

94. Qin Y, Santos HO, Khani V, et al. Effects of dehydroepiandrosterone (DHEA) supplementation on the lipid profile: a systematic review and dose-response meta-analysis of randomized controlled trials. Nutr Metab Cardiovasc Dis 2020;30:1465–75.

95. Li Y, Ren J, Li N, et al. A dose-response and meta-analysis of dehydroepiandrosterone (DHEA) supplementation on testosterone levels: perinatal prediction of randomized clinical trials. Exp Gerontol 2020. https://doi.org/10.1016/j.exger.2020.111110.

96. Lopresti AL, Drummond PD, Smith SJ. A randomized, double-blind, placebo-controlled, crossover study examining the hormonal and vitality effects of Ashwagandha (Withania somnifera) in aging, overweight males. Am J Mens Health 2019. https://doi.org/10.1177/1557988319835985.

97. Smith SJ, Lopresti AL, Teo SYM, et al. Examining the effects of herbs on testosterone concentrations in men: a systematic review. Adv Nutr 2021;12:744–65.

98. Auerbach JM, Khera M. Hypogonadism management and cardiovascular health. Postgrad Med 2020;132(sup4):35–41.

99. Bhasin S, Brito JP, Cunningham GR, et al. Testosterone therapy in men with hypogonadism: an Endocrine Society Clinical Practice Guideline. J Clin Endocrinol Metab 2018;103:1715–44.

100. Fantus RJ, Chang C, Hehemann MC, et al. The association between guideline-based exercise thresholds and low testosterone among men in the United States. Andrology 2020;8:1712–9.

Medical Treatment of Overactive Bladder

Justin Loloi, MD[a], Whitney Clearwater, MD, MPH[b], Alison Schulz, BS[c],
Sylvia O. Suadicani, PhD[a,c], Nitya Abraham, MD[a,*]

KEYWORDS

• Overactive bladder • Urge urinary incontinence • Pharmacotherapy • Antimuscarinic • Beta-agonist

KEY POINTS

- Antimuscarinic agents represent the most common pharmacologic therapy and act by inhibiting bladder smooth muscle contraction. These medications are associated with clinically-significant adverse effects including dry mouth, constipation and possible cognitive impairment with long-term use.
- Beta-3 agonists act on the detrusor smooth muscle, resulting in detrusor muscle relaxation and increased bladder capacity. Patients on this medicaiton should be closely monitored for adverse cardiovascular effects including worsening high blood pressure.
- Combination therapies may provide superior symptom control by targeting several components of the OAB pathophysiologic pathway.
- Anti-depressants may be used as an off-label treatment modality for OAB.
- There is ongoing research focused on novel therapeutic targets in the urothelium and lamina propria that are implicated in the pathophysiology of OAB.

INTRODUCTION

Overactive bladder (OAB) is a clinical condition affecting the bladder's ability to store urine that results in a sudden urge to urinate, often associated with increased frequency and nocturia, independent of urinary tract infections (UTIs) or other pathologic conditions. OAB is an exceedingly common clinical entity. In fact, it is estimated that approximately 20% of the world's population and 17% of the US population suffers from OAB.[1–3] OAB with urinary incontinence (UI) is often referred to as OAB-wet, whereas in the absence of UI, it is referred to as OAB-dry. OAB is typically viewed as resulting from abnormalities in bladder innervation or muscle function and often occurs in tandem with other chronic medical conditions such as constipation, diabetes, neurologic dysfunction, and depression, all of which can further contribute to the condition's considerable morbidity.[3] The impact of OAB on those who suffer from this condition is wide ranging, including decreased overall health, restriction of daily activities, decreased sexual function, social isolation, decreased quality of sleep, decreased self-esteem, poor mental health, and an overall decrease in quality of life, making it a condition of considerable clinical and social significance.[3]

Contributorship statement: J.L., W.C., A.S., S.S., and N.A. prepared the manuscript and figures. All authors approved the submitted manuscript.
Funding: None.
[a] Department of Urology, Montefiore Medical Center, Albert Einstein College of Medicine, 1250 Waters Place, Tower 1 PH, Bronx, NY 10461, USA; [b] Department of Obstetrics and Gynecology and Women's Health, Female Pelvic Medicine and Reconstructive Surgery, Montefiore Medical Center, 1250 Waters Place, Tower 2, 9th floor, Bronx, NY 10461, USA; [c] Albert Einstein College of Medicine, 1300 Morris Park Avenue, Bronx, NY 10461, USA
* Corresponding author.
E-mail address: nabraham@montefiore.org
Twitter: @nityaabraham (N.A.)

urologic.theclinics.com

The aim of this review is to provide a brief background on the epidemiology and cause of OAB, with a more comprehensive focus on OAB pathophysiology and the pharmacotherapy commonly used to manage OAB symptoms.

EPIDEMIOLOGY AND CAUSE

Although lower urinary tract symptoms (LUTS) occur in both men and women (10.8% men and 12.8% women worldwide, 16% men and women in the United States), the type of symptoms experienced differs significantly.[3–6] Specifically, women are more likely to experience storage symptoms such as increased frequency, nocturia, urgency, or UI, whereas men are more likely to have voiding symptoms such as intermittency, slow stream, and straining. Furthermore, women are much more likely to have OAB-wet.

Because men and women have different presentations of OAB, it stands to reason that the risk factors observed are also different. Women with a body mass index (BMI) greater than 30 are 2.2 times more likely to have OAB with UI compared with women with BMI less than 24.[5] A proposed reason for this finding is that a high BMI exposes pelvic muscles to increased intra-abdominal pressure and chronically stretches the pudendal nerve.[5] In men, the largest OAB risk factor is prostatic disease such as benign prostatic hypertrophy (BPH) or benign prostate enlargement (BPE).[3–5,7] About 50% of men with an obstructed bladder outlet due to BPE have detrusor overactivity.[8]

OAB prevalence tends to increase with age.[3,4] Although it is commonly seen in individuals older than 40 years, young people may also experience OAB, but bothersome symptoms generally increase in men and women older than 60 years.[7] Race has been shown to play a role in OAB risk; however, further investigation is warranted as to whether race/ethnicity is a proxy for other factors contributing to OAB.[4,5]

PATHOPHYSIOLOGY

OAB displays a complex pathophysiology involving changes in neurogenic, myogenic, and urotheliogenic mechanisms that control micturition.[9] Normal micturition relies on the proper function and intricate interplay between several key structures such as the cortex, pons, spinal cord, autonomic nervous system, and the lower urinary tract. During storage, the sympathetic system is active, which involves release of norepinephrine that activates beta-3 adrenergic receptors, resulting in detrusor muscle relaxation.

The parasympathetic system is inactive. Bladder filling activates stretch receptors in the bladder that subsequently send signals along myelinated fibers projecting to the midbrain. When a bladder volume threshold is reached and the frontal cortex processes that it is an appropriate time to void, the voiding reflex is initiated. During normal micturition, the detrusor muscle of the bladder contracts after relaxation of the urethra and striated urethral sphincter. Periaqueductal gray matter projects to the pontine micturition center (PMC), which then projects to the bladder via parasympathetic pathways in the sacral spinal cord. These parasympathetic neurons ultimately release acetylcholine causing bladder contraction due to stimulation of cholinergic M2 and M3 receptors thus initiating voiding.[10] The sympathetic system is inactive during voiding.

Micturition is also regulated locally by an elaborate signaling between the bladder urothelium, lamina propria, and afferent nerve fibers, with ATP being the main mediator in signal transmission.[8] Several receptors, channels, and transporters are involved in mechanisms of ATP release from the urothelium, which are activated in response to bladder distension, as it fills with urine.[6–8,11] In patients with OAB, ATP release is elevated, which indicates that mechanisms controlling these local responses during the storage phase are impaired.[7,8,11] Thus, therapeutic approaches targeting these mechanisms to decrease mechanosensitive ATP release and signaling show promise in reducing OAB symptoms.

The normal micturition pathway is disturbed in OAB. More specifically, decreased suprapontine inhibition of the micturition reflex (eg, stroke) leads to overactive contraction of the detrusor fibers. Other described pathophysiologic causes include damaged axonal paths in the spinal cord, loss of peripheral inhibition, and increased excitatory neurotransmission.[12] Furthermore, during aging or disease processes, the relative contribution of muscarinic activity in the regulation of bladder function may be altered and thereby affect mechanisms that would normally have little clinical importance but could then contribute to the pathophysiology of OAB.[13]

Several pathophysiologic factors may contribute to OAB. These include the metabolic syndrome, sex hormone deficiency, gastrointestinal functional disorders such as irritable bowel syndrome, and dysregulation of the autonomic nervous system.[14] Furthermore, there has been increased attention to the role psychiatric disorders may play in OAB; conditions such as depression and generalized anxiety disorder result from disruptions in the neurotransmitter serotonin, which has been shown to play a role in modulating bladder function.[15]

TREATMENTS

Classically, the standard first-line therapy for patients with OAB consists of behavioral modifications and physical therapy, including pelvic floor exercises, monitoring OAB symptoms with bladder diaries, strict restriction of bladder irritants such as caffeine, smoking cessation, and weight loss.[16] If these techniques fail to alleviate symptoms, second-line measures consist of pharmacologic intervention such as anticholinergic agents and beta-3 agonists.[11,17,18] Anticholinergic agents act on muscarinic receptors to prevent parasympathetic-mediated detrusor muscle contraction. Similarly, beta-3 agonists act on beta-3 adrenergic receptors in the bladder, which enhances the sympathetic inhibitory modulation of the detrusor muscle and thereby attenuates OAB contractions.[18] For those patients who do not respond to behavioral or pharmacologic treatment modalities, neuromodulation or chemodenervation may be considered.

ANTIMUSCARINICS/ANTICHOLINERGICS

Antimuscarinic/anticholinergic medications represent the most common pharmaceutical intervention in the treatment of OAB and have demonstrated efficacy against placebo in relieving the symptoms of OAB.[19,20] **Table 1** displays

Table 1
Antimuscarinics used for the treatment of overactive bladder

Drug	Dosing	Class	Mechanism of Action	Side Effects
Oxybutynin IR Oxybutynin XL	IR: 5 mg PO 3 times daily XL: 5, 10, or 15 mg PO daily	Nonselective anticholinergic antagonist	Competitive inhibitor of muscarinic receptor, inhibits detrusor contraction	• Constipation • Dry mouth • Dementia • Neurologic and psychiatric dysfunction
Tolterodine IR Tolterodine LA	IR: 2 mg PO twice daily LA: 2 or 4 mg PO daily	Selective anticholinergic antagonist	Competitive inhibitor of muscarinic receptor, inhibits detrusor contraction	• Constipation • Dry mouth
Solifenacin	5 or 10 mg PO once daily	Selective anticholinergic antagonist	Competitive inhibitor of M3 receptor of the bladder, inhibits detrusor contraction	• Constipation • Dry mouth
Darifenacin	7.5 or 15 mg PO once daily	Selective anticholinergic antagonist	Competitive inhibitor of M3 receptor of the bladder, inhibits detrusor contraction	• Constipation • Dry mouth
Trospium IR Trospium ER	IR: 20 mg PO twice daily ER: 60 mg PO daily	Nonselective anticholinergic antagonist	Competitive inhibitor of M1, M2, M3 receptors, inhibits detrusor contraction	• Constipation • Dry mouth
Fesoterodine	4 or 8 mg PO once daily	Anticholinergic antagonist	Prodrug that when activated, acts as muscarinic antagonist, inhibits detrusor contraction	• Constipation • Dry mouth

Abbreviations: ER, extended release; IR, immediate release; LA, long acting; XL, extended release PO, by mouth.

commonly used antimuscarinic agents along with their respective mechanism of action and associated adverse effects (see **Table 1**).

Oxybutynin (Ditropan) is a relatively nonselective antimuscarinic agent that has been used extensively in the management of OAB for several decades.[17] Oxybutynin is a tertiary amine that undergoes first-pass metabolism to form the active metabolite, N-desyl oxybutynin, which plays a large role in the action of the drug.[21] Oxybutynin is available in several forms including immediate- and extended-release oral formulations. In terms of pharmacologic action, oxybutynin has antispasmodic, anticholinergic, and local anesthetic properties. Oxybutynin competitively binds to muscarinic receptors present in the detrusor muscle, reducing acetylcholine-induced postganglionic muscarinic receptor stimulation, thus inhibiting bladder contraction.[22]

Despite its effectiveness and durability in managing the symptoms of OAB, oxybutynin harbors a considerable adverse effect profile, limiting its use in certain patients. Specifically, patients may experience the debilitating effects of the drug's anticholinergic properties such as constipation and dry mouth, which may lead to poor compliance.[23] Oxybutynin has the capability to pass the blood-brain barrier and thus may elicit neurologic and psychological effects.[24,25] More recently, there has been growing concern over the long-term safety profile of the anticholinergic drugs used for OAB, particularly oxybutynin, as it relates to its ability to cross the blood-brain barrier.[19,26] In fact, studies suggest that use of anticholinergic medications among patients with OAB was associated with an increased risk of new-onset dementia,[27–29] even when compared with other popular OAB medications such as the beta-3 agonists.[30]

Tolterodine is another pharmaceutical commonly used in the management of OAB. Tolterodine is a potent and competitive muscarinic receptor antagonist and was developed as the first antimuscarinic agent specifically for OAB treatment. Compared with its anticholinergic counterpart oxybutynin, tolterodine exhibits a higher bladder-selective profile[31] and lesser affinity for the salivary glands and parotid tissue.[32]

The side effects of tolterodine are similar to those observed in patients undergoing treatment with oxybutynin, with dry mouth reported in approximately 20% to 25% of patients.[33] Also, given the concern for exacerbation of urinary retention in men with bladder outlet obstruction undergoing OAB treatment with anticholinergic medications, tolterodine has been shown to not adversely affect urinary function in these men and can presumably be administered safely in men with BPE.[34]

Compared with placebo, tolterodine has been shown to have a statistically significant impact in improving health-related quality of life.[35]

Solifenacin is an oral antimuscarinic agent that was first marketed in Europe in 2014 and quickly gained international attention, now licensed for use in more than 40 countries.[36] This agent acts as a competitive antagonist of the muscarinic receptor and displays selectivity for the M3 receptor of the urinary bladder.[37] Multiple clinical trials have highlighted the drug's effectiveness in treating OAB.[38] With regard to its anticholinergic counterparts, in a randomized, 12-week double-blind trial comparing solifenacin to tolterodine in the treatment of OAB solifenacin was found to be at least as effective as tolterodine in reducing urinary frequency.[39] Furthermore, a meta-analyses of 7 placebo-controlled OAB studies demonstrated that solifenacin use led to a statistically significant reduction in the number of urgency episodes, greater than those observed with other antimuscarinic agents, including oxybutynin and tolterodine.[40]

Moreover, solifenacin has been regarded as a safer and more tolerable medication for OAB when compared with oxybutynin. Solifenacin has been shown to not only provide sustained (>40-week) improvement in incontinence, urgency, and micturition but also has a minimal adverse side effect profile that does not result in treatment discontinuation.[41]

Darifenacin, similar to solifenacin, is a once-daily M3 selective receptor antagonist; it is a potent drug that has been shown to have high affinity and selectivity for the M3 receptor in the bladder, along with low selectivity for the other types of muscarinic receptors.[42] Darifenacin has favorable safety, tolerability, and efficacy during the long-term treatment of OAB.[43] These results are sustained in studies evaluating darifenacin in the treatment of OAB in the elderly, where it was shown to confer significant improvement in all the major symptoms of OAB (including urinary frequency and urgency) with a small proportion of patients (<3%) withdrawing treatment due to side effects.[44]

Trospium chloride is an orally active, quaternary ammonium compound that binds specifically and with high affinity to muscarinic receptors.[45] This compound does not cross the blood-brain barrier in significant amounts and thus has minimal central anticholinergic activity.[45] In addition, trospium chloride does not interact with nicotinic acetylcholine receptors, and its affinity for the muscarinic receptor subtypes is greater than that of some of the other anticholinergics such as oxybutynin, tolterodine, darifenacin, and solifenacin.[46,47]

In a multicenter phase 3 clinical trial (total of 523 patients at 51 sites), trospium chloride was shown to have sustained effectiveness in decreasing the number of voids, and urge incontinence and urgency episodes, with an associated improvement in quality of life compared with placebo.[48] These results were further corroborated in a clinical trial randomizing patients with OAB to placebo versus trospium chloride. Patients receiving trospium experienced a statistically significant improvement in daily toilet voids, urgency severity, and urge UI compared with the placebo group. These patients experienced clinical benefit starting at the first week of the study that persisted the entire 12 week duration of the study.[49]

Patients may experience similar side effects observed with other anticholinergic medications such as dry mouth and constipation. However, the minimal central nervous system penetration of trospium chloride renders it an attractive option in treating elderly patients with OAB. Staskin and Harnett[50] were the first to investigate and show the lack of detectable central nervous system penetration of the drug in 65- to 75-year-old patients with OAB. In addition, further studies suggested that trospium chloride does not increase daytime sleepiness or somnolence or other central nervous system adverse effects in patients treated for OAB.[50]

Fesoterodine is a novel antimuscarinic agent that acts functionally as a prodrug. Once consumed, it is very rapidly hydrolyzed by nonspecific esterases to its active metabolite, 5-HMT, which is responsible for the antimuscarinic actions of fesoterodine.[51]

In several clinical trials, fesoterodine has been shown to convey efficacy and tolerability in the management of OAB. Specifically, in 2 randomized studies consisting of a total of 1681 subjects, treatment with fesoterodine when compared with placebo, was found to significantly improve all voiding diary variables in patients with OAB younger than 65 years, and all variables except for voided volume and urinary frequency in patients with OAB aged 65 to 75 years. Patients older than 75 years exhibited similar response to fesoterodine, with improvements in all voiding diary variables except voided volume.[52] Subsequent studies have further confirmed the beneficial effects of fesoterodine in improving symptoms related to OAB,[53,54] at both the 4 and 8 mg doses.[55] In fact, the 8 mg dose was shown to display superior efficacy over tolterodine extended release in reducing urinary urge incontinence episodes in patients with OAB.[56]

Fesoterodine is generally regarded as a well-tolerated drug. The most commonly observed adverse effects include dry mouth and constipation. A large majority of patients are able to tolerate fesoterodine without having to discontinue the medication.[57] In fact, studies investigating flexible dosing of fesoterodine on treatment satisfaction reveal that about half of patients opt for dose escalation with good tolerability and with significantly improved OAB symptoms, health-related quality of life, and treatment satisfaction.[58]

CONCERNS WITH LONG-TERM ANTICHOLINERGIC USE

The side effect profile of anticholinergic medications brings to light the importance of distinguishing between the various types of muscarinic receptors and the relevance of bladder selectivity for certain medications. Muscarinic receptors are expressed throughout the body. M1 receptors are located in exocrine glands and the central nervous system (CNS); M2 receptors in the lung, heart, and bladder; M3 receptors in blood vessels, lungs, and bladder; and M4 and M5 receptors in the CNS[59] (**Table 2**). Nonselective muscarinic receptor agonists thus result in side effects in these end organs. Drugs that are selective for M3 receptors in the urinary bladder have potential to alleviate symptoms of OAB without the adverse side

Table 2
Location and function of the various muscarinic receptors

	M1	M2	M3	M4	M5
Location	Exocrine glands, central nervous system	Lung, heart	Blood vessels, lungs, bladder	Central nervous system	Central nervous system
Function	Arousal, memory, gastric acid secretion	Decrease heart rate, decrease ventricular contractility	Smooth muscle contraction, vasodilation, bladder contraction	Memory, arousal, attention	Dopamine regulation in substantia nigra

effects experienced from antagonism of muscarinic receptors expressed in other organs and systems in the body.

Recently, there has been growing concern about the risk of long-term anticholinergics causing cognitive impairment, dementia, and Alzheimer disease leading to a 2021 Clinical Consensus Statement published by the American Urogynecologic Society advising to weigh the risks of anticholinergic use with benefits in quality of life, using the lowest effective anticholinergic dose, and avoiding anticholinergic medication in women older than 70 years.[60] Avoiding side effects due to medical therapy, specifically antimuscarinics, is an incredibly important notion given the concern for safety, particularly in the elderly population in whom the prevalence of OAB is high[61]; this coincides with the Choosing Wisely Campaign, an initiative founded to promote conversation between clinicians and patients to ensure high-quality evidence-based care and prevention of unnecessary testing or medication use.

Part of this campaign is a thorough medication review before initiating new drug therapy in vulnerable elderly patients.[62,63] Given the worrisome risk of the possible side effects of anticholinergic use, there is need for pharmaceuticals with an alternative mechanism of action and more desirable side effect profile.

BETA-3 AGONISTS

The beta-agonists represent an alternative second-line treatment option for OAB (grade B) (**Table 3**).[52] Beta-1 adrenergic receptors are located on the kidneys and heart, beta-2 receptors primarily in vascular smooth muscle, and beta-3 receptors in the bladder and fat cells (**Table 4**). The mechanism of action of beta-3 agonists is to activate the beta-3 adrenergic receptors on the detrusor smooth muscle resulting in detrusor muscle relaxation and increased bladder capacity.[64,65]

Mirabegron is a beta-3 agonist that has shown to significantly decrease daily urinary frequency

Table 3
Beta-3 adrenergic agonists and other drugs used for the treatment of overactive bladder

Drug Name	Dosing	Class	Mechanism of Action	Side Effects
Mirabegron	25 or 50 mg PO daily	Beta-3 agonist	Detrusor smooth muscle relaxation	• Avoid in severe uncontrolled hypertension (SBP > 180 and/or DBP > 110) • Avoid in cardiac arrhythmias • Drug interactions
Vibegron	75 mg PO daily	Beta-3 agonist	Detrusor smooth muscle relaxation	• Avoid in hepatic or renal impairment
Imipramine	10–75 mg PO daily	Tricyclic antidepressant	Inhibits muscarinic, adrenergic, and histamine receptors and inhibits reuptake of serotonin and norepinephrine in the bladder	• Increased risk of suicidal thinking • Arrhythmias • Heart block • Orthostatic hypotension • Constipation • Dry mouth
Duloxetine	20–40 mg PO twice daily	Selective serotonin norepinephrine reuptake inhibitor	Central inhibitor of serotonin and norepinephrine at Onuf nucleus	• Increased risk of suicidal thinking • Nausea • Vomiting • Dizziness
Desmopressin	27.7 µg sublingual daily or 0.05–0.1 mg PO daily	ADH analogue	Increases water permeability in renal tubular cells resulting in decreased urine volume and urine osmolality	• Hyponatremia

Abbreviations: ADH, antidiuretic hormone; DBP, diastolic blood pressure; PO, by mouth; SBP, systolic blood pressure

Table 4
Location and function of the various beta-adrenergic receptors

	Beta 1	Beta 2	Beta 3
Location	Kidneys, heart	Smooth muscle	Bladder, fat tissue, gall bladder
Function	Increase heart rate, increase contractility, renin secretion	Smooth muscle relaxation (bronchial, vascular, gastrointestinal, genitourinary)	Lipolysis, bladder relaxation

and incontinence episodes in patients with OAB.[66] This drug has demonstrated similar efficacy, improved side effect profile, and increased patient compliance when compared with anticholinergics.[30,67] However, it should be avoided in patients with uncontrolled hypertension (systolic blood pressure $\geq$ 180 and/or diastolic blood pressure $\geq$ 110)[68] or cardiac arrhythmia[69,70] due to potential worsening of these cardiovascular conditions.

Vibegron is a beta-3 receptor agonist, approved by the US Food and Drug Administration (FDA) in 2020 with selectivity for the beta-3 receptor. This drug was shown to significantly decrease frequency, urgency, and urge incontinence episodes and increase bladder capacity in patients with OAB when compared with placebo.[71] Vibegron has demonstrated efficacy in patients with OAB-dry; it also does not result in higher rates of incident hypertension or increase in blood pressure compared with placebo likely due to its selectivity for the beta-3 receptor and does not cause CYP2D6 drug interactions, potentially resulting in fewer drug interactions.[72] Insurance coverage and cost are similarly an issue for this newer medication.

ANTIDEPRESSANTS

The antidepressant class of medications has been used off label for OAB treatment given their peripheral and central actions.[73] Imipramine has been used to treat nocturnal enuresis. Imipramine is a tricyclic antidepressant that inhibits muscarinic, adrenergic, and histamine receptors and inhibits reuptake of serotonin and norepinephrine in the bladder, Onuf nucleus, and PMC.[74] In children with nocturnal enuresis, imipramine has demonstrated improvement in enuresis frequency with some children being dry at night[75]; TCAs have broad-spectrum targets and therefore can exhibit cardiac, anticholinergic, and antihistamine effects and can decrease seizure threshold in a dose-related response. Imipramine, like all antidepressants, has an FDA "black box" warning that it can increase risk of suicidal thinking and behavior in children, adolescents, and young adults (18–

24 years of age) with major depressive disorder and other psychiatric disorders. Imipramine may also cause orthostatic hypotension and sedation and therefore should be avoided in patients older than 65 years[76]; it also should be used with caution in the context of concurrent arrhythmia, heart block, seizure, fracture, bone marrow suppression, hyponatremia, decreased gastric motility, increased intraocular pressure, angle closure glaucoma, paralytic ileus, urinary retention, BPE, xerostomia, visual problems, and in concomitant monoamine oxidase inhibitor use.[77,78] Selective serotonin reuptake inhibitors may be more tolerable compared with imipramine due to the side effects of TCA.[77]

Duloxetine is a selective serotonin and norepinephrine reuptake inhibitor that acts on Onuf nucleus.[79] Antimuscarinics and beta-3 agonists act primarily on the peripheral pathways in OAB, whereas duloxetine acts primarily on the central pathway as demonstrated in an animal model.[80] Duloxetine significantly decreases urinary frequency and UI compared with placebo in women with OAB[81]; it has also been shown to decrease episodes of stress UI due to increased serotonin and noradrenaline at presynaptic motor neurons in Onuf nucleus located on the sacral segments of the spinal cord that control the urethral sphincter.[82] In animal models, duloxetine improves both OAB and depression symptoms.[79] Unfortunately, it has been shown to increase the risk of suicidal thinking and behavior in children, adolescents, and young adults (18–24 years of age) with major depressive disorder and other psychiatric disorders. Duloxetine should additionally be avoided in patients with uncontrolled narrow-angle glaucoma and concomitant monoamine oxidase inhibitor use; it may also cause nausea, vomiting, constipation, headache, dry mouth, fatigue, dizziness, and urinary retention.[83]

OTHER

Desmopressin is a synthetic analogue of the antidiuretic hormone (ADH) that works by increasing water permeability in renal tubular cells resulting in decreased urine volume and urine osmolality. Desmopressin has been shown to significantly decrease frequency and urgency during the first 8 hours of use[84] and to significantly improve quality of life when prescribed in combination with an anticholinergic for nocturnal enuresis.[85] Owing to its effect on the renal tubular cells it can cause hyponatremia, and electrolytes should be monitored while in use.[74] Desmopressin should be avoided in moderate to severe renal impairment (CrCl <50 mL/min), polydipsia, primary nocturnal enuresis, concomitant use of loop diuretics or glucocorticoids, syndrome of inappropriate ADH, gastroenteritis, salt wasting nephropathies, systemic infection, and heart failure.[86,87]

FUTURE PHARMACOLOGIC TREATMENTS AND COMBINATION THERAPIES

The goal of newer pharmacologic agents for OAB treatment is to increase their specificity to the bladder tissues to avoid unwanted systemic side effects.[88] Imidafenacin is an example of one of these potential novel drugs. Imidafenacin is an antimuscarinic antagonist with high specificity for the M1/M3 receptors but with greater specificity for the M3 receptor. Detrusor muscle contractions are almost exclusively controlled via the M3 receptor, so imidafenacin is postulated to have a more direct effect on the bladder, thus avoiding common side effects to the brain by M1 receptors and to the heart via M2 receptors. It has been shown to improve dry mouth and constipation while having no effects on the cardiovascular or neurologic systems.[88,89] Another selective M3 antagonist, tarafenacin has shown similar outcomes to imidafenacin.[88,90] After the success of vibregon, other beta-3 adrenoreceptor agonists such as ritobegron and solabegron are currently undergoing clinical trials to be approved for OAB treatment.[91,92] Solabegron showed a significant reduction in symptoms for women with moderate to severe OAB.[92]

COMBINATION THERAPY

OAB occurs through multiple pathways, and thus it is important to consider the combination of therapeutic agents with different targets. The most common combination for OAB treatment involves a beta-3 agonist with an anticholinergic agent.[93] The SYMPHONY (12 weeks' follow-up) and SYNERGY (12 months' follow-up) trials showed that daily solifenacin in combination with mirabegron significantly improved urinary frequency, urgency, and urge incontinence in OAB without an increase in adverse effects.[93,94] Other pharmacologic combinations under investigation include anticholinergic agents paired with a different anticholinergic agent such as trospium and solifenacin.[94]

NOVEL THERAPEUTIC TARGETS

Determining the pharmacologic target is important to achieve the intended therapeutic effect. Current therapies for OAB are mainly focused on targeting the detrusor muscle. However, the bladder is made up of various types of cells and extracellular components. An emerging treatment approach for OAB is targeting receptors on the transitional epithelium, or urothelium, and the lamina propria, which contains interstitial cells, vasculature, and nerve terminals.[95,96]

Changes in purine receptors have been shown to be involved in OAB. In a subset of patients with OAB, the purine P2X2 and P2X3 receptor subtypes are overexpressed on the bladder afferent nerves.[95,97] Activation of these receptors by ATP released from the urothelial cells in response to bladder distension, as it fills with urine, generates sensory signals to the brain that are essential for proper micturition. In this regard, increased activation of the bladder afferents can lead to detrusor overactivity. Similarly, ATP coreleased with acetylcholine from parasympathetic terminals activates P2X1 receptors expressed on detrusor muscle, and changes in levels of either released ATP or P2X1 expression can lead to increased contractility.[97] Potential therapeutic approaches for OAB can thereby involve attenuating P2X activation, downregulating P2X receptors, or inhibiting their signal transmission to reduce detrusor contractions.

Another purine receptor, P2Y, facilitates smooth muscle contractility and controls transfer of information from the urothelium to lamina propria myofibroblasts and afferent nerves.[97] Myofibroblasts are proposed to amplify the sensory response to bladder wall distension and the stretch-induced signaling from urothelial cells to the bladder afferent nerves.[97] Further research on myofibroblast function in physiologic and pathologic conditions is needed to determine their putative role as novel cellular targets in therapeutic interventions for OAB.

In addition to the muscarinic receptors, beta-3 adrenoceptors, and purinergic receptors, other receptors and channels expressed in the bladder are also emerging as potential molecular targets for novel pharmacologic interventions to manage OAB. Among these are the transient receptor potential (TRP) channels. Various animal models have shown that TRP channels are involved in

OAB, including TRPV1, TRPV4, TRPM8, and TRPA1.[95–98] Various studies have shown that TRPV1 levels are altered in OAB.[95,97] However, findings from previous clinical trials with TRPV1 antagonists were disappointing due to observations of marked and persistent hyperthermia in the TRPV1-treated subjects.[95] Current research involves desensitizing these receptors with intravesical instillation of capsaicin or other small molecule agonists, which suppress the activation of the bladder afferents and improve OAB symptoms.[96–98] TRPV4 has also been shown to be involved in bladder detrusor overactivity, and as such, TRPV4 antagonists could also help with OAB management.[96–98] Specifically, these channels have been shown to be upregulated in OAB and even more so in response to stress, which may explain why OAB symptoms often worsen during times of stress.[97] Similarly, TRPM8 channel abundance has been directly associated with voiding frequency.[96] However, in the urothelium, their expression is much lower than the expression of other TRP channels, which may imply that their therapeutic potential would be lower.[98] TRPA1 channels have been identified on urethral C-fiber afferents and urothelial and detrusor smooth muscle cells and have been shown to be upregulated in patients with bladder outlet obstruction.[96–98] These channels have been proposed to play a role in modulating signaling in the afferent limb of the micturition reflex, but there remains a large gap in the literature with respect to TRPA1 antagonists in OAB and detrusor overactivity in humans.[96,97]

Other ion channels of significant interest are the Ca^{2+}-activated K^+ channels with large or small unit ion conductance (BK and SK) expressed on detrusor muscle cells.[95,96,98,99] These channels hyperpolarize and repolarize the detrusor smooth muscle and are hypothesized to reduce detrusor overactivity.[95,96,98,99] In patients with OAB, there is reduced expression of these ion channels.[95,96,98] It was hypothesized that BK openers, which increase the activity of these channels, would be beneficial in OAB. One drug, nicorandil, is a BK opener with a nitric oxide donor property that shows potential as an OAB therapeutic by suppressing OAB from neurogenic and myogenic causes in animals.[95] However, these ion channels may be downregulated in OAB, which may explain how previous BK openers have shown little therapeutic benefit.[95,96,98] Therefore, a potential therapeutic approach is to increase the expression of BK channels through a gene therapy-based method with a plasmid vector.[96,99] Several preclinical in vivo studies have shown great promise and are being explored in clinical trials.[96,99]

Afferent fibers and sensory neurons are important in controlling detrusor activity. Gabapentin is a ligand that targets voltage-gated Ca^{2+} channels involved in afferent neuron activation[99]; it has been shown to reduce OAB symptoms in some studies. A more effective therapeutic, pregabalin, has shown increases in bladder capacity and improvement in OAB symptoms.[99]

Last, another important consideration for OAB treatment is bladder wall fibrosis. Many pathologic conditions that result in OAB involve fibrosis, or replacement of detrusor muscle with extracellular matrix (ECM).[96] The ECM is stiffer than muscle tissue, markedly reducing bladder compliance and impairing signal transmission and coordination of activity between muscle cells, leading to spontaneous contractions.[96] A key mediator in fibrotic signaling is transforming growth factor-β, and targeting this pathway has shown some promise in restoring normal bladder compliance and contractions.[96]

SUMMARY

OAB is a ubiquitous clinical entity with significant morbidity and impact on quality of life. OAB has a complex pathophysiology and is commonly comorbid with other chronic medical conditions. This review highlights and provides an overview of the several classes of pharmaceuticals geared toward the treatment of OAB, most notably the anticholinergics/antimuscarinics and beta-3 agonists, as well as off-label use of antidepressants. Future pharmaceutical agents should focus on bladder selectivity and broaden the focus to receptors and channels in the urothelium and lamina propria, with the goal of improving symptoms and minimizing side effects.

CLINICS CARE POINTS

- OAB is an exceedingly common clinical entity with considerable morbidity and negative impact on quality of life.
- Antimuscarinic agents represent the most common pharmacologic therapy and act by inhibiting bladder smooth muscle contraction.
- Antimuscarinic medications are associated with clinically significant adverse effects including dry mouth, constipation, and possible cognitive impairment with long-term use.
- Beta-3 agonists act on the detrusor smooth muscle, resulting in detrusor muscle relaxation and increased bladder capacity.

- Patients on certain beta-3 agonists should be closely monitored for adverse cardiovascular effects including worsening high blood pressure.
- Combination therapies may provide superior symptom control by targeting several components of the OAB pathophysiologic pathway.
- Antidepressants may be used as an off-label treatment modality for OAB.
- There is ongoing research focused on novel therapeutic targets in the urothelium and lamina propria that are implicated in the pathophysiology of OAB.

CONFLICTS OF INTEREST

NA Speakers Bureau: Urovant.

ACKNOWLEDGMENTS

None

REFERENCES

1. Latini JM, Giannantoni A. Pharmacotherapy of overactive bladder: epidemiology and pathophysiology of overactive bladder. Expert Opin Pharmacother 2011;12(7):1017–27.
2. Leron E, Weintraub AY, Mastrolia SA, et al. Overactive Bladder Syndrome: Evaluation and Management. Curr Urol 2018;11(3):117–25.
3. Eapen RS, Radomski SB. Review of the epidemiology of overactive bladder. Res Rep Urol 2016;8: 71–6.
4. Eapen RS, Radomski SB. Gender differences in overactive bladder. Can J Urol 2016;23(Suppl 1): 2–9.
5. Zhu J, Hu X, Dong X, et al. Associations Between Risk Factors and Overactive Bladder: A Meta-analysis. Female Pelvic Med Reconstr Surg 2019;25(3): 238–46.
6. Irwin DE, Abrams P, Milsom I, et al. Understanding the elements of overactive bladder: questions raised by the EPIC study. BJU Int 2008;101(11):1381–7.
7. Stewart WF, Van Rooyen JB, Cundiff GW, et al. Prevalence and burden of overactive bladder in the United States. World J Urol 2003;20(6):327–36.
8. Vuichoud C, Loughlin KR. Benign prostatic hyperplasia: epidemiology, economics and evaluation. Can J Urol 2015;22(Suppl 1):1–6.
9. Meng E, LIN WY, LEE WC, et al. Pathophysiology of overactive bladder. LUTS: Lower Urinary Tract Symptoms 2012;4:48–55.
10. Chu FM, Dmochowski R. Pathophysiology of overactive bladder. Am J Med 2006;119(3 Suppl 1):3–8.
11. Olivera CK, Meriwether K, El-Nashar S, et al. Nonantimuscarinic treatment for overactive bladder: a systematic review. Am J Obstet Gynecol 2016; 215(1):34–57.
12. Wein AJ, Rackley RR. Overactive bladder: a better understanding of pathophysiology, diagnosis and management. J Urol 2006;175(3 Pt 2):S5–10.
13. Banakhar MA, Al-Shaiji TF, Hassouna MM. Pathophysiology of overactive bladder. Int Urogynecol J 2012;23(8):975–82.
14. Peyronnet B, Mironska E, Chapple C, et al. A comprehensive review of overactive bladder pathophysiology: on the way to tailored treatment. Eur Urol 2019;75(6):988–1000.
15. Steers WD. Pathophysiology of overactive bladder and urge urinary incontinence. Rev Urol 2002; 4(Suppl 4):S7–18.
16. Bartley JM, Blum ES, Sirls LT, et al. Understanding clinic options for overactive bladder. Curr Urol Rep 2013;14(6):541–8.
17. Lam S, Hilas O. Pharmacologic management of overactive bladder. Clin Interv Aging 2007;2(3):337–45.
18. Robinson D, Cardozo L. Managing overactive bladder. Climacteric 2019;22(3):250–6.
19. Chancellor M, Boone T. Anticholinergics for overactive bladder therapy: central nervous system effects. CNS Neurosci Ther 2012;18(2):167–74.
20. Herbison P, Hay-Smith J, Ellis G, et al. Effectiveness of anticholinergic drugs compared with placebo in the treatment of overactive bladder: systematic review. Bmj 2003;326(7394):841–4.
21. Andersson KE, Chapple CR. Oxybutynin and the overactive bladder. World J Urol 2001;19(5): 319–23.
22. Jirschele K, Sand PK. Oxybutynin: past, present, and future. Int Urogynecol J 2013;24(4):595–604.
23. Getsios D, El-Hadi W, Caro I, et al. Pharmacological management of overactive bladder : a systematic and critical review of published economic evaluations. Pharmacoeconomics 2005;23(10):995–1006.
24. Andersson KE. Antimuscarinics for treatment of overactive bladder. Lancet Neurol 2004;3(1):46–53.
25. Gulsun M, Pinar M, Sabanci U. Psychotic disorder induced by oxybutynin: Presentation of two cases. Clin Drug Investig 2006;26(10):603–6.
26. Dmochowski RR, Thai S, Iglay K, et al. Increased risk of incident dementia following use of anticholinergic agents: A systematic literature review and meta-analysis. Neurourology and urodynamics 2021;40(1):28–37.
27. Gray SL, Anderson ML, Dublin S, et al. Cumulative use of strong anticholinergics and incident dementia: a prospective cohort study. JAMA Intern Med 2015;175(3):401–7.
28. Richardson K, Fox C, Maidment I, et al. Anticholinergic drugs and risk of dementia: case-control study. Bmj 2018;361:k1315.
29. Coupland CAC, Hill T, Dening T, et al. Anticholinergic Drug Exposure and the Risk of Dementia: A

Nested Case-Control Study. JAMA Intern Med 2019; 179(8):1084–93.

30. Welk B, McArthur E. Increased risk of dementia among patients with overactive bladder treated with an anticholinergic medication compared to a beta-3 agonist: a population-based cohort study. BJU Int 2020;126(1):183–90.

31. Van Kerrebroeck P, Kreder K, Jonas U, et al. Tolterodine once-daily: superior efficacy and tolerability in the treatment of the overactive bladder. Urology 2001;57(3):414–21.

32. Nilvebrant L, Andersson KE, Gillberg PG, et al. Tolterodine–a new bladder-selective antimuscarinic agent. Eur J Pharmacol 1997;327(2–3):195–207.

33. Ouslander JG. Management of overactive bladder. N Engl J Med 2004;350(8):786–99.

34. Abrams P, Kaplan S, De Koning Gans HJ, et al. Safety and tolerability of tolterodine for the treatment of overactive bladder in men with bladder outlet obstruction. J Urol 2006;175(3 Pt 1):999–1004.

35. Kelleher CJ, Reese PR, Pleil AM, et al. Health-related quality of life of patients receiving extended-release tolterodine for overactive bladder. Am J Manag Care 2002;8(19 Suppl):S608–15.

36. Cardozo L, Hessdörfer E, Milani R, et al. Solifenacin in the treatment of urgency and other symptoms of overactive bladder: results from a randomized, double-blind, placebo-controlled, rising-dose trial. BJU Int 2008;102(9):1120–7.

37. Maniscalco M, Singh-Franco D, Wolowich WR, et al. Solifenacin succinate for the treatment of symptoms of overactive bladder. Clin Ther 2006;28(9):1247–72.

38. Chapple CR, Cardozo L, Steers WD, et al. Solifenacin significantly improves all symptoms of overactive bladder syndrome. Int J Clin Pract 2006;60(8):959–66.

39. Chapple CR, Martinez-Garcia R, Selvaggi L, et al. A comparison of the efficacy and tolerability of solifenacin succinate and extended release tolterodine at treating overactive bladder syndrome: results of the STAR trial. Eur Urol 2005;48(3):464–70.

40. Michel MC, de la Rosette JJ. Role of muscarinic receptor antagonists in urgency and nocturia. BJU Int 2005;96(Suppl 1):37–42.

41. Wagg A, Wyndaele JJ, Sieber P. Efficacy and tolerability of solifenacin in elderly subjects with overactive bladder syndrome: a pooled analysis. Am J Geriatr Pharmacother 2006;4(1):14–24.

42. Newgreen DT, Anderson CWP, Carter AJ, et al. Darifenacin—a novel bladder-selective agent for the treatment of urge incontinence. Neurourol Urodyn 1995;14:555–7.

43. Haab F, Corcos J, Siami P, et al. Long-term treatment with darifenacin for overactive bladder: results of a 2-year, open-label extension study. BJU Int 2006; 98(5):1025–32.

44. Foote J, Glavind K, Kralidis G, et al. Treatment of overactive bladder in the older patient: pooled analysis of three phase III studies of darifenacin, an M3 selective receptor antagonist. Eur Urol 2005;48(3):471–7.

45. Rovner ES. Trospium chloride in the management of overactive bladder. Drugs 2004;64(21):2433–46.

46. Pak RW, Petrou SP, Staskin DR. Trospium chloride: a quaternary amine with unique pharmacologic properties. Curr Urol Rep 2003;4(6):436–40.

47. Uckert S, Stief CG, Odenthal KP, et al. Responses of isolated normal human detrusor muscle to various spasmolytic drugs commonly used in the treatment of the overactive bladder. Arzneimittelforschung 2000;50(5):456–60.

48. Zinner N, Gittelman M, Harris R, et al. Trospium chloride improves overactive bladder symptoms: a multicenter phase III trial. J Urol 2004;171(6 Pt 1):2311–5.

49. Rudy D, Cline K, Harris R, et al. Multicenter phase III trial studying trospium chloride in patients with overactive bladder. Urology 2006;67(2):275–80.

50. Staskin DR, Harnett MD. Effect of trospium chloride on somnolence and sleepiness in patients with overactive bladder. Curr Urol Rep 2004;5(6):423–6.

51. Nitti VW, Dmochowski R, Sand PK, et al. Efficacy, safety and tolerability of fesoterodine for overactive bladder syndrome. J Urol 2007;178(6):2488–94.

52. Kraus SR, Ruiz-Cerdá JL, Martire D, et al. Efficacy and tolerability of fesoterodine in older and younger subjects with overactive bladder. Urology 2010; 76(6):1350–7.

53. Khullar V, Rovner ES, Dmochowski R, et al. Fesoterodine dose response in subjects with overactive bladder syndrome. Urology 2008;71(5):839–43.

54. Chapple C, Van Kerrebroeck P, Tubaro A, et al. Clinical efficacy, safety, and tolerability of once-daily fesoterodine in subjects with overactive bladder. Eur Urol 2007;52(4):1204–12.

55. Michel MC. Fesoterodine: a novel muscarinic receptor antagonist for the treatment of overactive bladder syndrome. Expert Opin Pharmacother 2008;9(10):1787–96.

56. Herschorn S, Swift S, Guan Z, et al. Comparison of fesoterodine and tolterodine extended release for the treatment of overactive bladder: a head-to-head placebo-controlled trial. BJU Int 2010;105(1):58–66.

57. Dmochowski RR, Peters KM, Morrow JD, et al. Randomized, double-blind, placebo-controlled trial of flexible-dose fesoterodine in subjects with overactive bladder. Urology 2010;75(1):62–8.

58. Wyndaele JJ, Goldfischer ER, Morrow JD, et al. Effects of flexible-dose fesoterodine on overactive bladder symptoms and treatment satisfaction: an open-label study. Int J Clin Pract 2009;63(4):560–7.

59. Haab F, Stewart L, Dwyer P. Darifenacin, an M3 selective receptor antagonist, is an effective and well-tolerated once-daily treatment for overactive bladder. Eur Urol 2004;45(4):420–9.

60. American Urogynecologic Society Guidelines Committee. Clinical consensus statement: association of anticholinergic medication use and cognition in women with overactive bladder. Female Pelvic Med Reconstr Surg 2021;27(2):69–71.

61. Tyagi P, Tyagi V, Qu X, et al. Association of inflammaging (inflammation + aging) with higher prevalence of OAB in elderly population. Int Urol Nephrol 2014;46(5):871–7.

62. Reppas-Rindlisbacher CE, Fischer HD, Fung K, et al. Anticholinergic Drug Burden in Persons with Dementia Taking a Cholinesterase Inhibitor: The Effect of Multiple Physicians. J Am Geriatr Soc 2016; 64(3):492–500.

63. Lightner DJ, Gomelsky A, Souter L, et al. Diagnosis and Treatment of Overactive Bladder (Non-Neurogenic) in Adults: AUA/SUFU Guideline Amendment 2019. J Urol 2019;202(3):558–63.

64. Takeda M, Obara K, Mizusawa T, et al. Evidence for beta3-adrenoceptor subtypes in relaxation of the human urinary bladder detrusor: analysis by molecular biological and pharmacological methods. J Pharmacol Exp Ther 1999;288(3):1367–73.

65. Igawa Y, Yamazaki Y, Takeda H, et al. Functional and molecular biological evidence for a possible beta3-adrenoceptor in the human detrusor muscle. Br J Pharmacol 1999;126(3):819–25.

66. Nitti VW, Khullar V, van Kerrebroeck P, et al. Mirabegron for the treatment of overactive bladder: a prespecified pooled efficacy analysis and pooled safety analysis of three randomised, double-blind, placebo-controlled, phase III studies. Int J Clin Pract 2013;67(7):619–32.

67. Escobar CM, Falk KN, Mehta S, et al. Rethinking Second-Line Therapy for Overactive Bladder to Improve Patient Access to Treatment Options. Obstet Gynecol 2021;137(3):454–60.

68. Sebastianelli A, Russo GI, Kaplan SA, et al. Systematic review and meta-analysis on the efficacy and tolerability of mirabegron for the treatment of storage lower urinary tract symptoms/overactive bladder: Comparison with placebo and tolterodine. Int J Urol 2018;25(3):196–205.

69. Cui Y, Zong H, Yang C, et al. The efficacy and safety of mirabegron in treating OAB: a systematic review and meta-analysis of phase III trials. Int Urol Nephrol 2014;46(1):275–84.

70. Chapple CR, Kaplan SA, Mitcheson D, et al. Randomized double-blind, active-controlled phase 3 study to assess 12-month safety and efficacy of mirabegron, a β(3)-adrenoceptor agonist, in overactive bladder. Eur Urol 2013;63(2):296–305.

71. Staskin D, Frankel J, Varano S, et al. International Phase III, Randomized, Double-Blind, Placebo and Active Controlled Study to Evaluate the Safety and Efficacy of Vibegron in Patients with Symptoms of Overactive Bladder: EMPOWUR. J Urol 2020; 204(2):316–24.

72. Edmondson SD, Zhu C, Kar NF, et al. Discovery of Vibegron: A Potent and Selective β3 Adrenergic Receptor Agonist for the Treatment of Overactive Bladder. J Med Chem 2016;59(2):609–23.

73. Albayrak S, Solmaz V, Gencden Y, et al. Assessment of overactive bladder in women antidepressant users. Int Urol Nephrol 2015;47(9):1479–84.

74. Jayarajan J, Radomski SB. Pharmacotherapy of overactive bladder in adults: a review of efficacy, tolerability, and quality of life. Res Rep Urol 2013;6:1–16.

75. Gepertz S, Nevéus T. Imipramine for therapy resistant enuresis: a retrospective evaluation. J Urol 2004;171(6 Pt 2):2607–10.

76. American Geriatrics Society 2019 Updated AGS Beers Criteria® for Potentially Inappropriate Medication Use in Older Adults. J Am Geriatr Soc 2019; 67(4):674–94.

77. Anderson IM, Ferrier IN, Baldwin RC, et al. Evidence-based guidelines for treating depressive disorders with antidepressants: a revision of the 2000 British Association for Psychopharmacology guidelines. J Psychopharmacol 2008;22(4): 343–96.

78. Ray WA, Meredith S, Thapa PB, et al. Cyclic antidepressants and the risk of sudden cardiac death. Clin Pharmacol Ther 2004;75(3):234–41.

79. Thor KB, Katofiasc MA. Effects of duloxetine, a combined serotonin and norepinephrine reuptake inhibitor, on central neural control of lower urinary tract function in the chloralose-anesthetized female cat. J Pharmacol Exp Ther 1995;274(2):1014–24.

80. Wróbel A, Serefko A, Woźniak A, et al. Duloxetine reverses the symptoms of overactive bladder coexisting with depression via the central pathways. Pharmacol Biochem Behav 2020;189:172842.

81. Steers WD, Herschorn S, Kreder KJ, et al. Duloxetine compared with placebo for treating women with symptoms of overactive bladder. BJU Int 2007;100(2):337–45.

82. Di Rezze S, Frasca V, Inghilleri M, et al. Duloxetine for the treatment of overactive bladder syndrome in multiple sclerosis: a pilot study. Clin Neuropharmacol 2012;35(5):231–4.

83. Faure Walker N, Brinchmann K, Batura D. Linking the evidence between urinary retention and antipsychotic or antidepressant drugs: A systematic review. Neurourol Urodyn 2016;35(8):866–74.

84. Hashim H, Malmberg L, Graugaard-Jensen C, et al. Desmopressin, as a "designer-drug," in the treatment of overactive bladder syndrome. Neurourol Urodyn 2009;28(1):40–6.

85. Han YK, Lee WK, Lee SH, et al. Effect of desmopressin with anticholinergics in female patients with overactive bladder. Korean J Urol 2011;52(6):396–400.

86. Nevéus T, Fonseca E, Franco I, et al. Management and treatment of nocturnal enuresis-an updated standardization document from the International Children's Continence Society. J Pediatr Urol 2020; 16(1):10–9.

87. Song P, Huang C, Wang Y, et al. Comparison of desmopressin, alarm, desmopressin plus alarm, and desmopressin plus anticholinergic agents in the management of paediatric monosymptomatic nocturnal enuresis: a network meta-analysis. BJU Int 2019;123(3):388–400.

88. Painter CE, Suskind AM. Advances in pharmacotherapy for the treatment of overactive bladder. Curr Bladder Dysfunct Rep 2019;14(4):377–84.

89. Wu JP, Peng L, Zeng X, et al. Is imidafenacin an alternative to current antimuscarinic drugs for patients with overactive bladder syndrome? Int Urogynecol J 2021;32(5):1117–27.

90. Song M, Kim JH, Lee KS, et al. The efficacy and tolerability of tarafenacin, a new muscarinic acetylcholine receptor M3 antagonist in patients with overactive bladder; randomised, double-blind, placebo-controlled phase 2 study. Int J Clin Pract 2015;69(2):242–50.

91. Ellsworth P, Fantasia J. Solabegron: a potential future addition to the β-3 adrenoceptor agonist armamentarium for the management of overactive bladder. Expert Opin Investig Drugs 2015;24(3): 413–9.

92. Ohlstein EH, von Keitz A, Michel MC. A multicenter, double-blind, randomized, placebo-controlled trial of the β3-adrenoceptor agonist solabegron for overactive bladder. Eur Urol 2012;62(5):834–40.

93. Kasman A, Stave C, Elliott CS. Combination therapy in overactive bladder-untapped research opportunities: A systematic review of the literature. Neurourol Urodyn 2019;38(8):2083–92.

94. Abrams P, Kelleher C, Staskin D, et al. Combination treatment with mirabegron and solifenacin in patients with overactive bladder: efficacy and safety results from a randomised, double-blind, dose-ranging, phase 2 study (Symphony). Eur Urol 2015;67(3):577–88.

95. Cerruto MA, Asimakopoulos AD, Artibani W, et al. Insight into new potential targets for the treatment of overactive bladder and detrusor overactivity. Urol Int 2012;89(1):1–8.

96. Fry CH, Chakrabarty B, Hashitani H, et al. New targets for overactive bladder-ICI-RS 2109. Neurourol Urodyn 2020;39(Suppl 3). S113-s21.

97. Merrill L, Gonzalez EJ, Girard BM, et al. Receptors, channels, and signalling in the urothelial sensory system in the bladder. Nat Rev Urol 2016;13(4): 193–204.

98. Araki I, Du S, Kobayashi H, et al. Roles of mechanosensitive ion channels in bladder sensory transduction and overactive bladder. Int J Urol 2008;15(8): 681–7.

99. Lin CT, Chiang BJ, Liao CH. Perspectives of medical treatment for overactive bladder. Urol Sci 2020;31: 91–8.

Chemodenervation in Urology

Meera Ganesh, BA[a], Nicole Handa, MD[b], Stephanie Kielb, MD[b],*

KEYWORDS

- Botox • Overactive bladder • Bladder injections • Detrusor overactivity • Intradetrusor injection

KEY POINTS

- Botulinum toxin A exerts multiple effects in the bladder, which contributes to its therapeutic efficacy.
- The primary effect of botulinum toxin A in the bladder is inhibition of sensory innervation.
- Onabotulinum toxin A is currently FDA approved as a third-line treatment of overactive bladder and a fourth-line treatment of interstitial cystitis/bladder pain syndrome.
- Botulinum toxin A can be administered in an inpatient or outpatient setting.
- Detailed evaluation of patient comorbidities before procedure is important to prevent complications.

 Video content accompanies this article at http://www.urologic.theclinics.com.

BACKGROUND

The therapeutic utility of botulinum toxin was elucidated through the contributions of 3 scientists: Christian Kerner, a physician who isolated the substance from poisoned sausages in the early 1800s; Emile van Ermengem, a bacteriologist who isolated the bacteria that produced the toxin in 1897; and Alan B Scott, an ophthalmologist who successfully used the substance in a patient to treat strabism.[1] The first successful use of botulinum A toxin in the lower urinary tract was injections in the urethral sphincter to treat detrusor-sphincter dyssynergia.[2]

There are multiple botulinum toxins that are clinically available, predominantly based on serotype A1: onabotulinumtoxin A (Botox/Vistabel), abobotulinumtoxinA (Dysport/Azzalure), and incobotulinumtoxinA (Xeomin/Bocouture).[3] Multiple studies have compared the effectiveness of onabotulinumtoxin A and abobotulinumtoxinA at their respective standard doses and found no difference in the clinical effectiveness of the 2 preparations.[4,5] This article refers mainly to onabotulinumtoxin A (BTXA) when discussing use and indications because this is the best studied and only Food and Drug Administration (FDA)-approved toxin in use in the United States.

STRUCTURE OF BOTULINUM TOXIN

Botulinum A toxin (BoNT/A) is the most therapeutically relevant of the 7 types of botulinum toxins produced by the gram-positive anaerobic bacterium, *Clostridium botulinum*.[6,7] BoNT/A is synthesized in its inactive form as a single-chain polypeptide (approximately 150 kDa) and is activated when cleaved into a dichain structure (approximately 100 and 50 kDa) held together by a disulfide bond (**Fig. 1**).[8] This active structure binds to nontoxic elements, which enhance its ability to resist denaturation and proteolysis.[9]

Financial Disclosures: none.
Conflicts of Interest: none.

[a] Northwestern University, Feinberg School of Medicine, 420 E Superior Street, Chicago, IL 60611, USA;
[b] Department of Urology, Feinberg School of Medicine, Northwestern University, 675 N St Clair Street, Suite 20-150, Chicago, IL 60611, USA
* Corresponding author.
E-mail address: stephanie.kielb@nm.org

Urol Clin N Am 49 (2022) 263–272
https://doi.org/10.1016/j.ucl.2021.12.009
0094-0143/22/© 2022 Elsevier Inc. All rights reserved.

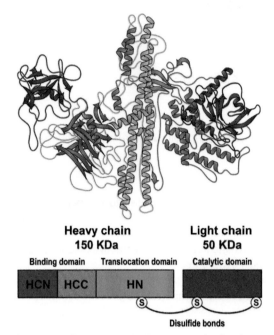

Heavy chain
150 KDa

Light chain
50 KDa

Binding domain　Translocation domain　Catalytic domain

HCN	HCC	HN	

Disulfide bonds

Fig. 1. Botulinum A toxin is composed of a heavy chain and a light chain held together by a disulfide bond. The chains are further divided into the binding, translocation, and catalytic domains, each of which has a specific function.

The light chain (LC) of BoNT/A contains the consensus sequence HEXXH, which is characteristic of a Zn-dependent endopeptidase.[10] The heavy chain (HC) is composed of 3 distinct domains: the alpha-helical domain (H_N) and another 50-kDa domain further subdivided into 2 25-kDa domains (H_{CN} and H_{CC}).[11]

MECHANISM OF ACTION

There are distinct stages in the mechanism of action for BoNT/A: binding/internalization and intracellular effects.

Binding/Internalization

The HC of BoNT/A is responsible for the internalization of the toxin into the cell. The 25-kDa H_{CC} domain of the HC binds to a complex of gangliosides on the presynaptic membrane.[12] BoNT/A subsequently binds to the synaptic vesicle glycoprotein 2 (SV2) and synaptotagmin, which are functional in vesicle exocytosis. The SV2 is then able to bind the H_{CC} and the H_{CN} regions more specifically to endocytose the toxin into the presynaptic vesicle.[13] The LC is then translocated into the synaptic vesicle through a protein-conducting channel, under cell-specific pH threshold.[14]

Acetylcholine Release

Synaptic vesicles in the presynaptic cells are loaded with acetylcholine that will be released into the synaptic membrane via calcium-regulated exocytosis.[15] For vesicle exocytosis to occur, the vesicle-associated membrane protein (VAMP) synaptobrevin, which is attached to the vesicle, must complex with syntaxin, another VAMP, and synaptosomal protein-25 (SNAP-25), which are present on the nerve plasmalemma. This ternary complex binds to N-ethylmaleimide sensitive factor attachment protein to form the SNARE complex, which facilitates membrane fusion for exocytosis.[15] The LC of BoNT/A binds and cleaves the SNAP-25 substrate of the SNARE complex to prevent neurotransmitter release (**Fig. 2**).[16]

EFFECT OF BOTULINUM TOXIN
Bladder Specific

The efficacy of botulinum toxin in causing bladder paralysis was initially thought to be a result of acetylcholine release inhibition. However, the persistence of cleaved SNAP-25 in bladder smooth muscle beyond the established duration in striated muscle suggests another possible explanation for the mechanism of action of BoNT/A.[17]

One proposed mechanism is the effect of BoNT/A on sensory transmission. Afferent nerves innervating the detrusor smooth muscle in the bladder detect bladder stretching and carry this information to the central nervous system. The distention results in neurotransmitter release of ATP, nerve growth factor (NGF), acetylcholine, and nitric oxide (NO).[18] BoNT/A inhibits the function of these neurotransmitters by normalizing the balance of ATP and NO and inhibiting the effect of NGF, dampening the excitability of the afferent neurons and bladder overactivity.[18,19] Another potential contribution to the efficacy of BoNT/A in the bladder is the concentrated distribution of SV2 and SNAP-25 receptors in the human parasympathetic fibers and some sensory fibers.[20] Both receptors have a high affinity for BoNT/A allowing for increased inhibition in bladder activity.

Another important finding is the reduction in the vanilloid receptor TRPV1 and ATP-gated receptor $P2X_3$. Both receptors (TRPV1 and $P2X_3$) are important in normal mechanical bladder function.[21,22] Decreased expression of the TRPV1 and $P2X_3$ immunoreactive fibers has been observed in patients with detrusor overactivity following BoNT/A injections.[23] BoNT/A likely causes this through inhibition of TRPV1 translocation to the plasma membrane via inhibition of protein kinase C induction of TRPV1.[24] The effect of BoNT/A on NGF

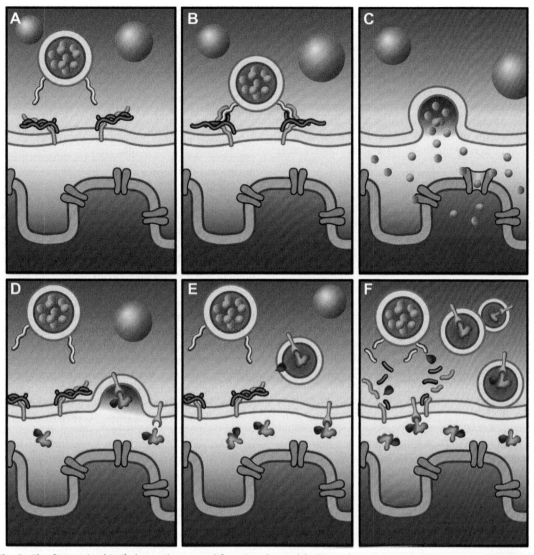

Fig. 2. The first series (*A–C*) shows the normal functional acetylcholine release at a synaptic junction. Presynaptic vesicles loaded with acetylcholine bind to the plasma membrane via the interaction of the VAMP synaptobevin (*light blue*) and proteins syntaxin (pink) and SNAP-25 (purple) to form the SNARE complex, which allows for vesicle fusion to the membrane and acetylcholine release. The second series (*D–F*) shows the effect of BoNT/A at the synaptic junction. The HC of BoNT/A (*orange*) binds to a ganglioside complex (*green*) to internalize the toxin. The LC (red) is then translocated to the vesicle where it cleaves SNAP-25 preventing formation of the SNARE complex and acetylcholine release.

could also play a role in the downregulation of neuronal receptors.[18,25] Reduction in these receptors causes reduction in detrusor overactivity.[26,27]

Pain Reduction

Chemodenervation of the bladder through BoNT/A has been investigated as a treatment of bladder pain due to its effects on the sensory pathways within the bladder. Unmyelinated C-fibers and partially myelinated A δ-fibers are responsible for pain perception in the bladder.[28]

NGF plays a role in excitability of C-fibers, and inhibition through BoNT/A injection can reduce pain nociception.[25,29] BoNT/A has been shown to also inhibit other nociceptive neuropeptides such as calcitonin gene-related peptide and substance P that are released by C-fibers in patients with bladder pain syndrome (BPS).[18] BoNT/A also reduces the upper and lower pain thresholds in both A δ-fibers and C-fibers through inhibition of ATP release and increase of NO to limit pain perception.[18,30]

Prostate

Injections of BoNT/A in the prostate have shown to reduce prostate size and improve lower urinary tract symptoms (LUTS) for patients with benign prostatic hyperplasia (BPH) refractory to medical therapy.[31] In rat models, BoNT/A reduced prostatic volume via selective denervation and prostatic atrophy.[32] Although much of the bladder mechanism of BoNT/A action in the bladder is through parasympathetic nerves, the innervation of the prostate is primarily sympathetic,[33] suggesting an alternate mechanism of action for BoNT/A in the prostate than in the bladder. Studies in rat models suggest that prostate atrophy is likely a result of sympathetic denervation,[34] which likely follows from acetylcholine inhibition, a well-described mechanism of action of BoNT/A.[8]

CLINICAL USAGE
Overactive Bladder

BTXA is a neuromuscular blocker that has been approved by the FDA for multiple conditions including both neurogenic and nonneurogenic overactive bladder (OAB) refractory to conservative management as well as urinary incontinence from detrusor overactivity from neurogenic causes (Fig. 3).[35] There is variability in epidemiologic estimates of OAB due to the nuances in the definition of OAB and its presentation with concurrent urge incontinence (UI). In the United States, OAB estimates range from 16.5% to 35.6%, with higher prevalence in females and the elderly.[36] The OAB population under Medicare is estimated to be 3.4 million individuals by 2027.[37]

According to the guidelines put forth by the American Urologic Association (AUA) and the Society of Urodynamics, Female Pelvic Medicine, and Urogenital Reconstruction, BTXA treatment of OAB is currently a third-line treatment, after a patient fails behavioral and pharmacologic management.[38] The efficacy of BTXA in OAB treatment has been widely demonstrated to reduce UI episodes and to improve urodynamic and quality-of-life parameters.[39,40] The major side effects of BTXA injections are an increased risk for urinary tract infections (UTIs) due to increased postvoid residuals (PVRs).[40,41] BTXA has also been shown to be more efficacious than some pharmacotherapies for OAB.[42] Sacral neuromodulation is another third-line treatment of OAB than BTXA, which causes a larger reduction in UI episodes; however, studies have suggested that BTXA could be more cost effective in the long term.[43,44]

Interstitial Cystitis and Bladder Pain

According to the AUA guidelines, intradetrusor BTXA treatment is a fourth-line treatment of interstitial cystitis (ICS)/BPS (Fig. 4).[45] Previous studies have shown improvement in patient-reported outcome measures such as the Interstitial Cystitis Symptom and Problem Index [46] and has also been shown to be more efficacious than other pharmacologic treatments including bacillus Calmette-

Overactive Bladder Treatment Guidelines			
1st Line	**2nd Line**	**3rd Line**	**4th Line**
Behavioral Therapy Bladder training Bladder control strategies Pelvic floor muscle training Fluid management	**Pharmacologic Management** Oral anti- muscarinics Oral β_3- adrenoreceptor agonists Transdermal oxybutynin patch Combination medical therapy	**Neuromodulation** Onabotulinumtoxin A Peripheral tibial nerve simulation (PTNS) Sacral neuromodulation (SNS)	**Surgical Management** Augmented Cystoplasty Urinary Diversion

Fig. 3. OAB treatment guidelines.

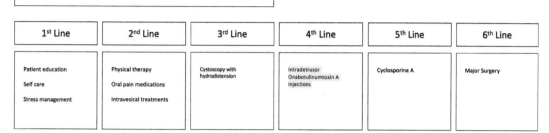

Fig. 4. Interstitial cystitis and bladder pain treatment guidelines.

Guérin, resiniferatoxin, lidocaine, chondroitin sulfate, oxybutynin, and pentosan polysulfate.[47] However, the heterogeneity in the types of studies conducted, confounding variables, and bias make BTXA treatment recommendations for ICS/BPS untenable and necessitate further research to determine the best treatment course for these patients.[46,48]

Benign Prostatic Hyperplasia

Treatment with BTXA has been considered for detailed management of BPH, although it is not currently FDA approved for this indication. For patients who have continued LUTS after medical management who are not undergoing interventional therapy, BTXA injections can be considered with careful monitoring.[49] BTXA injections can be administered in the prostate via the transperineal, transurethral, or transrectal routes.[50] Randomized controlled trials have shown BTXA injections to be efficacious in reducing LUTS for patients with BPH compared with standard medical management,[51] whereas others conclude that BTXA may have no effect compared with placebo in the treatment of BPH,[31] indicating further investigation is necessary to determine use in this setting.

Detrusor-Sphincter Dyssynergia

For patients with neurogenic detrusor-sphincter dyssynergia, BTXA injection is a common off-label treatment modality following pharmacologic therapy and clean intermittent catheterization.[52] One of the first uses of BTXA injections for lower urinary tract diseases was external urinary sphincter BTXA injections for patients with spinal cord injury with detrusor-sphincter dyssynergia.[53] Since this first application, BTXA has been effective in reducing detrusor-sphincter dyssynergia when administered in neurogenic patients with bladder symptoms through various routes: transurethral, transperineal.[54] For these patients the lower degree of dyssynergia, absence of bladder

neck dyssynergia, and presence of detrusor contractions all predict success of treatment.[55]

ADMINISTRATION

The official FDA recommendations state an onabotulinumtoxin A dose of 100 U for OAB treatment and 200 U for neurogenic detrusor overactivity.[35] In OAB treatment, BTXA doses of 100 U optimize effectiveness of treatment and prevention of high PVR levels which would necessitate intermittent catheterization.[56,57] Studies have compared doses of 200 and 300 U for treatment of neurogenic detrusor overactivity and found no significant difference between the 2 doses.[58]

Bladder BTXA injection procedures can be outpatient or inpatient depending on the available resources and the clinical needs of the patient. In all patients, 2% lidocaine should be administered before injection. For patients with autonomic dysreflexia, providers should be familiar with management to prevent autonomic dysreflexia provocation, continually monitor blood pressure, and have access to nitroglycerin ointment during treatment.[59] In these patients, continual blood pressure monitoring requirements may make the operating room more suitable for the procedure.

A flexible or rigid scope can be used for injection (Video 1). Flexible cystoscope needle tip lengths vary from 2 to 5 mm. For rigid cystoscopy, needle tip lengths vary from 2 to 8 mm. There are cystoscopes of both types that have options with adjustable needles.[60] Recommendations for neurogenic OAB include 6.7 to 10 U/mL at each site of injection with approximately 20 to 30 injections sparing the trigone area (**Fig. 5**). For idiopathic OAB, recommendations include 5 to 10 U/mL at each side with fewer injections overall.[61] Most recently, a pilot study by Avallone and colleagues[62] demonstrated comparable efficacy in as few as 1, 2, and 3 injection sites with equal dosage of the toxin for patients with idiopathic detrusor overactivity (IDO) and neurogenic detrusor overactivity (NDO). This effectiveness is likely

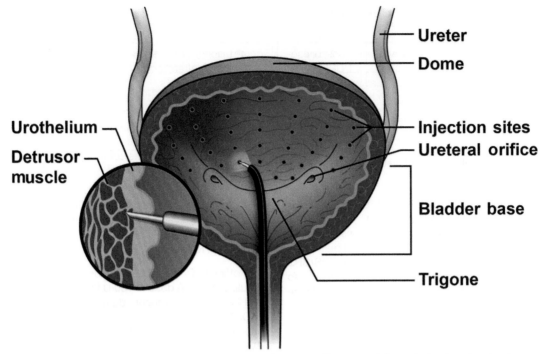

Fig. 5. A flexible cystoscope is inserted through the urethra. A needle is passed through the sheath. Injections can be made on the posterior wall in a trigone-sparing manner.

attributed to the ability of onabotulinumtoxin A to diffuse through the extracellular space of the detrusor muscle.[63] In delayed contrast MRI, toxin diffusion is evident in human bladders.[64] The official recommendation for injection depth is 2 mm into the intradetrusor muscle.[35] Comparison of injection into detrusor, suburothelial, and bladder base layers shows no difference in efficacy.[65] Although there is no difference in effectiveness in trigone versus trigone-sparing injections, there is a higher incidence of UTIs and voiding difficulties with trigone injections.[66]

SIDE EFFECTS AND CONSIDERATIONS
Urinary Tract Infections

UTIs are a well-documented side effect of bladder injections of BTXA for OAB.[39,40] Recent data show that a urine dip before procedure may not be indicated in asymptomatic patients because adverse events between those with positive and negative urine dips is not statistically significant.[67] A European consensus statement by Giannantoni and colleagues[68] recommended oral antibiotic prophylaxis 30 minutes before the procedure, to be continued for 2 to 3 days. However, recent investigations show that whereas asymptomatic bacteriuria does increase the risk of UTI, it does not

increase the risk of urosepsis, hospitalization, and therapy failure, thus preprocedure antibiotic prophylaxis may not be indicated for the asymptomatic population.[69] Postprocedural antibiotic prophylaxis may have some reduced rates of UTI; however, more research is necessary to standardize prophylaxis treatments and routes of administration.[70] Male patients with a retained prostate and female patients are at increased risk for UTIs following BTXA injections, which should inform preprocedural diagnostic medical decision making.[71]

Urinary Retention

Increased PVR is another detrimental side effect of BTXA injections for OAB.[40] Although rates of urinary retention requiring catheterization are low (1.6%),[72] careful evaluation of patient risk factors such as age, number of vaginal deliveries, and increased preoperative PVR should be made before recommendation for BTXA procedures.[73,74] Elderly patients with frailty—defined as age greater than 65 years and 3 of the following: unintentional weight loss, exhaustion, weakness, or reduced physical activity—and male patients also have higher risk for postprocedure voiding dysfunction requiring catheterization.[71] For complicated patients, uroflowmetry with PVR before the procedure is recommended.[68]

Repeat Injections

Another consideration for patients undergoing BTXA injections is the need for reinjection.[75] The therapeutic effect of BTXA injection is estimated to last approximately 2 to 4 months.[54,76] At 6 months postinjection, the effect of the toxin is diminished.[65] For patients who do not show improvement after a single procedure or have recurrence of symptoms, repeat BTXA injection is a treatment option. Studies have found BTXA injections to be clinically efficacious up to 4 injections.[77] There has also been preliminary success in using fewer injection sites at higher doses for reinjection in patients who were refractory to the primary procedure.[78]

Systemic Risks

Systemic botulism toxicity is a rare but potential complication of BTXA injections. BTXA has demonstrated retrograde axonal transport capability, which can contribute to inhibition of neurotransmission at other locations.[79] Serious adverse events from botulism toxicity resulting in death can occur from respiratory arrest, myocardial infarction, cerebrovascular accident, pulmonary embolism, and pneumonia among other causes.[80] Patients with systemic toxicity can present with diffuse muscle weakness and inspiratory difficulties.[81] Treatment of toxicity is urgent administration of BTXA antitoxin.[82] In pediatric patients, case reports of pyridostigmine have successfully reversed adverse effects of BTXA injection.[83] To prevent such complications, it is important to thoroughly evaluate patient history before administration of injection. Important considerations include prior BTXA injections (dosage and location) and concurrent ongoing BTXA treatment. If patients are undergoing multiple treatments, timing treatments to prevent overdosing is necessary. For adults the maximum recommended dose is 400 U over a 3-month period.[35] In pediatric patients, the maximum recommended dose is the lesser of 10 U/kg or 340 U over a 3-month period.[35]

SUMMARY

Overall, BTXA is a clinically efficacious tool for treating a myriad of urologic pathologies. The inhibitory effects on neurotransmission can alleviate bladder hyperactivity and LUTS in patients. Although treatment guidelines have specific indications for BTXA injections, there is ongoing investigation into novel urologic uses for the toxin. The ease of outpatient administration of BTXA contributes to its attractiveness as a therapeutic. Although there are some key considerations of patient history that will affect medical decision making with regard to injection, botulinum toxin will continue to be a quintessential component of the urologist toolbox.

CLINICS CARE POINTS

- BTXA injections can be used for a variety of pathologies: OAB, interstitial cystitis/bladder pain, BPH, and detrusor-sphincter dyssynergia
- There are a few key side effects to be cognizant of the most prevalent being UTI and urinary retention
- Repeat injections may be necessary to prevent recurrence of symptoms as the toxin wears off
- Dosage should be monitored to avoid systemic toxicity

ACKNOWLEDGMENTS

Sheila Macomber

SUPPLEMENTARY DATA

Supplementary data related to this article can be found online at https://doi.org/10.1016/j.ucl.2021.12.009.

REFERENCES

1. Cruz F. Targets for botulinum toxin in the lower urinary tract. Neurourol Urodyn 2014;33(1):31–8.
2. Dykstra DD, Sidi AA. Treatment of detrusor-sphincter dyssynergia with botulinum A toxin: a double-blind study. Arch Phys Med Rehabil 1990;71(1):24–6.
3. Pirazzini M, Rossetto O, Eleopra R, et al. Botulinum Neurotoxins: Biology, Pharmacology, and Toxicology. Pharmacol Rev 2017;69(2):200–35.
4. Ravindra P, Jackson BL, Parkinson RJ. Botulinum toxin type A for the treatment of non-neurogenic overactive bladder: does using onabotulinumtoxinA (Botox((R))) or abobotulinumtoxinA (Dysport((R))) make a difference? BJU Int 2013;112(1):94–9.
5. Peyronnet B, Castel-Lacanal E, Roumiguie M, et al. Intradetrusor injections of onabotulinum toxin A (Botox(R)) 300 U or 200 U versus abobotulinum toxin A (Dysport(R)) 750 U in the management of neurogenic detrusor overactivity: A case control study. Neurourol Urodyn 2017;36(3):734–9.
6. Chancellor MB, Smith CP. Biology and mechanism of action. Botulinum toxin in Urology. Berlin Heidelberg: Springer; 2011. p. 13–26.

7. Aronson JK, Dukes MNG. Meyler's side effects of drugs : the international encyclopedia of adverse drug reactions and interactions. 15th edition. Elsevier; 2006.

8. Simpson LL. The origin, structure, and pharmacological activity of botulinum toxin. Pharmacol Rev 1981;33(3):155–88.

9. Wagman J. Isolation and sedimentation study of low molecular weight forms of type A botulinus toxin. Arch Biochem Biophys 1954;50(1):104–12.

10. Li Binz T, Niemann H, Singh BR. Probing the mechanistic role of glutamate residue in the zinc-binding motif of type A botulinum neurotoxin light chain. Biochemistry 2000;39(9):2399–405.

11. Lalli G, Herreros J, Osborne SL, et al. Functional characterisation of tetanus and botulinum neurotoxins binding domains. J Cell Sci 1999;112(Pt 16): 2715–24.

12. Burns JR, Lambert GS, Baldwin MR. Insights into the mechanisms by which clostridial neurotoxins discriminate between gangliosides. Biochemistry 2017;56(20):2571–83.

13. Rummel A. Two feet on the membrane: uptake of clostridial neurotoxins. In: Barth H, editor. Uptake and trafficking of protein toxins. Springer International Publishing; 2017. p. 1–37. https://doi.org/10.1007/82_2016_48.

14. Fischer A, Mushrush DJ, Lacy DB, et al. Botulinum neurotoxin devoid of receptor binding domain translocates active protease. Plos Pathog 2008;4(12):e1000245.

15. Dolly O. Synaptic transmission: inhibition of neurotransmitter release by botulinum toxins. Headache 2003;43(s1):16–24.

16. Breidenbach MA, Brunger AT. Substrate recognition strategy for botulinum neurotoxin serotype A. Nature 2004;432(7019):925–9.

17. Schulte-Baukloh H, Zurawski TH, Knispel HH, et al. Persistence of the synaptosomal-associated protein-25 cleavage product after intradetrusor botulinum toxin A injections in patients with myelomeningocele showing an inadequate response to treatment. BJU Int 2007;100(5):1075–80.

18. Yeh TC, Chen PC, Su YR, et al. Effect of Botulinum Toxin A on Bladder Pain-Molecular Evidence and Animal Studies. Toxins (Basel) 2020;12(2). https://doi.org/10.3390/toxins12020098.

19. Yoshimura N, Bennett NE, Hayashi Y, et al. Bladder overactivity and hyperexcitability of bladder afferent neurons after intrathecal delivery of nerve growth factor in rats. J Neurosci 2006;26(42):10847–55.

20. Coelho A, Dinis P, Pinto R, et al. Distribution of the high-affinity binding site and intracellular target of botulinum toxin type A in the human bladder. Eur Urol 2010;57(5):884–90.

21. Birder LA, Nakamura Y, Kiss S, et al. Altered urinary bladder function in mice lacking the vanilloid receptor TRPV1. Nat Neurosci 2002;5(9):856–60.

22. Cockayne DA, Hamilton SG, Zhu Q-M, et al. Urinary bladder hyporeflexia and reduced pain-related behaviour in P2X3-deficient mice. Nature 2000; 407(6807):1011–5.

23. Apostolidis A, Popat R, Yiangou Y, et al. Decreased sensory receptors P2X$_3$ and TRPV1 in suburothelial nerve fibers following intradetrusor injections of botulinum toxin for human detrusor overactivity. J Urol 2005;174(3):977–83.

24. Morenilla-Palao C, Planells-Cases R, García-Sanz N, et al. Regulated exocytosis contributes to protein kinase C potentiation of vanilloid receptor activity. J Biol Chem 2004;279(24):25665–72.

25. Giannantoni A, Stasi SMD, Nardicchi V, et al. Botulinum-A toxin injections into the detrusor muscle decrease nerve growth factor bladder tissue levels in patients with neurogenic detrusor overactivity. J Urol 2006;175(6):2341–4.

26. Brady CM, Apostolidis AN, Harper M, et al. Parallel changes in bladder suburothelial vanilloid receptor TRPV1 and pan-neuronal marker PGP9.5 immunoreactivity in patients with neurogenic detrusor overactivity after intravesical resiniferatoxin treatment. BJU Int 2004;93(6):770–6.

27. Brady CM, Apostolidis A, Yiangou Y, et al. P2X3-immunoreactive nerve fibres in neurogenic detrusor overactivity and the effect of intravesical resiniferatoxin. Eur Urol 2004;46(2):247–53.

28. Takeda M, Mochizuki T, Yoshiyama M, et al. Sensor mechanism and afferent signal transduction of the urinary bladder: special focus on transient receptor potential ion channels. Low Urin Tract Symptoms 2010;2(2):51–60.

29. Seki S, Sasaki K, Fraser MO, et al. Immunoneutralization of nerve growth factor in lumbosacral spinal cord reduces bladder hyperreflexia in spinal cord injured rats. J Urol 2002;168(5):2269–74.

30. Collins VM, Daly DM, Liaskos M, et al. OnabotulinumtoxinA significantly attenuates bladder afferent nerve firing and inhibits ATP release from the urothelium. BJU Int 2013;112(7):1018–26.

31. Hsu YC, Wang HJ, Chuang YC. Intraprostatic botulinum neurotoxin type A injection for benign prostatic hyperplasia-A spotlight in reality. Toxins (Basel) 2016;8(5). https://doi.org/10.3390/toxins8050126.

32. Doggweiler R, Zermann D-H, Ishigooka M, et al. Botox-induced prostatic involution. The Prostate 1998; 37(1):44–50.

33. Ganzer R, Stolzenburg J-U, Wieland WF, et al. Anatomic study of periprostatic nerve distribution: immunohistochemical differentiation of parasympathetic and sympathetic nerve fibres. Eur Urol 2012; 62(6):1150–6.

34. Silva J, Pinto R, Carvallho T, et al. Mechanisms of prostate atrophy after glandular botulinum neurotoxin type a injection: an experimental study in the rat. Eur Urol 2009;56(1):134–40.

35. FDA. BOTOX (onabotulinumtoxinA) for injection, for intramuscular, or intradermal use. Food and Drug Administration; 2017.

36. Eapen RS, Radomski SB. Review of the epidemiology of overactive bladder. Res Rep Urol 2016;8: 71–6.

37. Puckrein GWD, Xu L, Congdon P, et al. The prevalence and forecast prevalence of overactive bladder in the medicare population. Clin Med Insights: Urol 2019;12.

38. Lightner DJ GA, Souter L et al. Diagnosis and Treatment of Non-Neurogenic Overactive Bladder (OAB) in Adults: an AUA/SUFU Guideline (2019). Vol. 202. 2019:548. AUA/SUFU Guideline Ammendment. Accessed 2021.

39. Lopez Ramos H, Torres Castellanos L, Ponce Esparza I, et al. Management of Overactive Bladder With OnabotulinumtoxinA: Systematic Review and Meta-analysis. Urology 2017;100:53–8.

40. Chibelean C, Nechifor-Boila IA. Botulinum neurotoxin A for overactive bladder treatment: advantages and pitfalls. Can J Urol 2015;22(2):7681–9.

41. Cui Y, Zhou X, Zong H, et al. The efficacy and safety of onabotulinumtoxinA in treating idiopathic OAB: A systematic review and meta-analysis. Neurourol Urodyn 2015;34(5):413–9.

42. Lozano-Ortega G, Walker D, Rogula B, et al. The relative efficacy and safety of mirabegron and onabotulinumtoxina in patients with overactive bladder who have previously been managed with an antimuscarinic: a network meta-analysis. Urology 2019;127:1–8.

43. Harvie HS, Amundsen CL, Neuwahl SJ, et al. Cost-Effectiveness of Sacral Neuromodulation versus OnabotulinumtoxinA for Refractory Urgency Urinary Incontinence: Results of the ROSETTA Randomized Trial. J Urol 2020;203(5):969–77.

44. Lo CW, Wu MY, Yang SS, et al. Comparing the Efficacy of OnabotulinumtoxinA, Sacral Neuromodulation, and Peripheral Tibial Nerve Stimulation as Third Line Treatment for the Management of Overactive Bladder Symptoms in Adults: Systematic Review and Network Meta-Analysis. Toxins (Basel) 2020;12(2). https://doi.org/10.3390/toxins12020128.

45. Hanno PM ED, Moldwin R et al. Diagnosis and Treatment Interstitial Cystitis/Bladder Pain Syndrome (2014). Vol. 193. 2015:1545. AUA Guideline Ammendment. Accessed 2021.

46. Giannantoni A, Gubbiotti M, Bini V. Botulinum Neurotoxin A Intravesical Injections in Interstitial Cystitis/Bladder Painful Syndrome: A Systematic Review with Meta-Analysis. Toxins (Basel) 2019;11(9). https://doi.org/10.3390/toxins11090510.

47. Zhang W, Deng X, Liu C, et al. Intravesical treatment for interstitial cystitis/painful bladder syndrome: a network meta-analysis. Int Urogynecol J 2017; 28(4):515–25.

48. Parsons BA, Goonewardene S, Dabestani S, et al. The benefits and harms of botulinum toxin-A in the treatment of chronic pelvic pain syndromes: a systematic review by the European Association of Urology Chronic Pelvic Pain Panel. Eur Urol Focus 2021. https://doi.org/10.1016/j.euf.2021.01.005.

49. Kevin T. McVary M, Chair; Claus G. Roehrborn, MD, Co-Chair; Andrew L. Avins, MD, MPH; Michael J. Barry, MD; Reginald C. Bruskewitz, MD; Robert F. Donnell, MD; Harris E. Foster, Jr., MD; Chris M. Gonzalez, MD; Steven A. Kaplan, MD; David R. Penson, MD; James C. Ulchaker, MD; John T. Wei, MD. Management of Benign Prostatic Hyperplasia. 2014. Benign Prostatic Hyperplasia (BPH) Guideline. Accessed 2021.

50. Ng LG. Botulinum toxin and benign prostatic hyperplasia. Asian J Urol 2018;5(1):33–6.

51. Delongchamps NB, Benard A, Azzouzi R, et al. 1079 A randomized clinical trial comparing prostatic injection of botulinum neurotoxin type A (Botox®) to optimized medical therapy in patients with BPH-related LUTS: End-of-study results of the PROTOX trial. Eur Urol Supplements 2016;15(3):e1079a.

52. Li H, Nahm N, Borchert A, et al. Contemporary treatment of detrusor sphincter dyssynergia: a systematic review. Curr Bladder Dysfunct Rep 2018;13(4): 206–14.

53. Dykstra DD, Sidi AA, Scott AB, et al. Effects of Botulinum a Toxin On Detrusor-Sphincter Dyssynergia In Spinal Cord Injury Patients. J Urol 1988;139(5): 919–22.

54. Schurch B, Hauri D, Rodic B, et al. Botulinum-A Toxin as a Treatment of Detrusor-Sphincter Dyssynergia: A Prospective Study in 24 Spinal Cord Injury Patients. J Urol 1996;155(3):1023–9.

55. Soler JM, Previnaire JG, Hadiji N. Predictors of outcome for urethral injection of botulinum toxin to treat detrusor sphincter dyssynergia in men with spinal cord injury. Spinal Cord 2016;54(6):452–6.

56. Dmochowski R, Chapple C, Nitti VW, et al. Efficacy and safety of onabotulinumtoxinA for idiopathic overactive bladder: a double-blind, placebo controlled, randomized, dose ranging trial. J Urol 2010;184(6): 2416–22.

57. Birk S. Botox may boost QOL in overactive bladder: treatment with 100 U 'may be the best dose in terms of balancing efficacy and safety. Ob gyn news 2009; 44(9):16.

58. Li GP, Wang XY, Zhang Y. Efficacy and Safety of OnabotulinumtoxinA in Patients With Neurogenic Detrusor Overactivity Caused by Spinal Cord Injury: A Systematic Review and Meta-analysis. Int Neurourol J 2018;22(4):275–86.

59. Fougere RJ, Currie KD, Nigro MK, et al. Reduction in Bladder-Related Autonomic Dysreflexia after OnabotulinumtoxinA Treatment in Spinal Cord Injury. J Neurotrauma 2016;33(18):1651–7.

60. Jr JAS, Howards SS, Preminger GM, et al. Hinman's Atlas of urologic Surgery. Elsevier; 2016.

61. Karsenty G, Baverstock R, Carlson K, et al. Technical aspects of botulinum toxin type A injection in the bladder to treat urinary incontinence: reviewing the procedure. Int J Clin Pract 2014;68(6):731–42.

62. Avallone MA, Sack BS, El-Arabi A, et al. Less is more-A pilot study evaluating one to three intradetrusor sites for injection of OnabotulinumtoxinA for neurogenic and idiopathic detrusor overactivity. Neurourol Urodyn 2017;36(4):1104–7.

63. Ramirez-Castaneda J, Jankovic J, Comella C, et al. Diffusion, spread, and migration of botulinum toxin. Mov Disord 2013;28(13):1775–83.

64. Alsinnawi M, Torreggiani W, Sheikh M, et al. Delayed contrast-enhanced MRI to localize Botox after cystoscopic intravesical injection. Int Urol Nephrol 2015; 47(6):893–8.

65. Kuo HC. Comparison of effectiveness of detrusor, suburothelial and bladder base injections of botulinum toxin a for idiopathic detrusor overactivity. J Urol 2007;178(4 Pt 1):1359–63.

66. El-Hefnawy AS, Elbaset MA, Taha D-E, et al. Trigonal-sparing versus trigonal-involved Botox injection for treatment of idiopathic overactive bladder: A randomized clinical trial. Low Urin Tract Symptoms 2021;13(1):22–30.

67. Derisavifard S, Giusto LL, Zahner P, et al. Safety of Intradetrusor OnabotulinumtoxinA (BTX-A) Injection in the Asymptomatic Patient With a Positive Urine Dip. Urology 2020;135:38–43.

68. Giannantoni A, Carbone A, Carone R, et al. Real-life clinical practice of onabotulinum toxin A intravesical injections for overactive bladder wet: an Italian consensus statement. World J Urol 2017;35(2): 299–306.

69. Leitner L, Sammer U, Walter M, et al. Antibiotic prophylaxis may not be necessary in patients with asymptomatic bacteriuria undergoing intradetrusor onabotulinumtoxinA injections for neurogenic detrusor overactivity. Scientific Rep 2016;6(1):33197.

70. Eckhardt SE, Takashima Y, Handler SJ, et al. Antibiotic regimen and route of administration do not alter rates of urinary tract infection after intravesical botulinum toxin injection for overactive bladder. Int Urogynecol J 2021. https://doi.org/10.1007/s00192-021-04691-4.

71. Abrar M, Pindoria N, Malde S, et al. Predictors of Poor Response and Adverse Events Following Botulinum Toxin A for Refractory Idiopathic Overactive Bladder: A Systematic Review. Eur Urol Focus 2020. https://doi.org/10.1016/j.euf.2020.06.013.

72. Patel DN, Jamnagerwalla J, Houman J, et al. What is the true catheterization rate after intravesical onabotulinumtoxinA injection? Int Urogynecol J 2018; 29(7):1005–9.

73. Davis NF, Burke JP, Redmond EJ, et al. Trigonal versus extratrigonal botulinum toxin-A: a systematic review and meta-analysis of efficacy and adverse events. Int Urogynecol J 2015;26(3):313–9.

74. Osborn DJ, Kaufman MR, Mock S, et al. Urinary retention rates after intravesical onabotulinumtoxinA injection for idiopathic overactive bladder in clinical practice and predictors of this outcome. Neurourol Urodyn 2015;34(7):675–8.

75. Shepherd JP, Carter-Brooks CM, Chermanksy C. A cost-effectiveness analysis of Onabotulinumtoxin A as first-line treatment for overactive bladder. Int Urogynecol J 2018;29(8):1213–9.

76. Karsenty G, Reitz A, Lindemann G, et al. Persistence of therapeutic effect after repeated injections of botulinum toxin type A to treat incontinence due to neurogenic detrusor overactivity. Urology 2006; 68(6):1193–7.

77. Ni J, Wang X, Cao N, et al. Is repeat Botulinum Toxin A injection valuable for neurogenic detrusor overactivity—A systematic review and meta-analysis. Neurourol Urodyn 2018;37(2):542–53.

78. Martínez-Cuenca E, Bonillo MA, Morán E, et al. Onabotulinumtoxina Re-Injection for Refractory Detrusor Overactivity Using 3-4 Injection Sites: Results of a Pilot Study. Urology 2020;137:50–4.

79. Restani L, Novelli E, Bottari D, et al. Botulinum neurotoxin A impairs neurotransmission following retrograde transynaptic transport. Traffic 2012; 13(8):1083–9.

80. Cote TR, Mohan AK, Polder JA, et al. Botulinum toxin type A injections: adverse events reported to the US Food and Drug Administration in therapeutic and cosmetic cases. J Am Acad Dermatol 2005;53(3): 407–15.

81. Bensen GP, Rutherford CC, Gardner TB. Systemic Botulism Toxicity Caused by Pyloric Botox Injection to Treat Gastroparesis. Case Rep Gastroenterol 2020;14(2):373–6.

82. Jones RGA, Corbel MJ, Sesardic D. A review of WHO International Standards for botulinum antitoxins. Biologicals 2006;34(3):223–6.

83. Boerner RM, Young DL, Gnagi SH, et al. Pyridostigmine for the Reversal of Severe Adverse Reactions to Botulinum Toxin in Children. J Pediatr 2018;194: 241–3.

Pharmacologic Management of Interstitial Cystitis/Bladder Pain Syndrome

Christopher J. Chermansky, MD[a],*, Marina O. Guirguis, MD[b]

KEYWORDS

- Interstitial cystitis • Bladder pain syndrome • Pharmacology • Intravesical treatment

KEY POINTS

- Interstitial cystitis/bladder pain syndrome (IC/BPS) is defined as persistent or chronic discomfort perceived to be related to the urinary bladder accompanied by urinary urgency or frequency.
- Pharmacotherapies used to treat IC/BPS include both oral, intravesical agents, and intradetrusor drugs.
- Oral therapies include amitriptyline, hydroxyzine, cyclosporine A, and pentosan polysulfate sodium (PPS), although the recent finding of pigmented maculopathy (and the disabling symptoms of prolonged dark adaptation and difficulty reading) with chronic PPS is very concerning and must be discussed with patients, many of whom will choose to either come off this medicine or not even start it.
- Intravesical therapies usually involve a mixture of multiple agents in a "cocktail," most commonly alkalinized lidocaine and heparin.
- Intradetrusor OnabotulinumtoxinA 100U can be used to treat refractory IC/BPS symptoms.

INTRODUCTION

Interstitial cystitis/bladder pain syndrome (IC/BPS) is defined by International Continence Society (ICS) as persistent or chronic pelvic pain, pressure, or discomfort perceived to be related to the urinary bladder accompanied by an urgent need to void or urinary frequency.[1] This is diagnosed in the absence of any identifiable pathology which could explain these symptoms. The pelvic/suprapubic pain associated with IC/BPS is frequently characterized by painful urgency and pain with bladder filling.[2] Recently, the chronic pelvic pain working group of the ICS has classified IC/BPS into either hypersensitive bladder with no identifiable pathology explaining the symptoms or IC with Hunner's lesions (HL) identified on the basis of cystoscopy.[3] Though IC/BPS was first described in the late 19th and early 20th centuries,[4,5] the etiology of IC/BPS

is still unclear. Many women who suffer from IC/BPS also struggle with chronic fatigue syndrome, other pain disorders such as endometriosis, pelvic floor dysfunction, and fibromyalgia, as well as anxiety and depression.[6–9] We will briefly discuss some of the possible causes of IC/BPS and, more importantly, the pathophysiology behind them.

The bladder is lined with urothelium, a specialized transitional epithelium that typically forms a barrier protecting the bladder wall. This is accompanied by a urothelial glycosaminoglycan (GAG) layer, which is thought to contribute to the barrier function.[10] In patients with IC/BPS, structural and molecular changes in the urothelium have been observed.[7] The urothelial cells can be activated to release mediators by mechanical, thermal, or chemical stimuli leading to epithelial dysfunction. As such, the integrity of the barrier is difficult to

[a] Chief of Urology UPMC Magee Womens Hospital, 300 Halket Street, Suite 2541, Pittsburgh, PA 15213, USA;
[b] Division of Urogynecology, Department of Obstetrics and Gynecology, Magee Womens Hospital, 300 Halket Street, Pittsburgh, PA 15213, USA
* Corresponding author.
E-mail address: chermanskycj2@upmc.edu
Twitter: @MGuirguisMD (M.O.G.)

Urol Clin N Am 49 (2022) 273–282
https://doi.org/10.1016/j.ucl.2022.01.003
0094-0143/22/© 2022 Elsevier Inc. All rights reserved.

maintain. Another contributor to IC/BPS is neurogenic inflammation, which is a result of the release of proinflammatory neuropeptides including substance P and nerve growth factor. These mediators are released by the peripheral sensory nerves, and they induce mast cell degranulation within the bladder, which provokes the release of more mediators. Some have suggested that this leads to persistent afferent nerve sensitization and local bladder inflammation which aggravates mast cell degranulation. This results in changes in neural plasticity and sensitization within the spinal cord and dorsal root ganglia, which promotes continued pain symptoms.[11]

As mentioned earlier, it is common for women with IC/BPS to have other pain syndromes such as fibromyalgia and vulvodynia. Functional pain syndromes are frequently marked by hyperalgesia or allodynia, which suggests a problem with sensory processing within the central nervous system in these patients.[12] Hypersensitivity may additionally contribute to persistent activation of dorsal horn neurons, which result in changes that mediate pain well after any local insult within the bladder.[2]

ORAL PHARMACOTHERAPIES
Pentosan Polysulfate Sodium

Pentosan polysulfate sodium (PPS) is a heparin analog that is currently the only US FDA-approved oral medication for the treatment of IC/BPS. It is thought that PPS corrects the deficiency in the GAG layer associated with IC/BPS.[1] This medication has been studied more than any other medication in terms of treating IC/BPS. Five trials have been performed comparing PPS to placebo, of which 4 were randomized control trials (RCTs).[1] In one multicenter RCT comparing PPS 100 mg TID to placebo in 148 patients, Parsons and colleagues[13] reported at 3 months that 32% of the patients on PPS showed significant improvement compared with 16% on placebo ($P = .01$). In another double-blind, placebo-controlled study, there was again a statistically significant difference in symptom improvement favoring those receiving PPS 100 mg TID (28%) compared with those receiving placebo (13%).[14] By contrast, another prospective double-blinded multicenter study of 115 patients revealed no difference between those receiving PPS 200 mg BID for 4 months (56%) and those receiving placebo (49%).[15] In addition, Nickel and colleagues[16] performed a randomized double-blind placebo-controlled study in 368 adults comparing PPS 100 mg daily, PPS 100 mg TID, or matching placebo for 24 weeks. The O'Leary-Sant Interstitial Cystitis Symptom

Index (ICSI) was administered at baseline, and at weeks 4, 8, 12, 18, and 24. There was no statistically significant difference between the PPS group and the placebo group or between the 2 PPS groups for the primary end point, defined as responder achieving a 30% or greater reduction from the baseline ICSI total score at study end. This primary end point was achieved by 40.7% taking placebo, 39.8% taking PPS 100 mg daily, and 42.6% taking PPS TID. This trial, sponsored by Johnson & Johnson, was terminated early for lack of efficacy. A meta-analysis of the 5 trials that included PPS and placebo arms revealed a statistically significant but clinically somewhat weak relative risk ratio of 1.69 (95% confidence interval [CI], 1.16–2.46). The rates of adverse events in the placebo-controlled RCTs of PPS were relatively low (10%–20% of patients), generally not serious, and similar bewteen treatment and placebo groups.

Although the AEs specific to PPS have traditionally included headache, nausea, diarrhea, and changes in liver function and platelet counts, a newer and much more concerning AE reported with chronic PPS use is the finding of maculopathy associated with chronic PPS use. Pearce and colleagues[17] reported his initial retrospective series of 6 adults on chronic PPS that were diagnosed with pigmented maculopathy. The authors identified 38 patients at the Emory Eye Center who were on chronic PPS, and the 6 patients with maculopathy constituted 16% of this group. The patients with maculopathy reported a mean of PPS use of 15.5 years, and they reported difficulty reading and prolonged dark adaptation. The authors stated that it remained unclear whether drug cessation would halt or alter the course of the retinal disease. The following year, the same authors examined the charts of 219 IC/BPS patients, and all the patients underwent eye examination.[18] PPS exposure, documented in 80 of 219 subjects (36.5%), was the sole statistically significant predictor of pigmentary maculopathy with an odds ratio of 11.25 (95% CI, 3.69–34.33, $P < .0001$). The authors found evidence of the maculopathy in 14 of 80 patients (17.8%), and the median duration of PPS intake was 18.3 years (range, 3–21.9 years). Furthermore, there were no cases of maculopathy in the 139 patients who did not have exposure to PPS. Based on these findings, they suggested that PPS exposure is directly linked to the maculopathy as a medication toxicity.

Ludwig undertook a large, multicenter, retrospective cohort study of commercially insured patients to further study PPS exposure and maculopathy.[19] Although they did not find an association at 5 years of PPS exposure, they did note higher risk in a small number of patients with extended exposure of carrying a diagnosis of a hereditary maculopathy. It should be noted that in this study, the mean duration of PPS use was less than 1 year, and only 130 patients (0.26%) had ≥5 years of PPS use. In addition, across all PPS users in the study, only 29% had an eye examination, and this examination may have occurred at any time, not necessarily at the end of the observation period. Jain and colleagues[20] performed another claims-based analysis using data from a large US medical claims database. A total of 3012 and 1604 PPS users were compared with 15,060 and 8017 matched controls at 5 and 7 years, respectively. At 5 years, multivariate analysis showed no significant association ($P > .13$). Yet, at 7 years, PPS users had significantly increased odds of having maculopathy (OR = 1.41, 95% CI, 1.09–1.83, $P = .009$).

Recent prospective analysis supported the association between PPS and maculopathy and further delineated at-risk exposure levels. Vora and colleagues[21] evaluated data available in the Kaiser Permanente Northern California system and screened 117 of 138 IC/BPS patients on PPS identified as having at least 500 g of exposure. The overall prevalence of maculopathy in this population of patients was 23.1%. Furthermore, subgroup analysis demonstrated maculopathy in 12.7% of patients with 500 to 999 g of exposure versus 41.7% of patients with greater than 1500 g of exposure ($P = .01$). As for screening patients taking PPS, Sadda and colleagues[22] recommend screening at 500 g of exposure (approximately 4.5 years with a standard daily dose of 100 mg TID) and annually thereafter, labeling those with exposure of greater than 1500 g as high risk.

In summary, PPS maculopathy is increasingly recognized in literature. Several studies indicate an increased risk of maculopathy with higher cumulative exposure, with an average prevalence of 20% among patients with >3 to 5 years of daily exposure. Those providers who prescribe oral PPS for IC/BPS should strongly consider the risk of maculopathy. Annual retinal screening should be performed on patients with 500 g over 5 years of PPS exposure, and baseline retinal examination should be done before medication commencement.

Amitriptyline

Amitriptyline is a tricyclic antidepressant that is another of the oral second-line treatments for IC/BPS as recommended in the AUA guideline.[1] Amitriptyline is thought to improve urgency by blocking anticholinergic and histamine receptors, and it improves pain by inhibiting the reuptake of serotonin and norepinephrine. Multiple studies have been done supporting the improvement of symptoms with the use of amitriptyline. Van Ophoven and colleagues[23] published an RCT comparing amitriptyline to placebo. Patients (44 women and 6 men) were treated for 4 months with a self-titration protocol that allowed them to escalate drug dosage in 25 mg increments in 1 week intervals (maximum dosage 100 mg). The change from baseline in the O'Leary-Sant IC symptom and problem index was the primary outcome parameter. They found that 63% of the amitriptyline group significantly improved compared with 4% of the placebo group. Furthermore, the mean symptom score decreased from 26.9 to 18.5 in the amitriptyline group compared with 27.6 to 24.1 in the placebo group ($P = .005$). The same authors performed an observational study with similar dosing and that also revealed improvement of 50% to 64% in individuals taking amitriptyline.[24]

Foster and colleagues performed a multicenter, randomized, double-blind, placebo-controlled clinical trial of amitriptyline.[25] A total of 271 subjects were randomized, and 231 (85%) provided a global response assessment (GRA) at 12 weeks of follow-up. In an intent to treat analysis, the response rates of subjects reporting moderate or marked improvement from baseline in the amitriptyline and placebo groups were 55% and 45%, respectively ($P = .12$). Yet, of the 160 subjects on amitriptyline who achieved a dose of 50 mg per day, the responder rate was 77% in the amitriptyline group compared with 53% in the placebo group ($P < .001$).

Owing to its adverse effects, amitriptyline is always titrated when initiated. The most common side effects are fatigue and malaise. As such, bedtime dosing is used to mitigate this side effect. Other side effects include dizziness, dry mouth, and constipation.

Hydroxyzine

Hydroxyzine is another of the oral second-line treatments for IC/BPS as recommended in the AUA guideline.[1] Hydroxyzine is a histamine (H1) receptor antagonist that decreases mast cell activation. Given that increased mast cells have been found within the urothelium of some patients with IC/BPS, antihistamines such as hydroxyzine have been found to improve bladder storage symptoms.[1] Sant and colleagues[26] performed an RCT randomizing patients to either oral hydroxyzine (10 mg daily titrated to 50 mg daily over several weeks if tolerated) or placebo. A total of 121 participants (89% of goal) were randomized over 18 months and 79% provided complete follow-up data. The response rate for hydroxyzine was 31% for those treated and 20% for those not treated (*P* = .26). Another study that was observational reported that 92% of patients experienced clinically significant improvement (25 mg daily titrated up to 75 mg daily over several weeks); however, the patients in this study all had systemic allergies, and these patients may represent a subset that is more likely to respond to hydroxyzine.[27] AEs from hydroxyzine include short-term sedation and weakness, and dosing should begin at 25 mg and titrated up.[1]

Although one RCT demonstrated a 31% rate of response to hydroxyzine 50 mg,[26] another study demonstrated a response to hydroxyzine 75 mg of up to 55% in patients with an allergy history.[27] Hydroxyzine is also typically titrated up starting with a 25 mg dosage because of patient somnolence.[1,26,27]

Cyclosporine A

The AUA recommends oral Cyclosporine (CyA) as fifth-line therapy for IC/BPS.[1] Cyclosporine (CyA) is a selective immunosuppressive agent that inhibits calcineurin, which is necessary for the activation of T cells. CyA has been successful in the treatment of several autoimmune diseases such as psoriasis and rheumatoid arthritis. To explore a possible autoimmune etiology for IC, immunosuppressants like CyA have been tested in the treatment of IC.

Forsell and colleagues[28] first reported on the use of CyA for 3 to 6 months in 11 patients (10 women and 1 man) with IC. The patients were started at a dose of 2.5 to 5 mg/kg daily, and the dose was decreased to 1.5 to 3 mg/kg daily after 2 to 3 weeks. Because potential AEs from CyA use include impaired renal function and hypertension, serum creatinine and blood pressure were monitored regularly. Bladder pain, measured subjectively by patient report and not by validated questionnaires, did decrease after 6 weeks in 10 patients. Urinary frequency decreased (*P* < .01), and maximum voided volume increased (*P* < .01). Serum creatinine did not change, and mild hypertension occurred in 2 patients and resolved after the CyA dose was lowered. After treatment ended, symptoms recurred in most patients within 2 months. The same authors reported long-term outcomes with CyA in 23 IC patients (20 women and 3 men).[29] The mean follow-up was 60.8 ± 35.7 months. After a year of CyA treatment, urinary frequency decreased from 20.8 ± 6.3 voids/d before treatment to 10.2 ± 3.8 voids/d (*P* < .001), maximal bladder capacity increased from 161.8 ± 74.6 mL to 360.7 ± 99.3 mL

(*P* < .001), and mean voided volume increased from 101.4 ± 42.7 mL to 246.4 ± 97.9 mL (*P* < .001). Bladder pain resolved in 20 of the 23 patients, and 11 of the patients eventually stopped treatment after remaining asymptomatic for at least a year; however, bladder pain recurred in 9 patients within 3 months. No nephrotoxicity was seen in any of the patients, and hypertension was reported in 3 patients and required antihypertensive therapy. AEs included gingival hyperplasia and facial hair growth. The authors concluded that long-term CyA was safe and effective.

Sairanen and colleagues[30] undertook a prospective open-label RCT comparing CyA to oral PPS in IC/BPS. A total of 64 patients were randomized to either CyA 1.5 mg/kg twice daily or PPS 100 mg TID for 6 months. The primary end point was reduction in daily micturition frequency, and secondary end points included mean voided volume, number of nocturia episodes, O'Leary-Sant symptom score, visual analog scale (VAS) for pain, and subjective GRA. There was no difference in baseline patient characteristics between the groups. HL were seen on cystoscopy in 15 of 64 patients, with 5 patients in the CyA group and 10 in the PPS group. Reduction in daily micturition frequency of greater than 50% was seen in 11 patients (34%) in the CyA group and no patients in the PPS group (*P* < .001). Furthermore, the clinical response rate (according to GRA) was 75% for CyA compared with 19% for PPS (*P* < .001). Also, AEs were higher in the CyA arm (94%) than in the PPS arm (56%), with 3 serious AEs in the CyA arm (increased blood pressure, increased serum creatinine) and 1 serious AE in the PPS arm (gross hematuria). At 6 months, a total of 19 patients continued CyA treatment and only 4 patients continued PPS treatment. In this study, CyA showed superior efficacy over PPS in patients with IC/BPS.

Forrest, Payne, and Erickson pooled their findings on the response rate of CyA for IC/BPS in a retrospective study of 44 patients (30 women and 14 men) followed a mean of 15 to 30 months.[31] Most patients (34/44 or 77%) had IC with confirmed HL. The starting daily dose of CyA was 3 mg/kg in 2 divided doses with a maximum of 300 mg daily. After establishing good symptom relief, the dose was tapered as tolerated. Meaningful response was defined as markedly improved on the 7-point GRA or a ≥50% decrease in ICSI score. Overall, 59% of the patients reported a meaningful response; however, success rates with CyA were much higher (29/34 or 85%) among those IC patients with HL compared with those without HL (3/10 or 30%). Furthermore, those IC patients without HL who had improvement did not improve to the same degree as those IC patients with HL. For all responders, the response was seen within 4 months, and improvements were maintained if CyA was maintained. AEs included increased serum creatinine in 9 patients (managed by either decreasing dose in 4 or discontinuing in 5), hypertension in 3 patients (managed with anti-hypertensive meds), alopecia in 1, mouth ulcers in 2, and acute gout in 1. Of the 85% of IC patients with HL who saw efficacy with CyA, 6 patients stopped the medication because of AEs, leaving a final success rate of 68% (23/34) in IC patients with HL. The authors concluded that CyA outcomes were much better for IC patients with HL than for those without HL, and they stressed that AEs are common with CyA, and close monitoring is mandatory.

Ehren and colleagues[32] evaluated CyA response in 10 IC patients with HL for 4 months (3 mg/kg daily for 3 months and then reduced dosage for the last month). An aim of this study was to evaluate whether the measurement of luminal nitric oxlde (NO) could be used as an objective marker of response to CyA. ICSI scores decreased from a baseline score of 16 to 8 after 3 months of CyA, and the scores rose to 12 after CyA was discontinued. All 10 patients exhibited elevated bladder NO levels of 489 $\pm$ 141 ppb at baseline, and these levels decreased dramatically to 16 $\pm$ 6 ppb after 2 weeks of CyA therapy and continued to decrease during the first 2 months of the study. After the CyA dose was reduced to 0.75 mg/kg/d at 3 months, NO levels increased to 144 $\pm$ 70 ppb at 4 months. Two weeks after CyA was discontinued, NO levels returned to 478 $\pm$ 187 ppb, the same as baseline levels. As for AEs, none of the patients experienced elevation of serum creatinine or a rise in blood pressure. The authors concluded that the measurement of luminal NO was a reliable and easy way to evaluate anti-inflammatory treatments in IC patients with HL.

Crescenze and Shoskes conducted an open-label study of 26 IC/BPS patients treated with CyA 3 mg/kg divided twice daily for 3 months.[33] Of the 26 patients, 7 (27%) had HL. The primary end point was moderate or marked improvement of GRA or greater than 50% improvement on the ICSI at 3 months. At 3 months, 22 of the 26 patients completed follow-up, 31% (8/26) improved by GRA, and 15% (4/26) had greater than 50% improvement in the ICSI score. Yet, IC patients with HL were the most responsive to CyA therapy with 42% of the patients with HL reporting greater than 50% improvement in ICSI scores versus 11% for patients without HL (P = .01). AEs, including hypertension and decline in renal function, were seen and prompted either dose reduction or drug cessation in a small number of patients. The authors concluded that a longer follow-up was needed to determine the duration of the medication effect and to optimize treatment protocols.

In summary, the data on CyA as treatment for IC/BPS suggest sustained efficacy in patients with HL or with active bladder inflammation; however, because of the relatively small number of patients treated, the lack of long-term follow-up data on large numbers of patients, and the potential for serious AEs, physicians must weigh the risk-to-benefit ratio and manage patient expectations. Although the therapeutic benefit of CyA in IC/BPS patients with HL supports inflammation as an etiology, the exact mechanism by which CyA facilitates healing and improves bladder pain remains unclear.

INTRAVESICAL PHARMACOTHERAPIES

Intravesical pharmacotherapies are used to treat the local effects of IC/BPS within the bladder wall. Bladder instillations are thought to restore the urothelium and GAG layer and decrease the permeability seen in some patients with IC/BPS.[1] The frequency of bladder instillations can vary, but they are typically delivered every 1 to 4 weeks for a total of 4 to 6 instillations.[1] These instillations are typically a "cocktail" of multiple medications.

Dimethyl Sulfoxide (DMSO)

Dimethyl sulfoxide (DMSO) is second-line treatment for IC/BPS as recommended in the AUA guideline, and it is the only FDA-approved intravesical treatment used as a single agent, although it is often combined with other medications such as heparin and lidocaine.[1] DMSO promotes smooth muscle relaxation through nerve blockade, inhibits collagen, and has anti-inflammatory effects. Perez-Marrero and colleagues[34] performed a controlled crossover study of DMSO in 33 IC patients. The medication was administered intravesically every 2 weeks for 2 sessions of 4 treatments each. Response was assessed 1-month post-treatment. Blinded evaluators used urodynamic and voiding parameters to rate patient improvement and patients rated global improvement. The evaluators found that improvement was seen in 93% in the DMSO group and 35% in the placebo group. The patients reported that 87% in the DMSO group were better and 59% in the placebo group were better. More recently, Yoshimura and colleagues[35] sought to evaluate the efficacy and safety of intravesical KRP-116D, 50% DMSO, compared with placebo. A total of 96 patients were randomized to receive either KRP-116D (n = 49) or placebo (n = 47). The intravesical study drug was administered every 2 weeks for 12 weeks. The change in the O'Leary Sant ICSI score from baseline to week 12 was −5.2 in the KRP-116D group and −3.4 in the placebo group (P = .0188). As for AEs, the incidence of garlic-like breath in this study was very low (4.1%). The instillation dwell time for DMSO should be limited to 15 to 20 minutes because longer periods of holding are associated with significant pain.

Lidocaine

The chronic pain seen with IC/BPS is thought to result from sensitized bladder afferents. Lidocaine is a local anesthetic that has been used as an intravesical treatment for IC/BPS either alone or combined with other medications.[1] Because lidocaine is a weak base and because urine is usually acidic (pH 5–6), there is concern that much of the intravesical lidocaine remains ion trapped within the urine. As such, efforts have been undertaken to alkalinize the lidocaine to aid in urothelial penetration. Nickel and colleagues[36] performed a phase 2, multicenter, double-blind RCT within the US and Canada. They randomized 102 patients (99 women) to either 10 cc of intravesical alkalinized lidocaine (a combination of 200 mg lidocaine alkalinized with 8.4% sodium bicarbonate) or placebo. The patients received the treatment for 5 consecutive days. Efficacy was assessed by changes in the GRA, Likert scales for bladder pain, and validated O'Leary-Sant ICSI and ICPI scales. At 3 days after the last treatment, moderate or marked improvement in the GRA was seen in 30% of patients receiving the alkalinized lidocaine compared with only 9.6% of patients receiving placebo (P = .012); however, these differences were not statistically significant at 10 days after the last treatment. Although no studies have directly compared lidocaine concentrations, one study did see an increase in success rate when the lidocaine was increased from 1% to 2%.[37] In this open-label trial, the lidocaine was combined with 40,000 units heparin and 3 cc of 8.4% sodium bicarbonate. The success rate increased from 75% to 94% after increasing the lidocaine concentration from 1% to 2%, respectively. AEs from intravesical lidocaine are typically not serious but include dysuria, urethral irritation, and bladder pain.

Heparin

Intravesical heparin is another second-line treatment for IC/BPS as recommended in the AUA guideline, and it was initially evaluated as monotherapy; however, it has more recently been combined with other intravesical agents like alkalinized lidocaine.[1] It is thought to mimic the GAG layer of the bladder, and it is involved in proliferation of fibroblasts and smooth muscles as well as angiogenesis. Parsons and colleagues[38] treated 48 patients with 10,000 IU heparin in 10 cc sterile water 3 times per week for 3 months with retention of 1 hour. At the 3-month assessment, 27 of 48 patients (56%) reported clinically significant improvement. Of the 23 patients who elected continued therapy, 20 continued in remission, and of the 16 patients who continued out to 1 year, 15 remained in remission. Kuo also evaluated the efficacy of intravesical heparin in 40 women with IC/BPS.[39] These women received 25,000 IU heparin in 5 cc water twice per week for 3 months. Symptom score improvement of greater than 50% was seen in 29 of 40 patients (72.5%) at 3 months, and 8 of those with less than 50% improvement did report improved nocturia. Nomiya evaluated the efficacy of 32 women with IC/BPS given 20,000 IU heparin, 5 cc of 4% lidocaine, and 25 cc of 7% sodium bicarbonate.[40] This intravesical combination was given weekly for 12 consecutive weeks. Efficacy was measured with O'Leary and Sant's ICSI and ICPI scales, GRA, and VAS for pain. The proportion of responders after completion of all instillations rose from 33.3% at week 1 to 90% at 1 month and then diminished to 16.7% by 6 months after the last instillation. AEs from intravesical heparin are infrequent and minor. Although there have been no good placebo-controlled studies, intravesical heparin either alone or in combination with other agents does appear to benefit some IC/BPS patients.

Pentosan Polysulfate Sodium

Pentosan polysulfate sodium (PPS), as discussed earlier, is a heparin analog that has been used orally to treat symptoms of IC/BPS. The intravesical administration of PPS has been studied with the goal of mimicking the GAG layer of the urothelium. Daha and colleagues[41] performed an open-label study of 29 women with IC/BPS who received 300 mg of intravesical PPS twice a week for 10 weeks and thereafter a voluntary maintenance therapy once a month for 3 months. Treatment response was assessed by VAS for quality of life and O'Leary-Sant Symptom and Problem Index (OSPI), and both improved from baseline to 1 week, 3, 6, and 12 months after treatment ended. Davis and colleagues[42] randomized 41 women with IC/BPS to either intravesical PPS and oral PPS or intravesical placebo and oral PPS for 6 weeks. Patients continued oral PPS for another 12 weeks. The primary outcome was the change in the OSPI from baseline to weeks 6, 12, and 18. At week 12, those patients receiving both intravesical and oral PPS saw a 46% reduction in the OSPI from baseline, and the patients who received only oral PPS (and intravesical placebo) saw a 24% reduction in the OSPI ($P = .04$). No studies have been published to date evaluating pigmented maculopathy in patients given intravesical PPS.

INTRADETRUSOR ONABOTULINUM TOXIN A

Intradetrusor onabotulinum toxin A (BoNTA) is currently listed in the AUA guideline as a fourth-line treatment for IC/BPS.[1] Kuo and Chancellor performed an RCT in IC/BPS patients comparing hydrodistention with either 100 U or 200 U doses of BoNTA versus hydrodistention alone.[43] Of the 67 patients, 44 received either BoNTA 200 U (n = 15) or 100 U (n = 29) followed by hydrodistention 2 weeks later and 23 received hydrodistention alone. At 3 months, the bladder pain VAS, functional bladder capacity, and GRA significantly improved only in the BoNTA groups versus the control group ($P = .002$). The 200 U dose did not provide better efficacy compared with 100 U, and AEs were higher with BoNTA 200 U. These authors concluded that BoNTA 100 U followed by hydrodistention was efficacious in IC/BPS. Chung and colleagues[44] also combined BoNTA 100 U with hydrodistention, and they reported significant improvement in virtually all measured outcomes with a GRA-based success rate of 52.2% at 6 months of follow-up. About one-third of patients had dysuria but there were no cases of urinary retention.

Regarding efficacy with repeated BoNTA as a treatment for IC/BPS, Pinto and colleagues[45] injected BoNTA 100 U into the trigone with retreatment upon symptom return. They recruited 34 IC/BPS patients, and they were followed for up to 3 years. At baseline, the VAS pain score was 5.9 ± 0.8 and the OSPI score was 28.8 ± 6.3. One month after the first treatment, the VAS pain score decreased to 2.7 ± 0.7 ($P < .05$) and the OSPI score decreased to 16.1 ± 3.2 ($P < .05$). The duration of these improvements was 9 to 10 months after each treatment. With respect to AEs, nearly one-third of patients had UTIs, and there were no cases of urinary retention.

Lee and Kuo[46] compared the treatment outcomes of BoNTA injections for treatment of each IC/BPS type. They prospectively enrolled 44 patients who were classified as having either HL (n = 10) or no HL (n = 30) based on cystoscopy. All patients received 4 sets of intravesical BoNTA injections 100 U every 6 months. The primary end point was the GRA 6 months after the 4th set of BoNTA injections, and secondary end points

included changes in ICSI, ICPI, VAS pain scores, and urinary frequency episodes. After 4 BoNTA treatments, 15 of 30 patients (50%) with no HL saw success with scores ≥ 2, and none of the 10 patients (0%) with HL had success. None of the patients with HL had significant changes in the secondary end points. Thus, intradetrusor BoNTA did not benefit any patient with HL.

PHARMACOTHERAPIES IN CLINICAL DEVELOPMENT
Certolizumab Pegol

Tumor necrosis factor-alpha (TNFα), a proinflammatory cytokine, results in excess inflammation and organ injury in autoimmune diseases. Patients with IC/BPS have been shown to have elevated levels of TNFα in urine. Certolizumab pegol is a novel anti-TNF agent that treats autoimmune diseases such as Crohn's disease and rheumatoid arthritis. Bosch[47] evaluated the efficacy and safety of certolizumab pegol compared with placebo in women with IC/BPS refractory to oral and intravesical treatments. In this phase 2 study, a total of 42 women were randomized to receive either subcutaneous certolizumab pegol 400 mg (n = 28) and or placebo with sterile saline (n = 14) at weeks 0, 2, 4, and 8. Patients were monitored at weeks 10, 14, and 18. The primary end point was the difference in GRA between certolizumab pegol and placebo at week 2, and the GRA analysis at week 2 did not show a statistically significant difference between certolizumab pegol and placebo; however, there was a statistically significant improvement at week 18 for certolizumab pegol compared with placebo in change from baseline for ICSI of −3.6 (95% CI, −6.9 to −0.29, $P = .03$) and ICPI of −3.0 (95% CI, −6.1 to 0.12, $P = .042$). The most common AE reported was UTI in 7 taking certolizumab pegol and 4 taking placebo ($P > .99$). Women with moderate to severe refractory IC/BPS were more likely to experience significant improvement in symptoms with certolizumab pegol compared with placebo. Limitations of the study included no proper sample size calculation, no intent-to-treat analysis, and the omission of cystoscopy in determining if these patients had HL. The authors admitted the need for a larger, longer, multicenter, RCT to further investigate certolizumab pegol as a treatment for IC/BPS.

META-ANALYSIS OF PHARMACOTHERAPIES FOR IC/BPS

Di and colleagues[48] compared the efficacy and safety of pharmacotherapies for IC/BPS with a

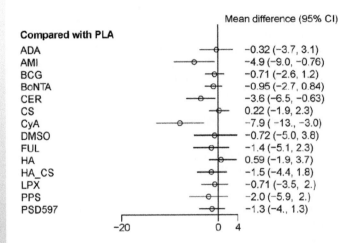

Mean difference (95% CI)

Compared with PLA

ADA	−0.32 (−3.7, 3.1)
AMI	−4.9 (−9.0, −0.76)
BCG	−0.71 (−2.6, 1.2)
BoNTA	−0.95 (−2.7, 0.84)
CER	−3.6 (−6.5, −0.63)
CS	0.22 (−1.9, 2.3)
CyA	−7.9 (−13., −3.0)
DMSO	−0.72 (−5.0, 3.8)
FUL	−1.4 (−5.1, 2.3)
HA	0.59 (−1.9, 3.7)
HA_CS	−1.5 (−4.4, 1.8)
LPX	−0.71 (−3.5, 2.)
PPS	−2.0 (−5.9, 2.)
PSD597	−1.3 (−4., 1.3)

−20   0 4

Fig. 1. Analysis of the O'Leary Sant Interstitial Cystitis Symptom Index (ICSI) using forest plot. ADA, adalimumab; AMI, amitriptyline; BCG, bacillus Calmette–Guérin; BoNTA, botulinum toxin A; CER, certolizumab pegol; CS, chondroitin sulfate; CyA, cyclosporine A; DMSO, dimethyl sulfoxide; FUL, fulranumab; HA, hyaluronic acid; HA/CS, hyaluronic acid plus chondroitin sulfate; LPX, lipotoxin; PLA, placebo; PPS, pentosan polysulfate; PSD597, alkalinized lidocaine.

systematic review and Bayesian network meta-analysis of evidence from RCTs. They identified a total of 23 RCTs with 1871 participants. The efficacy outcomes they evaluated included ICSI, ICPI, VAS, and Likert score for pain. The ICSI was significantly reduced in the CyA group (MD = −7.9, 95% CI, −13.0 to 3.0), the amitriptyline group (MD = −4.9, 95% CI, −9.0 to −0.76), and the certolizumab pegol group (MD = −3.6, 95% CI, −6.5 to −0.63) compared with placebo groups (**Fig. 1**). For ICPI, CyA showed superior benefit compared with placebo (MD = −7.6, 95% CI, −13 to −2.3). VAS score improved significantly in CyA compared with PPS (MD = 3.09, 95% CI, 0.13 to 6.07). In terms of safety outcomes, AEs for BoNTA were the only variate higher than chondroitin sulfate (MD = −2.02, 95% CI, −4.99 to 0.66) and placebo (MD = −1.60, 95% CI, −3.83 to 0.17).

SUMMARY

The AUA guideline on the diagnosis and treatment of IC/BPS provides a basic framework for clinicians to build a management regimen. Yet, individualizing treatment based on a patient's phenotype is important in aiding the effective treatment of IC/BPS. We believe that patients should be first clinically phenotyped, and then multimodal therapy directed to each positive domain should be initiated. If the etiology appears to be organ specific, such as pain specific to bladder filling, using amitriptyline and/or a combination intravesical treatment including alkalinized lidocaine has been successful as second-line treatments. Given the recent finding of pigmented maculopathy (and the disabling symptoms of prolonged dark adaptation and difficulty reading) in those patients exposed to chronic oral PPS use, those providers who prescribe oral PPS for IC/BPS must strongly consider the risk of maculopathy and discuss with patients the risks and the need to monitor for maculopathy during treatment. Because greater than 50% of IC/BPS patients have pelvic floor muscle spasticity on presentation, these patients should be treated concurrently with pelvic floor muscle physical therapy, which as a second-line treatment is a standard of care.[1] For the subset of IC/BPS patients with HL, we believe that cystoscopy and fulguration should be the first step of their care path. For those who fail fulguration, low-dose CyA should be strongly considered. In the recently published meta-analysis, CyA was shown to have superior over other pharmacologic treatments in the treatment of IC/BPS with HL.

DISCLOSURE

CJC: For Cook Myosite, I am a Study Site PI on Phase 3 Multicenter, Randomized, Double-blind, Randomized, Placebo-controlled Trial Comparing Autologous Muscle Derived Cells with Placebo in Women with Stress Urinary Incontinence.

CLINICS CARE POINTS

- When deciding on therapeutic options for treatment of IC/BPS, one must be aware of and counsel patients on potential adverse effects of pharmacologic therapies.

- Amitriptyline and hydroxyzine are both typically titrated to mitigate the side effect of drowsiness.

- Pentosan polysulfate sodium has recently been associated with pigmented maculopathy, and patients must be counseled about

- the disabling symptoms of prolonged dark adaptation and difficulty reading that occur with this AE.
- Cyclosporine A, although effective in IC/BPS patients with HL, is associated with hypertension and renal abnormalities, and patients on this therapy must be monitored.

REFERENCES

1. Hanno PM, Erickson D, Moldwin R, et al. American urological association. Diagnosis and treatment of interstitial cystitis/bladder pain syndrome: AUA guideline amendment. J Urol 2015;193:1545–53.
2. Lai HH, Krieger JN, Pontari MA, et al. Painful bladder filling and painful urgency are distinct characteristics in men and women with urological chronic pelvic pain syndromes: a MAPP research network study. J Urol 2015;194(6):1634–41.
3. Doggweiler R, Whitmore KE, Meijlink JM, et al. A standard for terminology in chronic pelvic pain syndromes: A report from the chronic pelvic pain working group of the international continence society. Neurourol Urodyn 2017;36(4):984–1008.
4. Skene AJC. Diseases of the bladder and urethra in women. Am J Psychiatry 1879;35(4):574–6.
5. Hunner GL. A rare type of bladder ulcer in women. South Med J 1915;8(5):410.
6. Nickel JC, Tripp DA, Pontari M, et al. Interstitial cystitis/painful bladder syndrome and associated medical conditions with an emphasis on irritable bowel syndrome, fibromyalgia and chronic fatigue syndrome. J Urol 2010;184(4):1358–63.
7. Birder LA. Pathophysiology of interstitial cystitis. Int J Urol 2019;26(S1):12–5.
8. Krieger JN, Stephens AJ, Landis JR, et al. Relationship between chronic nonurological associated somatic syndromes and symptom severity in urological chronic pelvic pain syndromes: Baseline evaluation of the MAPP study. J Urol 2015;193(4):1254–62.
9. Lai HH, Shen B, Rawal A, et al. The relationship between depression and overactive bladder/urinary incontinence symptoms in the clinical OAB population. BMC Urol 2016;16(1):1–8.
10. Birder L, Andersson KE. Urothelial signaling. Physiol Rev 2013;93(2):653–80.
11. Akiyama Y, Luo Y, Hanno PM, et al. Interstitial cystitis/bladder pain syndrome: the evolving landscape, animal models and future perspectives. Int J Urol 2020;27(6):491–503.
12. Clauw DJ. Fibromyalgia and related conditions. Mayo Clin Proc 2015;90(5):680–92.
13. Parsons CL, Benson G, Childs SJ, et al. A quantitatively controlled method to study prospectively interstitial cystitis and demonstrate the efficacy of pentosanpolysulfate. J Urol 1993;150(3):845–8.
14. Mulholland SG, Sant GR, Hanno P, et al. Pentosan polysulfate sodium for therapy of interstitial cystitis. A double-blind placebo-controlled clinical study. Urology 1990;35(6):552–8.
15. Holm-Bentzen M, Jacobsen F, Nerstrom B, et al. A prospective double-blind clinically controlled multicenter trial of sodium pentosanpolysulfate in the treatment of interstitial cystitis and related painful bladder disease. J Urol 1987;138:503–7.
16. Nickel JC, Herschorn S, Whitmore KE, et al. Pentosan polysulfate sodium for treatment of interstitial cystitis/bladder pain syndrome: Insights from a randomized, double-blind, placebo controlled study. J Urol 2015;193:857–62.
17. Pearce WA, Chen R, Jain N. Pigmentary maculopathy associated with chronic exposure to pentosan polysulfate sodium. Opthalmology 2018;125:1793–802.
18. Hanif AM, Shah R, Yan J, et al. Strength of association between pentosan polysulfate and a novel maculopathy. Ophthalmology 2019;126:1464–6.
19. Ludwig CA, Vail D, Callaway NF, et al. Pentosan polysulfate sodium exposure and drug-induced maculopathy in commercially insured patients in the United States. Ophthalmology 2020;127:535–43.
20. Jain N, Li AL, Yu Y, et al. Association of macular disease with long-term use of pentosan polysulfate sodium: findings from a US cohort. Br J Ophthalmol 2020;104:1093–7.
21. Vora RA, Patel AP, Melles R. Prevalence of maculopathy associated with long-term pentosan polysulfate therapy. Ophthalmology 2020;127:835–6.
22. Sadda SR. A path to the development of screening guidelines for pentosan maculopathy. Can J Ophthalmol 2020;55:1–2.
23. van Ophoven A, Pokupic S, Heinecke A, et al. A prospective, randomized, placebo controlled, double-blind study of amitriptyline for the treatment of interstitial cystitis. J Urol 2004;172:533–6.
24. van Ophoven A, Hertle L. Long-term results of amitriptyline treatment for interstitial cystitis. J Urol 2005;174:1837–40.
25. Foster HE Jr, Hanno PM, Nickel JC, et al, Interstitial Cystitis Collaborative Research Network. Effect of amitriptyline on symptoms in treatment naïve patients with interstitial cystitis/painful bladder syndrome. J Urol 2010;183:1853–8.
26. Sant GR, Propert KJ, Hanno PM, et al. A pilot clinical trial of oral pentosan polysulfate and oral hydroxyzine in patients with interstitial cystitis. J Urol 2003;170:810–5.
27. Theoharides TC, Sant GR. Hydroxyzine therapy for interstitial cystitis. Urology 1997;49:108–10.
28. Forsell T, Ruutu M, Isoniemi H, et al. Cyclosporine in severe interstitial cystitis. J Urol 1996;155:1591–3.

29. Sairanen J, Forsell T, Ruutu M. Long-term outcome of patients with interstitial cystitis treated with low dose cyclosporine A. J Urol 2004;171:2138–41.

30. Sairanen J, Tammela TL, Leppilahti M, et al. Cyclosporine A and pentosan polysulfate sodium for the treatment of interstitial cystitis: a randomized comparative study. J Urol 2005;174:2235–8.

31. Forrest JB, Payne CK, Erickson DR. Cyclosporine A for refractory interstitial cystitis/bladder pain syndrome: experience of 3 tertiary centers. J Urol 2012;188:1186–91.

32. Ehrén I, Hallén Grufman K, Vrba M, et al. Nitric oxide as a marker for evaluation of treatment effect of cyclosporine A in patients with bladder pain syndrome/interstitial cystitis type 3C. Scand J Urol 2013;47:503–8.

33. Crescenze IM, Tucky B, Li J, et al. Efficacy, side effects, and monitoring of oral cyclosporine in interstitial cystitis-bladder pain syndrome. Urology 2017; 107:49–54.

34. Perez-Marrero R, Emerson LE, Feltis J. A controlled study of dimethyl sulfoxide in interstitial cystitis. J Urol 1988;140:36–9.

35. Yoshimura N, Homma Y, Tomoe H, et al. Efficacy and safety of intravesical instillation of KRP-116D (50% dimethyl sulfoxide solution) for interstitial cystitis/ bladder pain syndrome in Japanese patients: A multicenter, randomized, double-blind, placebo-controlled, clinical study. Int J Urol 2021;28:545–53.

36. Nickel JC, Moldwin R, Lee S, et al. Intravesical alkalinized lidocaine (PSD597) offers sustained relief from symptoms of interstitial cystitis and painful bladder syndrome. BJU Int 2009;103:910–8.

37. Parsons CL. Successful downregulation of bladder sensory nerves with combination of heparin and alkalinized lidocaine in patients with interstitial cystitis. Urology 2005;65:45–8.

38. Parsons CL, Housley T, Schmidt JD, et al. Treatment of interstitial cystitis with intravesical heparin. Br J Urol 1994;73:504–7.

39. Kuo HC. Urodynamic results of intravesical heparin therapy for women with frequency urgency syndrome and interstitial cystitis. J Formos Med Assoc 2001;100:309–14.

40. Nomiya A, Naruse T, Niimi A, et al. On- and post-treatment symptom relief by repeated instillations of heparin and alkalized lidocaine in interstitial cystitis. Int J Urol 2013;20:1118–22.

41. Daha LK, Lazar D, Simak R, et al. The effects of intravesical pentosanpolysulfate treatment on the symptoms of patients with bladder pain syndrome/ interstitial cystitis: preliminary results. Int Urogynecol J Pelvic Floor Dysfunct 2008;19:987–90.

42. Davis EL, El Khoudary SR, Talbott EO, et al. Safety and efficacy of the use of intravesical and oral pentosan polysulfate sodium for interstitial cystitis: a randomized double-blind clinical trial. J Urol 2008;179:177–85.

43. Kuo HC, Chancellor MB. Comparison of intravesical botulinum toxin type A injections plus hydrodistention with hydrodistention alone for the treatment of refractory interstitial cystitis/painful bladder syndrome. BJU Int 2009;104:657–61.

44. Chung SD, Kuo YC, Kuo HC. Intravesical onabotulinumtoxin A injections for refractory painful bladder syndrome. Pain Physician 2012;15:197–202.

45. Pinto R, Lopes T, Silva J, et al. Persistent therapeutic effect of repeated injections of onabotulinum toxin a in refractory bladder pain syndrome/interstitial cystitis. J Urol 2013;189:548–53.

46. Lee CL, Kuo HC. Intravesical botulinum toxin a injections do not benefit patients with ulcer type interstitial cystitis. Pain Physician 2013;16:109–16.

47. Bosch PC. A randomized, double-blind, placebo-controlled trial of certolizumab pegol in women with refractory interstitial cystitis/bladder pain syndrome. Eur Urol 2018;74:623–30.

48. Di XP, Luo DY, Jin X, et al. Efficacy and safety comparison of pharmacotherapies for interstitial cystitis and bladder pain syndrome: a systematic review and Bayesian network meta-analysis. Int Urogynecol J 2021;32:1129–41.

Medical Treatment for Urinary Tract Infections

James Ross, MD[a], Duane Hickling, MD, MSc[b],*

KEYWORDS

- Urinary tract infection • Antimicrobials • Nonantimicrobial treatment • Prophylaxis

INTRODUCTION

Urinary tract infection (UTI) is a common cause of infection in humans. UTIs can be classified based on the segment of the urinary tract involved. Infection of the lower urinary tract (bladder) is referred to as cystitis, whereas the infection of the upper urinary tract (kidneys) is referred to as pyelonephritis.[1] Symptoms of cystitis are localized and can include dysuria, urinary urgency and frequency, cloudy and foul-smelling urine, and supra-pubic pain or discomfort. Patients with pyelonephritis typically present more unwell with fever, flank pain, and potentially other systemic signs and symptoms of sepsis such as hemodynamic instability.

For the majority of UTIs, uropathogens are introduced, in an ascending manner, into the lower urinary tract from extraurinary reservoirs including periurethra tissue, vagina, perineum, and distal gut. The diagnosis of UTI is confirmed by the presence of positive urine culture and symptoms as described above. If classical UTI symptoms are present, the widely accepted definition of a positive urine culture is 10^2 colony forming units (CFU) per milliliter of a known uropathogenic organism taken from a midstream urine specimen.[3]

Antimicrobials have long been the mainstay of treatment of UTIs. The antimicrobial used as well as the route and duration of administration depends on individual patient risk factors, the localization of infection to the lower or upper urinary tract, hemodynamic stability of the patient, and is tailored to culture results including antimicrobial sensitivities. In recent years, the emergence of antimicrobial resistance has led to more judicial use of antimicrobials in the treatment of UTIs as well as the search for effective and safe nonantimicrobial alternatives.[4] This article will provide readers with a comprehensive review of pharmacologic treatment and prevention of UTI with both antimicrobial and nonantimicrobial-based therapies.

EPIDEMIOLOGY

UTIs are a common cause of morbidity for people of all ages. In the United States alone, UTIs affect 11 million people annually, with an estimated cost for the evaluation and treatment of $2 to 3.5 billion USD per year.[1,5] The incidence of UTI is generally higher in women than in men. Using a self-reported UTI history, The National Health and Nutrition Examination Survey (NHANES) estimated the annual incidence of UTI for women 18 years of age or older at 12.6% compared with 3% for men.[6] Women aged 15 to 29 have the highest frequency of infection (approximately 20% per year).[7] Approximately 60% of women will experience symptomatic acute bacterial cystitis in their lifetime. Of these women, 20% to 40% will experience more than one infectious episode.[3,8] UTIs are also common among hospitalized and institutionalized patients. Approximately 1 million cases of nosocomial UTIs occur annually in the United States, of which 80% are attributable to catheter use.[1,9]

[a] Department of Surgery, Division of Urology, Functional and Reconstructive Urology, University of Ottawa, 1053 Carling Avenue, Ottawa, Ontario K1Y4E9, Canada; [b] Department of Surgery, Division of Urology, Female Pelvic Medicine and Reconstructive Surgery, University of Ottawa, 1053 Carling Avenue, Ottawa, Ontario K1Y4E9, Canada
* Corresponding author.
E-mail address: dhickling@toh.ca

Urol Clin N Am 49 (2022) 283–297
https://doi.org/10.1016/j.ucl.2021.12.004
0094-0143/22/© 2022 Elsevier Inc. All rights reserved.

urologic.theclinics.com

PATHOPHYSIOLOGY

The development of a UTI is dependent on a series of complex interactions between the microorganism causing infection and the host being infected. The ascending route of infection is the most common. In this route, peri-urethral colonization of bacteria from the distal gut results in the colonization of the urethra and eventual migration to the bladder and possibly the upper urinary tract. Hematogenous and lymphatic spread to the urinary tract are also possible but much less common.[7]

The key initiating step of UTI is bacterial adherence to the urothelial lining of the urethra and bladder. Common infectious organisms such as uropathogenic *E. coli* (UPEC) express adhesion molecules that allow the organism to attach to urinary tract tissues. Type 1 pilli is an adhesin molecule commonly expressed on UPEC organisms and is composed of a helical rod of repeating subunits with a distal tip containing the adhesin FimH. FimH has the ability to bind to proteins called uroplakins on the surface of urothelial cells. The interactions between FimH and uroplakins in bladder urothelium are the initial step in the series of events leading to UTI.[10] P pili are another form of adhesin molecules that have a specific affinity for the kidneys and are found in a high number of UPEC strains causing pyelonephritis.[11]

Following attachment to the urothelium, the UPEC organisms are taken up into the urothelial cells whereby they are protected from host defense mechanisms. Within the urothelial cells, these organisms rapidly grow and divide forming biofilm-like clusters of bacteria referred to as intracellular bacterial communities (IBCs).[12] Bacterial cells along the edges of IBCs are able to escape host cells and reinvade other superficial urothelial cells leading to secondary IBC formations. After a few days of replication, the bacterial cell reproduction slows and enters a dormant state and is referred to as quiescent intracellular reservoirs (QIRs).[13] These reservoirs of intracellular bacteria within the bladder urothelium are proposed to play a role in the development of recurrent UTIs in susceptible patients.

UNCOMPLICATED VERSUS COMPLICATED URINARY TRACT INFECTIONS

UTIs can be further categorized as uncomplicated or complicated based on the presence or absence of certain risk factors. An uncomplicated UTI is defined as those occurring in otherwise healthy, nonpregnant women with a normal urinary tract and may include simple cystitis, pyelonephritis, or recurrent cystitis with prompt response to first-line antimicrobial therapy.[2,14] The identification of risk factors for complicated UTIs is important as these infections may require further work-up and specific antimicrobials with longer courses of treatment.

Risk Factors for Uncomplicated Urinary Tract Infections

- Female sex
- Previous UTI
- Sexual intercourse
- Spermicide use
- Genetic susceptibility

Risk Factors for Complicated Urinary Tract Infections

- Anatomic or functional abnormality of the urinary tract
- Renal insufficiency
- Foreign body (ie, catheter, stent, nephrostomy tube)
- Transplantation
- Antimicrobial-resistant organism(s)
- Recent antimicrobial use within the last 3 months
- Elderly
- Male
- Recurrent UTIs
- Pregnancy
- Recent urologic procedure or manipulation of the genito-urinary system
- Symptoms greater than 14 days
- Immunocompromised host

TREATMENT OF SYMPTOMATIC URINARY TRACT INFECTIONS
Antimicrobials

Antimicrobials are substances produced either synthetically or by living organisms that confer bacterial cytotoxic properties. They can be broadly divided into 2 primary groups—bactericidal or bacteriostatic. Bactericidal antimicrobials refer to those causing irreversible death of bacteria. Bacteriostatic antimicrobials inhibit bacterial replication without causing death (**Table 1**). Despite the intuitive notion that bactericidal antimicrobials may confer a greater antibacterial effect, a recent systematic review found no clinical difference in the use of bactericidal versus bacteriostatic antimicrobials in the treatment of serious bacterial infection.[15]

Antimicrobials exert their effects via the inhibition of cellular processes involved in growth and reproduction or by the breakdown of critical

Table 1
Bactericidal versus bacteriostatic antimicrobials

Anti-Bacterial Effect	Antimicrobial Class
Bacteriostatic	Chloramphenicol
	Clindamycin
	Macrolides
	Sulfonamides
	Tetracycline
Bactericidal	Aminoglycosides
	Quinolones
	Beta-lactams
	Vancomycin

cellular defenses. They can be further classified based on mechanism of action (**Table 2**).[4]

TREATMENT OF UNCOMPLICATED URINARY TRACT INFECTIONS

The Infectious Diseases Society of America (IDSA) Guidelines for Treatment of Acute Uncomplication Cystitis and Pyelonephritis in Women (2010 Update) recommends the following for first-line treatments[16]:

Simple Cystitis

1) Nitrofurantoin 100 mg PO twice daily x 5 days (avoid if pyelonephritis suspected)

OR.

2) Trimethoprim-sulfamethoxazole (TMP-SMX) 160/800 mg (1 double-strength tablet) PO twice daily x 3 days (avoid if local resistance patterns exceed 20% resistance or if used to treat UTI within the previous 3 months)

OR.

3) Fosfomycin 3g PO x one dose (avoid if pyelonephritis suspected)

Alternative options:

4) Fluoroquinolones (ciprofloxacin, ofloxacin, levofloxacin) are highly efficacious but can cause significant side effects and have high resistance in some areas; these should be reserved as alternative treatments to first-line therapy

OR.

5) Beta-Lactams (amoxicillin-clavulanate, cefdinir, cefaclor, and cefpodoxime-proxetil) generally have inferior results and more adverse effects and should be used as an alternative

to first-line therapy. Amoxicillin or ampicillin should not be used as empirical therapy due to poor efficacy

Acute Pyelonephritis

Patients NOT requiring hospitalization

1) Ciprofloxacin 500 mg PO twice daily x 7 days if local fluoroquinolone resistance </ = 10%

OR.

2) Once daily dose of fluoroquinolone (ciprofloxacin 1000 mg PO once daily x 7 days or levofloxacin 750 mg PO once daily x 5 days) if local fluoroquinolone resistance </ = 10%
   a. If the local prevalence of fluoroquinolone resistance is greater than 10% an initial one-time dose of a long-acting parenteral antimicrobial (ceftriaxone 1g intravenous x one dose or a consolidated 24-h dose of intravenous aminoglycoside) is recommended

OR.

3) Trimethoprim-sulfamethoxazole 160/800 mg (1 double-strength tablet) PO twice daily x 14 days if uropathogen known to be susceptible
   a. If susceptibility is unknown an initial intravenous dose of a long-acting parenteral antimicrobial (ceftriaxone 1g intravenous x 1 or a consolidated 24-h dose of intravenous aminoglycoside) is recommended

OR.

4) Oral beta-lactam agents are an option but are less effective than other available agents; if used an initial intravenous dose of a long-acting parenteral antimicrobial (ceftriaxone 1g intravenous x one dose or a consolidated 24-h dose of intravenous aminoglycoside) is recommended

Patients requiring hospitalization

1) Should be initially treated with an intravenous antimicrobial regimen:
   a. Fluoroquinolone
      OR.
   b. Aminoglycoside ± ampicillin
      OR.
   c. Extended-spectrum cephalosporin or penicillin ± an aminoglycoside
      OR.
   d. Carbapenem
2) Patient can be stepped down to targeted oral therapy once afebrile and clinically stable with appropriate sensitivities available.

Table 2
Mechanism of action and side effects of common antimicrobials (antibacterial and antifungal) used in the treatment of urinary tract infection

Antimicrobial Class	Mechanism of Action	Examples	Common Side Effects
Anti-Bacterial Beta-Lactams	Inhibits bacterial cell wall synthesis via the binding of penicillin-binding proteins	1. Penicillins (ie, Amoxi-cillin, Ampicillin) 2. Cephalosporins (1st, 2nd, 3rd, and 4th generation) 3. Aztreonam	• Hypersensitivity • GI upset • Maculopapular rash • Decreased platelet aggregation • Acute interstitial nephritis (especially methicillin)
Aminoglycosides	Inhibition of protein synthesis via the binding of 30s ribosomal subunit	1. Tobramycin 2. Gentamycin 3. Neomycin 4. Streptomycin	• Ototoxicity • Nephrotoxicity • Neuromuscular blockade at high concentrations *Avoid in:* • Pregnancy • Impaired renal/hepatic function *Caution in:* • Myasthenia gravis • HIV/AIDS
Sulfonamides and Trimethoprim	Inhibition of enzymes involved in folic acid metabolism	1. Trimethoprim-Sulfamethoxazole	• Hypersensitivity • Rash • GI upset • Hematologic toxicity *Avoid in:* • Pregnancy *Caution in:* • Patients on warfarin
Fluoroquinolones	Inhibits DNA replication via inhibition of DNA gyrase enzyme	1. Ciprofloxacin 2. Levofloxacin 3. Moxifloxacin 4. Ofloxacin 5. Gemifloxacin	• Tendinopathy • Neuropathy • GI upset • QT prolongation • Photosensitivity *Caution in:* • Concomitant antacid, iron, zinc, or sucralfate use – decreases antimicrobial absorption • Concomitant theophylline or warfarin use – can alter drug metabolism *Avoid in:* • Children – arthropathic effects • Pregnant – arthropathic effect on fetus • Epilepsy – may lower seizure threshold

(*continued on next page*)

Table 2
(continued)

Antimicrobial Class	Mechanism of Action	Examples	Common Side Effects
Nitrofurantoin	Reactive metabolic intermediates that inactivate a number of bacterial enzyme pathways	NA	• GI upset • Peripheral neuropathy • Hemolysis in patients with G6PD deficiency • Pulmonary toxicity *Avoid in:* • Low creatinine clearance (<50 mL/min) – adequate urine concentrations not achieved • Concomitant probenecid, magnesium, or quinolone use – can alter drug activity/clearance
Fosfomycin	Inhibition of bacterial cell wall synthesis	NA	• Headache • GI upset • Vaginitis
Vancomycin	Inhibition of bacterial cell wall synthesis by prevention of binding of peptidoglycans of the cell wall to penicillin-binding proteins	NA	• Red-man syndrome • fever, chills, rash, hypotension • Nephrotoxicity • Ototoxicity *Caution in:* • Concomitant use of other ototoxic or nephrotoxic drugs
Anti-Fungal			
Fluconazole	Inhibits fungal cell wall synthesis through the inhibition of enzyme required in the creation of ergosterol		• Headache • GI upset • Dizziness • Rash • Altered taste • Hepatotoxicity • Arrhythmia *Caution in:* • Drugs metabolized by cytochrome p450 system including coumadin • Preexisting hepatic insufficiency • Preexisting renal insufficiency • Arrhythmias *Avoid in:* • Pregnancy

(continued on next page)

Table 2
(continued)

Antimicrobial Class	Mechanism of Action	Examples	Common Side Effects
Flucytosine	Possibly from the inhibition of purine and pyrimidine uptake into fungal cells and metabolism of 5-fluorouracil		• GI upset • Hepatotoxicity • Myelosuppression *Caution in:* • Preexisting hepatotoxicity • Preexisting renal insufficiency • Neutropenia *Avoid in:* • Pregnancy and breastfeeding
Amphotericin B	Forms pores in fungal cell membrane leading to leakage of ions and fungal cell death		• GI upset • Joint pain • Fatigue • Shortness of breath • Rash • Hepatotoxicity • Renal toxicity • Anemia • Cardiac arrhythmias *Caution in:* • Preexisting hepatotoxicity • Preexisting renal insufficiency

TREATMENT OF COMPLICATED URINARY TRACT INFECTIONS

There is a lack of specific guidelines for the treatment of complicated UTIs. Therapy is usually continued for 10 to 14 days on culture-specific antimicrobials and switched from parenteral to oral therapy when the patient is afebrile and clinically stable. Repeat urine cultures should be performed if the patient fails to respond to therapy.[17] Antimicrobial treatment and duration should be tailored to the specific patient based on culture results and baseline comorbidities.

Catheter-associated UTIs (CAUTIs) is a common cause of complicated UTI, particularly among hospitalized and institutionalized patients. Bacterial biofilm formation and catheter encrustation may act to shield bacteria from antimicrobial treatment; therefore, upon diagnosis of CAUTI, the patient's catheter should be changed with careful, aseptic technique.[18] In addition to other benefits, the use of clean intermittent catheterization has been found to reduce the instance of UTI in comparison to indwelling catheters and is recommended as the standard method of bladder drainage for patients with incomplete bladder emptying who are physically able to pass their own catheter.[19]

TREATMENT OF FUNGAL URINARY TRACT INFECTIONS

The 2016 IDSA guidelines for the treatment of candida-cystitis and pyelonephritis recommend the following as first-line treatments[20]:

Treatment of Candida-Cystitis

1. For fluconazole-susceptible organisms (*Candida albicans*):
   a. Fluconazole 200 mg (3 mg/kg) PO once daily for 2 weeks
2. For fluconazole-resistant organisms (ie, *Candida glabrata, Candida krusei*):
   a. Amphotericin B deoxycholate 0.3 to 0.6 mg/kg once daily for one to 7 days
      OR.
   b. Flucytosine 25 mg/kg PO four times daily for 7 to 10 days (*Candida glabrata* only)
      OR.
   c. Amphotericin B deoxycholate bladder irrigation 50 mg/L of sterile water once daily for 5 days

3. Removal of indwelling catheter is recommended if feasible

Treatment of Candida-Pyelonephritis

1. For fluconazole-susceptible organisms *(Candida albicans)*:
   a. PO fluconazole 200 to 400 mg (3–6 mg/kg) once daily for 2 weeks
2. For fluconazole-resistant organisms
   a. Amphotericin B deoxycholate 0.3 to 0.6 mg/kg once daily for one to 7 days *(Candida krusei)*
      OR.
   b. Flucytosine 25 mg/kg PO four times daily for 7 to 10 days *(Candida glabrata)*
3. Elimination of urinary tract obstruction is strongly recommended
4. For patients who have nephrostomy tubes or stents in place, consider removal or replacement

ASYMPTOMATIC BACTERIURIA

Asymptomatic bacteriuria is defined as the presence of $>/ = 1$ species of bacteria in the urine at $>/ = 10^5$ CFU/mL in the absence of signs or symptoms of UTI. Asymptomatic bacteriuria is common in many populations, particularly in those with abnormalities of the genitourinary tract associated with difficulties voiding and/or catheterization.

The IDSA recommends against screening for or treating asymptomatic bacteriuria in most patients. Specific patient groups that should be screened for asymptomatic bacteriuria include pregnant women and patients due to undergo a urologic procedure in which mucosal trauma is anticipated. For pregnant women, it is recommended that they be screened for asymptomatic bacteriuria at one of the initial visits during early pregnancy and if cultures are positive they should be treated with 4 to 7 days of culture-sensitive antimicrobials. Special attention should be paid to select antimicrobials that are deemed safe in pregnancy. For patients due to undergo a urologic procedure, a shorter course of antimicrobials (1 or 2 doses) is recommended for positive cultures in asymptomatic individuals.[21]

For patients with asymptomatic candiduria, treatment with an antifungal agent is not recommended unless patients belong to a group at high risk for dissemination including neutropenic patients, newborns with very low birth weight (<1500g), and patients due to undergo urologic manipulation.[20]

ANTIMICROBIAL RESISTANCE

Although antimicrobials have been proven very effective in the treatment of UTIs, years of inappropriate and over-use have inevitably resulted in the emergence of further antimicrobial resistance among infectious organisms.[22] Bacteria have developed a number of mechanisms of resistance to specific antimicrobials including the production of enzymes that break down or alter the antimicrobial, mutations in the antimicrobial receptor, as well as the production of cellular transport molecules that actively secrete the antimicrobial out of the cell.[5] In 2015 the World Health Organization released a report on the 'Global Action Plan on Antimicrobial Resistance' to help bring further attention to this serious issue.[23] As a result, there has been a recent shift in focus to the study of other nonantimicrobial alternatives to the treatment and prevention of UTI.

NONANTIMICROBIAL TREATMENT OF ACUTE URINARY TRACT INFECTION
Nonsteroidal Antiinflammatories

One randomized control trial (RCT) of 248 women with acute cystitis symptoms randomized to ibuprofen for 3 days versus Fosfomycin 3g x one dose. The number of courses of antimicrobials prescribed was significantly lower in the ibuprofen group and 2/3rds of patients treated symptomatically with ibuprofen recovered without the use of any antimicrobials. However, patients randomized to the ibuprofen group were found to have overall worse symptom scores, longer duration of symptoms (5.6 days vs 4.6 days; $P < .05$), and a trend toward higher incidence of pyelonephritis ($P = .12$).[24] Another study randomized 253 women with symptomatic cystitis to diclofenac or norfloxacin. Diclofenac was found to decrease courses of antimicrobials prescribed (62% with diclofenac vs 98% with norfloxacin; $P < .001$) but was found to be inferior to norfloxacin for symptomatic relief and was also associated with increased risk of pyelonephritis (**Table 3**).[25]

Phenazopyridine

Phenazopyridine (pyridium) is an Azo dye that is excreted mostly unchanged into the urine and produces a local anesthetic effect. One case series of 118 patients with UTI symptoms who were given phenazopyridine 500 mg three times daily found a complete improvement of symptoms in 55.1% and almost all patients reported some improvement. Common reported side effects were mild and included headache, rash, dizziness, and fever (see **Table 3**).[26] More serious side effects, including methemoglobinemia, myelosuppression, hemolytic anemia, renal/hepatic failure, and anaphylaxis have been reported but are rare.[27,28]

Table 3
Nonantimicrobial treatment of acute cystitis

Intervention	Evidence	Adverse Effects
Nonsteroidal Antiinflammatories	Ibuprofen: • RCT Comparison: Fosfomycin • 2/3rds of patients recovered without antibiotics Diclofenac: • RCT comparison: Norfloxacin • 62% recovered without antibiotics	• Worse symptoms scores, longer duration of symptoms, trend toward higher risk of pyelonephritis
Phenzopyridine	• Case series: • 55.1% reported the resolution of symptoms • Almost all patients reported at least some improvement in symptoms	• Common: headache, rash, dizziness, and fever • Uncommon: methemoglobinemia, myelosuppression, hemolytic anemia, renal/hepatic failure, and anaphylaxis
Urinary Alkalinisation	• No RCT data • Systematic review inconclusive	• None reported

Urinary Alkalinization

Urinary alkalizers work to raise urine pH which is thought to provide some symptomatic relief from cystitis-related symptoms. A Cochrane review found no RCTs for the use of urinary alkalinization in the treatment of UTI-related symptoms and as such was unable to draw any conclusions regarding its efficacy (see **Table 3**).[29] Despite anecdotal reports of good efficacy, an observational study of 128 women with uncomplicated UTIs found no correlation between reported symptoms of UTI and urine pH.[30]

URINARY TRACT INFECTION PREVENTION
Antimicrobial Prophylaxis

Recurrent UTI (rUTI) is defined as at least 3 UTIs within the last 12 months or 2 within the last 6 months. Antimicrobial prophylaxis, including low-dose continuous prophylaxis and postcoital prophylaxis have all been shown to be efficacious in UTI prevention.[31] Self-start antimicrobial treatment has also been shown to be effective and safe in appropriately selected patients with rUTI. No specific antimicrobial has been shown to be superior for prophylaxis.[32] When considering starting antimicrobial prophylaxis, antimicrobial choice and schedule should be based on patient-specific factors including allergies/intolerance, risk factors, cause and frequency of infection, reliability, and patient motivation.

Low-Dose Continuous Antimicrobial Prophylaxis

A Cochrane review including 19 randomized controlled trials (RCTs) with 1120 women found that antimicrobial prophylaxis for 6 to 12 months reduced the rate of UTI during prophylaxis compared with placebo (risk ratio (RR): 0.21; 95% confidence interval (CI): 0.13–0.34). Antimicrobial prophylaxis was associated with a higher risk of adverse events compared with placebo (RR: 1.78) and after prophylaxis was complete, no further benefit was noted.[31] No antimicrobial has been found to be superior in the prevention of recurrent UTI with prophylaxis (**Table 4**).[22]

Postcoital Antimicrobial Prophylaxis

A single double-blind, placebo-controlled RCT randomized 16 women with recurrent UTIs to postcoital trimethoprim-sulfamethoxazole and 11 to placebo. Postcoital prophylaxis was found to decrease the incidence of UTI from 3.6/y to 0.3/y. Postcoital prophylaxis was found to be effective in reducing UTIs regardless of frequency of intercourse (**Table 5**).[33]

Selfstart Antimicrobial Treatment

A systematic review found no difference between intermittent dosing versus daily dosing in risk of rUTIs (RR: 1.15; 95% CI: 0.88–1.50).[22] Another prospective trial found that women with a history of rUTIs were able to self-diagnose a culture-positive UTI in 84% of cases.[34] Generally speaking, a self-start regimen should be reserved for patients who have documented culture-positive previous UTIs and who are motivated and compliant with instructions.[32]

Intravesical Antimicrobial Prophylaxis

Intravesical antimicrobial prophylaxis has been shown to be beneficial in both treatment and

Table 4
Recommended antimicrobial prophylaxis regimens according to AUA/SUFU/CUA guideline on recurrent uncomplicated UTI in women[22]

Antimicrobial	Dose
Trimethoprim	100 mg PO once daily
Trimethoprim-Sulfamethoxazole	40 mg/200 mg PO once daily
Trimethoprim-Sulfamethoxazole	40 mg/200 mg PO thrice weekly
Nitrofurantoin	50 mg PO once daily
Nitrofurantoin	100 mg PO once daily
Cephalexin	125 mg PO once daily
Cephalexin	250 mg PO once daily
Fosfomycin	3g PO every 10 d

Data from Anger J, Lee U, Ackerman AL, et al. Recurrent Uncomplicated Urinary Tract Infections in Women: AUA/CUA/SUFU Guideline. J Urol. 2019;202(2):282-289.

prophylaxis for patients with UTIs caused by resistant organisms, most notably in the context of patients with neurogenic bladder and those performing clean intermittent catheterization (**Table 6**). A prospective trial of 63 patients treated with intravesical gentamycin as treatment and prophylaxis for 6 months demonstrated a reduction in UTIs from 4.8 to 1.0 during treatment. Furthermore, the antimicrobial resistance rate of uropathogens isolated decreased from 78% to 23%.[35] A systematic review of intravesical antimicrobial prophylaxis noted a reduction in symptomatic UTIs in 78% of patients with intravesical antimicrobial prophylaxis. A change in the sensitivity of organisms was found in 23% to 30%.[36] In both studies, systemic absorption of antimicrobial and associated side effects was minimal.

NONANTIMICROBIAL PROPHYLAXIS
Cranberry

The American Cranberry (*Vaccinium macrocarpon*) has been extensively studied as a potential means

of preventing recurrent UTIs. Proanthocyanidin (PAC) is the chemical component of cranberry believed to confer a prophylactic benefit. PAC works by inhibiting type P fimbriae binding, thereby providing a dose-depending effect on *E. coli* adherence. A recent systematic review of 5 RCTs demonstrated an overall decreased risk of UTI recurrence (RR: 0.67; 95% CI: 0.54–0.83). No significant difference was noted between cranberry and antimicrobial prophylaxis in recurrent UTI prevention; however, this was based on low-quality evidence.[22] Of note, cranberry may come in different formulations, most commonly tablets or juice. The content of PAC may vary across brand and formulation. There is currently not enough evidence to suggest one formulation over another; however, the sugar content of juice may be prohibitive for some patients (**Table 7**).[37]

Methenamine Hippurate

Methenamine works via the production of formaldehyde as a by-product of metabolism which

Table 5
Recommended postcoital antimicrobial prophylaxis regimens according to AUA/SUFU/CUA guideline on recurrent uncomplicated UTI in women[22]

Antimicrobial	Dose
Trimethoprim-Sulfamethoxazole	40 mg/200 mg PO x 1 postintercourse
Trimethoprim-Sulfamethoxazole	80 mg/400 mg PO x 1 postintercourse
Nitrofurantoin	50 mg to 100 mg PO x 1 postintercourse
Cephalexin	250 mg PO x 1 postintercourse

Data from Anger J, Lee U, Ackerman AL, et al. Recurrent Uncomplicated Urinary Tract Infections in Women: AUA/CUA/SUFU Guideline. J Urol. 2019;202(2):282 to -289.

Table 6
Intravesical antimicrobial regimens used for prophylaxis[36]

Antimicrobial	Dose
Neomycin/Polymyxin	30–40 mg/mL/200,000 units twice daily x 8 wk
Gentamycin	80 mg in 10 mL saline nightly
Gentamycin	14.4–28.8 mg in 30–60 mL saline nightly
Gentamycin	80 mg in 20 mL of saline daily for 2 wk then once a week

Data from Pietropaolo A, Jones P, Moors M, Birch B, Somani BK. Use and Effectiveness of Antimicrobial Intravesical Treatment for Prophylaxis and Treatment of Recurrent Urinary Tract Infections (UTIs): a Systematic Review. Curr Urol Rep. 2018;19(10):78.

acts as a bacteriostatic agent. A Cochrane Review concluded that methanamine salts may be safe and effective when used for short-term prophylaxis (</ = 7 days) in patients with nonneurogenic bladders and normal urinary tract anatomy (RR: 0.53; 95% CI: 0.24–1.18). The use of longer intervals may not be associated with improvement in the incidence of UTI. Side effects are generally mild and include GI upset, dysuria, abdominal cramping, anorexia, rash, and stomatitis (see **Table 7**). Alternatives To prophylactic Antibiotics for the treatment of Recurrent UTI in women (ALTAR) trial is a multicentre, patient-randomized, noninferiority trial comparing methenamine hippurate, to standard daily low-dose antibiotics. Final results of this trial are pending at this time.[38]

D-Mannose/Mannosides

D-mannose acts by inhibiting Type 1 pili and FimH mediated uroepithelial cell adhesion of uropathogenic *E. coli*. One RCT randomized 308 women with recurrent UTI to (1) prophylaxis with 2g of D-mannose in 200 mL of water, (2) 50 mg of nitrofurantoin daily, or (3) no prophylaxis. Prophylaxis with either D-mannose or nitrofurantoin was associated with a significant reduction in UTI compared with placebo (*P* < .0001). Reduction in UTI was similar between D-mannose and nitrofurantoin; however, the incidence of side effects was less common with D-mannose (see **Table 7**).[39] Given the proposed mechanism of action, D-mannose may not be effective against strains of uropathogens that do not express type 1 pili and FimH.[40]

Probiotics

Probiotics are live microorganisms that provide health benefits.[41] Previous dogma suggests that the urinary tract is sterile, however, more recent research suggests that it contains a diverse microbiota.[42] Lactobacillus is the most common genus

of bacteria in both the vagina and urinary tract. Lactobacillus is believed to have an antimicrobial effect via a number of pathways, including the maintenance of an acidic environment via the production of lactic acid and hydrogen peroxide, prevention of biofilm formation, and competitive inhibition of uropathogens.[43,44]

A Cochrane review of oral Lactobacillus in the prevention of UTIs which included 9 RCTs and 735 patients found no significant reduction in the risk of recurrent symptomatic bacterial UTIs between patients treated with probiotics and placebo (RR: 0.82; 95% CI: 0.62–1.12). The authors concluded that a benefit of probiotics could not be absolutely ruled out, however, due to the overall poor quality of evidence available (see **Table 7**).[45] A double-blind, placebo-controlled RCT randomized women with a history of recurrent UTI to receive vaginal lactobacillus or placebo for 10 weeks and found a reduction in recurrent UTIs in patients receiving vaginal probiotics (RR: 0.5; 95% CI: 0.2–1.2).[46]

Vitamin C

It is believed that vitamin C can have bacteriostatic effects via the reduction of urinary nitrates to reactive nitrogen oxides. A weak association has been found between dietary vitamin C and a decreased risk of UTI in healthy young women and pregnant women (odds ratio (OR): 0.59, 95% CI: 0.35–0.98 - no prior UTI; OR: 0.85,95% CI: 0.58–1.25 - >/ = 1 prior UTI).[47,48] Vitamin C has not been found to decrease the incidence of UTI in patients with spinal cord injury (see **Table 7**).[49]

Estrogen

Hypo-estrogen states in postmenopausal women is a recognized risk factor for UTI.[1] A systematic review found that vaginal estrogen reduced the incidence of UTI recurrence in postmenopausal

Table 7
Type, proposed mechanism, and dosage of nonantimicrobial prophylaxis options for patients with recurrent UTIs

Intervention	Proposed Mechanism of Action	Evidence	Dosing
Cranberry	PAC inhibits type P fimbriae binding of uropathogenic *E. coli*	Systematic review: reduction in recurrent UTI (RR: 0.67; 95% CI: 0.54–0.83)	No standard; expert opinion minimum 36 mg of PAC once daily
Methanamine	Bacteriostatic effects of metabolic by-product (formaldehyde)	Systematic review: short-term reduction in recurrent UTI ($</ = 7$ d; RR: 0.53; 95% CI: 0.24–1.18)	1g PO once or twice daily
D-mannose/ mannosides	Inhibits Type 1 pili/Fim H mediated urothelial cell adhesion	RCT: Reduction in UTI compared with no prophylaxis; no different than nitrofurantoin	2g/200 mL of water daily
Probiotics	Maintenance of acidic environment; inhibits biofilm formation; competitive inhibition	Systematic review: unclear benefit for PO lactobacillus; Vaginal lactobacillus RCT reduction in recurrent UTIs (RR: 0.5; 95% CI: 0.2–1.2)	Multiple formulations available
Vitamin C	Reduction of urinary nitrates to reactive nitrogen oxides	Decreased UTI risk (OR: 0.59, 95% CI: 0.35–0.98 - no prior UTI; OR: 0.85,95% CI: 0.58–1.25 - $>/ = 1$ prior UTI)	100 mg PO once daily
Vaginal Estrogen	Prevent vaginal atrophy; maintenance of healthy vaginal flora in postmenopausal women	Systematic review: reduction in recurrent UTIs (RR: 0.25; 95% CI: 0.13–0.50)	1 Estriol cream 0.5 mg once daily x 2 wk then twice weekly 2 Vaginal ring 2 mg estradiol every 90 d 3 Vaginal tablet 10mcg dally x 2 wk then 2 to 3 times per week
Hydration	Dilution/flushing of uropathogenic bacteria	RCT: Reduction in recurrent UTIs (1.9 vs 3.2; difference of means 1.7; CI: 1.3–2.1; $P < .001$)	Increase to >1.5 L of water daily if baseline daily intake <1.5 L

women with a history of recurrent UTIs (RR: 0.25; 95% CI: 0.13–0.50). In the same review, oral estrogens did not reduce the incidence of recurrent UTI compared with placebo (RR: 1.08; 95% CI: 0.88–1.33). No conclusions could be made on a superior formulation of vaginal estrogen (ring vs tablet suppository vs cream) (see **Table 7**).[50] Vaginal estrogen delivers low-dose hormonal therapy to local vaginal tissues with minimal systemic absorption and data do not show an increased risk of cancer recurrence among women currently undergoing treatment of breast cancer or those with a personal history of breast cancer.[51]

Hydration

An RCT of 140 healthy premenopausal women with recurrent UTIs with a self-reported history of drinking less than 1.5 L of water per day were randomized to drink 1.5 L of water/day on top of normal fluid consumption versus continuing with normal fluid consumption. There was a significant decrease in the mean number of UTIs in the group randomized to greater than 1.5 L/d (1.7 vs 3.2; $P < .001$) (see **Table 7**).[52] The benefit of increased fluid intake in women consuming greater than 1.5 L of water daily at baseline is not clear.

FUTURE DIRECTIONS
Immunotherapy

The development of immunotherapy represents a novel form of UTI treatment and prevention. The mechanism of action involves the inoculation of inactivated bacteria or bacterial antigens and promotion of host immune response. Treatment takes the form of sublingual spray, oral tablet, vaginal suppository, or intramuscular injection. No form of immunotherapy is currently approved for widespread use in the United States or Canada.

Uromune is a sublingual vaccine spray composed of a glycerinated suspension of heat-inactivated bacteria of 4 common UTI-pathogens: E. coli, Klebsiella pneumoniae, Proteus vulgaris, and Enterococcus faecalis.[53] Two retrospective studies found that Uromune daily for 3 months significantly reduced UTI-recurrence (35% to 90%) compared with 6 months of antimicrobial prophylaxis.[54,55] Three prospective studies found UTI free rates ranged from 33% to 78% over 9 to 24 months.[56-58] No significant safety issues were identified.

Uro-Vaxom is a daily oral capsule containing 18 common E. coli strains. A systematic review demonstrated UTI-free rates from 52.6% to 87.5% compared with 50% in the placebo group.[59] Solco-Urovac is a vaginal suppository containing 10 uropathogenic bacterial strains. A systematic review of 4 studies demonstrated a reduction in UTI recurrence when given with a booster dose at 6, 10, and 14 weeks compared with placebo (OR: 0.23; 95% CI: 0.11–0.48). No benefit was demonstrated in Solco-Urovac given without booster dosing.[59]

ExPEC4 V is a tetravalent O-polysaccharide conjugate vaccine given as an intramuscular injection. It is composed of the O-antigens of 4 common uropathogenic E. coli strains. A multicentered phase 1b, placebo-controlled RCT randomized women with a history of recurrent UTI to a single injection of either intramuscular ExPEC4V or placebo. ExPEC4V induced significant IgG responses to all serotypes compared with baseline at 30 days. No difference was noted in vaccine serotype UTIs between the vaccine and placebo group (0.149 vs 0.146 mean episodes; $P = .522$). However, there was significantly fewer UTIs caused by E. coli of any serotype in the vaccine group compared with placebo (0.207 mean episodes vs 0.463 mean episodes; $P = .002$).[60]

Fecal Transplant

Fecal microbiome transplantation has been a recognized treatment of Clostridium difficile (C. difficile) infection. A decrease in UTIs in patients undergoing fecal transplant for C. diff has been noted in previous reports.[61] A prospective study of 11 patients undergoing fecal transplantation via retention enema for recurrent UTI resulted in a decrease in median UTIs from 3 to 1 over a 6 month period ($P = .055$). There was also a nonsignificant reduction in multi-drug resistant organisms as well as an increase in patient microbiome diversity after treatment.[62]

Prebiotics

A prebiotic is a substrate that is selectively used by host microorganisms to confer a health benefit. A double-blind, placebo-controlled RCT examined the efficacy and safety of an intravaginal prebiotic gel in the recovery of vaginal flora in women previously treated for bacterial vaginosis. Patients were randomized to receive intravaginal glucooligosaccharides-alpha prebiotic or placebo gel. After 8 days of treatment, all women who received prebiotic treatment had normal vaginal flora, while 33% of women in the control group did not completely restore normal vaginal flora. After 16 days of treatment, all women treated with the prebiotic gel maintained normal vaginal flora, whereas in the placebo group 24% had not completely restored vaginal flora.[63] Further study is required to clarify the role of prebiotics in the treatment and prevention of UTI.

SUMMARY

UTI is common and is associated with significant morbidity and health care cost. Antimicrobial therapy remains the mainstay treatment despite alarming trends in antimicrobial resistance. Health care providers must practice antimicrobial stewardship to avoid further resistance and should also consider evidence-based nonantimicrobial alternatives for UTI treatment and prevention.

CLINICS CARE POINTS

- Urinary tract infections are associated with significant morbidity and health care cost.
- Antimicrobials represent the mainstay of urinary tract infection treatment.
- The emergence of antimicrobial resistance represents a serious risk.

- Nonantimicrobial alternatives to urinary tract infection treatment and prevention is an ongoing area of research to reduce antimicrobial dependence and overuse.

CONFLICTS OF INTEREST

J. Ross – Nothing to Disclose. D. Hickling – has been an advisory board member for Pfizer; a speakers' bureau member for Allergan, Astellas, and Pfizer; has received grants/honoraria from Allergan, Astellas, and Pfizer; and has participated in clinical trials supported by Astellas.

REFERENCES

1. Foxman B. The epidemiology of urinary tract infection. Nat Rev Urol 2010;7(12):653–60.
2. Mazzulli T. Diagnosis and management of simple and complicated urinary tract infections (UTIs). Can J Urol 2012;19(51):42–8.
3. Foxman B. Urinary Tract Infection Syndromes: Occurrence, Recurrence, Bacteriology, Risk Factors, and Disease Burden. Infect Dis Clin North Am 2014;28(1):1–13.
4. Kapoor G, Saigal S, Elongavan A. Action and resistance mechanisms of antibiotics: A guide for clinicians. J Anaesthesiol Clin Pharmacol 2017;33(3):300–5.
5. O'Brien VP, Hannan TJ, Nielsen HV, et al. Drug and Vaccine Development for the Treatment and Prevention of Urinary Tract Infections. Microbiol Spectr 2016;4(1).
6. Johnson CC. Definitions, classification, and clinical presentation of urinary tract infections. Med Clin North Am 1991;75(2):241–52.
7. Foxman B, Brown P. Epidemiology of urinary tract infections: transmission and risk factors, incidence, and costs. Infect Dis Clin North Am 2003;17(2):227–41.
8. Geerlings SE. Clinical Presentations and Epidemiology of Urinary Tract Infections. Microbiol Spectr 2016;4(5).
9. Flores-Mireles A, Hreha TN, Hunstad DA. Pathophysiology, Treatment, and Prevention of Catheter-Associated Urinary Tract Infection. Top Spinal Cord Inj Rehabil 2019;25(3):228–40.
10. Thankavel K, Madison B, Ikeda T, et al. Localization of a domain in the FimH adhesin of Escherichia coli type 1 fimbriae capable of receptor recognition and use of a domain-specific antibody to confer protection against experimental urinary tract infection. J Clin Invest 1997;100(5):1123–36.
11. Mulvey MA. Adhesion and entry of uropathogenic Escherichia coli. Cell Microbiol 2002;4(5):257–71.
12. Justice SS, Hung C, Theriot JA, et al. Differentiation and developmental pathways of uropathogenic Escherichia coli in urinary tract pathogenesis. Proc Natl Acad Sci U S A 2004;101(5):1333–8.
13. Mysorekar IU, Hultgren SJ. Mechanisms of uropathogenic Escherichia coli persistence and eradication from the urinary tract. Proc Natl Acad Sci U S A 2006;103(38):14170–5.
14. Sabih A, Leslie SW. Complicated Urinary Tract Infections. In: StatPearls. StatPearls Publishing; 2021. Available at: http://www.ncbi.nlm.nih.gov/books/NBK436013/. Accessed July 2, 2021.
15. Nemeth J, Oesch G, Kuster SP. Bacteriostatic versus bactericidal antibiotics for patients with serious bacterial infections: systematic review and meta-analysis. J Antimicrob Chemother 2015;70(2):382–95.
16. Gupta K, Hooton TM, Naber KG, et al. International clinical practice guidelines for the treatment of acute uncomplicated cystitis and pyelonephritis in women: A 2010 update by the Infectious Diseases Society of America and the European Society for Microbiology and Infectious Diseases. Clin Infect Dis 2011;52(5):103–20.
17. Stamm WE, Hooton TM. Management of urinary tract infections in adults. N Engl J Med 1993;329(18):1328–34.
18. Schumm K, Lam TBL. Types of urethral catheters for management of short-term voiding problems in hospitalized adults. Cochrane Database Syst Rev 2008;2:CD004013.
19. Campeau L, Shamout S, Baverstock RJ, et al. Canadian Urological Association Best Practice Report: Catheter use. Can Urol Assoc J 2020;14(7):e281–9.
20. Pappas PG, Kauffman CA, Andes DR, et al. Clinical Practice Guideline for the Management of Candidiasis: 2016 Update by the Infectious Diseases Society of America. Clin Infect Dis Off Publ Infect Dis Soc Am 2016;62(4):e1–50.
21. Nicolle LE, Gupta K, Bradley SE, et al. Clinical Practice Guideline for the Management of Asymptomatic Bacteriuria: 2019 Update by the Infectious Diseases Society of America. Clin Infect Dis Off Publ Infect Dis Soc Am 2019;68(10):e83–110.
22. Anger J, Lee U, Ackerman AL, et al. Recurrent Uncomplicated Urinary Tract Infections in Women: AUA/CUA/SUFU Guideline. J Urol 2019;202(2):282–9.
23. Eurosurveillance editorial team. WHO member states adopt global action plan on antimicrobial resistance. Euro Surveill 2015;20(21).
24. Gágyor I, Bleidorn J, Kochen MM, et al. Ibuprofen versus fosfomycin for uncomplicated urinary tract infection in women: randomised controlled trial. BMJ 2015;351:h6544.
25. Kronenberg A, Bütikofer L, Odutayo A, et al. Symptomatic treatment of uncomplicated lower urinary tract infections in the ambulatory setting: randomised, double blind trial. BMJ 2017;359:j4784.

26. Gupta O, Aggarwal K. Role of Phenazopyridine in Urinary Tract Infections. Indian J Clin Pract 2012; 22(9):437–42.

27. Haigh C, Dewar JC. Multiple adverse effects of pyridium: a case report. South Med J 2006;99(1):90–2.

28. Nathan DM, Siegel AJ, Bunn HF. Acute methemoglobinemia and hemolytic anemia with phenazopyridine: possible relation to acute renal failure. Arch Intern Med 1977;137(11):1636–8.

29. O'Kane DB, Dave SK, Gore N, et al. Urinary alkalisation for symptomatic uncomplicated urinary tract infection in women. Cochrane Database Syst Rev 2016;2016(4):CD010745.

30. Brumfitt W, Hamilton-Miller JM, Cooper J, et al. Relationship of urinary pH to symptoms of "cystitis. Postgrad Med J 1990;66(779):727–9.

31. Albert X, Huertas I, Pereiró II, et al. Antibiotics for preventing recurrent urinary tract infection in nonpregnant women. Cochrane Database Syst Rev 2004;3:CD001209.

32. Aydin A, Ahmed K, Zaman I, et al. Recurrent urinary tract infections in women. Int Urogynecol J 2015; 26(6):795–804.

33. Stapleton A, Latham RH, Johnson C, et al. Postcoital antimicrobial prophylaxis for recurrent urinary tract infection. A randomized, double-blind, placebo-controlled trial. JAMA 1990;264(6):703–6.

34. Gupta K, Hooton TM, Roberts PL, et al. Patient-initiated treatment of uncomplicated recurrent urinary tract infections in young women. Ann Intern Med 2001;135(1):9–16.

35. Stalenhoef JE, van Nieuwkoop C, Menken PH, et al. Intravesical Gentamicin Treatment for Recurrent Urinary Tract Infections Caused by Multidrug Resistant Bacteria. J Urol 2019;201(3):549–55.

36. Pietropaolo A, Jones P, Moors M, et al. Use and Effectiveness of Antimicrobial Intravesical Treatment for Prophylaxis and Treatment of Recurrent Urinary Tract Infections (UTIs): a Systematic Review. Curr Urol Rep 2018;19(10):78.

37. Fu Z, Liska D, Talan D, et al. Cranberry Reduces the Risk of Urinary Tract Infection Recurrence in Otherwise Healthy Women: A Systematic Review and Meta-Analysis. J Nutr 2017;147(12):2282–8.

38. Forbes R, Ali A, Abouhajar A, et al. ALternatives To prophylactic Antibiotics for the treatment of Recurrent urinary tract infection in women (ALTAR): study protocol for a multicentre, pragmatic, patient-randomised, non-inferiority trial. Trials 2018;19(1): 616.

39. Kranjčec B, Papeš D, Altarac S. D-mannose powder for prophylaxis of recurrent urinary tract infections in women: a randomized clinical trial. World J Urol 2014;32(1):79–84.

40. van der Bosch JF, Verboom-Sohmer U, Postma P, et al. Mannose-sensitive and mannose-resistant adherence to human uroepithelial cells and urinary

virulence of Escherichia coli. Infect Immun 1980; 29(1):226–33.

41. Hill C, Guarner F, Reid G, et al. Expert consensus document. The International Scientific Association for Probiotics and Prebiotics consensus statement on the scope and appropriate use of the term probiotic. Nat Rev Gastroenterol Hepatol 2014;11(8):506–14.

42. Hilt EE, McKinley K, Pearce MM, et al. Urine is not sterile: use of enhanced urine culture techniques to detect resident bacterial flora in the adult female bladder. J Clin Microbiol 2014;52(3):871–6.

43. Vagios S, Hesham H, Mitchell C. Understanding the potential of lactobacilli in recurrent UTI prevention. Microb Pathog 2020;148:104544.

44. Osset J, Bartolomé RM, García E, et al. Assessment of the capacity of Lactobacillus to inhibit the growth of uropathogens and block their adhesion to vaginal epithelial cells. J Infect Dis 2001;183(3):485–91.

45. Schwenger EM, Tejani AM, Loewen PS. Probiotics for preventing urinary tract infections in adults and children. Cochrane Database Syst Rev 2015;12: CD008772.

46. Stapleton AE, Au-Yeung M, Hooton TM, et al. Randomized, placebo-controlled phase 2 trial of a Lactobacillus crispatus probiotic given intravaginally for prevention of recurrent urinary tract infection. Clin Infect Dis Off Publ Infect Dis Soc Am 2011;52(10): 1212–7.

47. Foxman B, Chi JW. Health behavior and urinary tract infection in college-aged women. J Clin Epidemiol 1990;43(4):329–37.

48. Ochoa-Brust GJ, Fernández AR, Villanueva-Ruiz GJ, et al. Daily intake of 100 mg ascorbic acid as urinary tract infection prophylactic agent during pregnancy. Acta Obstet Gynecol Scand 2007;86(7):783–7.

49. Castelló T, Girona L, Gómez MR, et al. The possible value of ascorbic acid as a prophylactic agent for urinary tract infection. Spinal Cord 1996;34(10): 592–3.

50. Perrotta C, Aznar M, Mejia R, et al. Oestrogens for preventing recurrent urinary tract infection in postmenopausal women. Obstet Gynecol 2008;112(3): 689–90.

51. Ponzone R, Biglia N, Jacomuzzi ME, et al. Vaginal oestrogen therapy after breast cancer: is it safe? Eur J Cancer Oxf Engl 1990 2005;41(17):2673–81.

52. Hooton TM, Vecchio M, Iroz A, et al. Effect of Increased Daily Water Intake in Premenopausal Women With Recurrent Urinary Tract Infections. JAMA Intern Med 2018;178(11):1509–15.

53. Nickel JC, Saz-Leal P, Doiron RC. Could sublingual vaccination be a viable option for the prevention of recurrent urinary tract infection in Canada? A systematic review of the current literature and plans for the future. Can Urol Assoc J 2020;14(8):281–7.

54. Lorenzo-Gómez MF, Padilla-Fernández B, García-Criado FJ, et al. Evaluation of a therapeutic vaccine

for the prevention of recurrent urinary tract infections versus prophylactic treatment with antibiotics. Int Urogynecol J 2013;24(1):127–34.

55. Lorenzo-Gómez MF, Padilla-Fernández B, García-Cenador MB, et al. Comparison of sublingual therapeutic vaccine with antibiotics for the prophylaxis of recurrent urinary tract infections. Front Cell Infect Microbiol 2015;5.

56. Yang B, Foley S. First experience in the UK of treating women with recurrent urinary tract infections with the bacterial vaccine Uromune. BJU Int 2018;121(2):289–92.

57. Ramírez Sevilla C, Gómez Lanza E, Manzanera JL, et al. Active immunoprophyilaxis with uromune® decreases the recurrence of urinary tract infections at three and six months after treatment without relevant secondary effects. BMC Infect Dis 2019;19(1):901.

58. Carrión-López P, Martínez-Ruiz J, Librán-García L, et al. Analysis of the Efficacy of a Sublingual Bacterial Vaccine in the Prophylaxis of Recurrent Urinary Tract Infection. Urol Int 2020;104(3–4):293–300.

59. Prattley S, Geraghty R, Moore M, et al. Role of Vaccines for Recurrent Urinary Tract Infections: A Systematic Review. Eur Urol Focus 2020;6(3):593–604.

60. Huttner A, Hatz C, van den Dobbelsteen G, et al. Safety, immunogenicity, and preliminary clinical efficacy of a vaccine against extraintestinal pathogenic Escherichia coli in women with a history of recurrent urinary tract infection: a randomised, single-blind, placebo-controlled phase 1b trial. Lancet Infect Dis 2017;17(5):528–37.

61. Tariq R, Pardi DS, Tosh PK, et al. Fecal Microbiota Transplantation for Recurrent Clostridium difficile Infection Reduces Recurrent Urinary Tract Infection Frequency. Clin Infect Dis Off Publ Infect Dis Soc Am 2017;65(10):1745–7.

62. Jeney SES, Lane F, Oliver A, et al. Fecal Microbiota Transplantation for the Treatment of Refractory Recurrent Urinary Tract Infection. Obstet Gynecol 2020;136(4):771–3.

63. Coste I, Judlin P, Lepargneur J-P, et al. Safety and efficacy of an intravaginal prebiotic gel in the prevention of recurrent bacterial vaginosis: a randomized double-blind study. Obstet Gynecol Int 2012;2012:147867.

Medical Treatment of Female Sexual Dysfunction

Rossella E. Nappi, MD, PhD[a,b,]*, Lara Tiranini, MD[a,b], Ellis Martini, MD[a,b], David Bosoni, MD[a,b], Alessandra Righi, MD[a,b], Laura Cucinella, MD[a,b]

KEYWORDS

- Female sexual dysfunction • Hypoactive sexual desire disorder
- Genitourinary syndrome of menopause • Estrogens • Androgens • Psychoactive drugs
- Vasoactive drugs

KEY POINTS

- Recognition of female sexual dysfunction (FSD) in the clinical setting should be universal, and counseling is an essential part of sexual health care.
- Health care providers (HCPs) should provide information on the full range of therapeutic options, from pharmacotherapies to psychosocial interventions, and on the importance to combine multiple strategies.
- Few pharmacologic therapies are approved for FSD. HCPs can address hypoactive sexual desire disorder by using two psychoactive agents (flibanserin and bremelanotide) in premenopausal women and transdermal testosterone in postmenopausal women.
- Other hormonal therapies (systemic and local) can be used to relieve genitourinary syndrome of menopause/vulvovaginal atrophy associated sexual pain and eventually improve other dimensions of sexual function.

INTRODUCTION

A sexual problem associated with personal distress in women qualifies as a female sexual dysfunction (FSD).[1] Although sexual symptoms are quite common across the life span, "true" dysfunction are less prevalent because many biopsychosocial determinants influence attitudes to reporting distressing problems with desire, arousal, orgasm, or experiences of sexual pain.[2] The Prevalence of Female Sexual Problems Associated with Distress and Determinants of Treatment Seeking demonstrated that 43.1% of women reported sexual symptoms but only 22.2% reported sexually related personal distress.[3] When distress was combined with a sexual problem, 12% experienced any FSD that were more common in women aged 45 to 64 years

(14.8%) than in younger (10.8%) or older (8.9%) women.[3]

Recognition of FSD in the clinical setting should be universal as virtual every medical condition and associated treatments may carry a multidimensional impairment of healthy sexual function and behavior.[4] However, motivation to seek help and assistance from health care providers (HCPs) may vary depending on a wide range of intrapersonal and interpersonal factors.[5] A proactive approach is needed to educate women on common changes related to hormonal fluctuations, for instance at menopause, and risk factors, such as mood disorders and urinary incontinence, that may affect sexual response.[6] However, it is essential to provide information on the full range of therapeutic options, from pharmacotherapies to psychosocial interventions,[7] and on the

a Research Center for Reproductive Medicine, Gynecological Endocrinology and Menopause, IRCCS S. Matteo Foundation, Pavia, Italy; b Department of Clinical, Surgical, Diagnostic and Pediatric Sciences, University of Pavia, Pavia, Italy
* Corresponding author. Research Centre for Reproductive Medicine, IRCCS Policlinico San Matteo, Piazzale Golgi 2, Pavia 27100, Italy.
E-mail address: renappi@tin.it

Urol Clin N Am 49 (2022) 299–307
https://doi.org/10.1016/j.ucl.2022.02.001
0094-0143/22/© 2022 Elsevier Inc. All rights reserved.

importance to combine multiple strategies or involve the partner under some circumstances.[8]

At present, the International Society for the Study of Women's Sexual Health, the International Consultation of Sexual Medicine, and the American Foundation of Urologic Diseases published evidence-based consensus guidelines on definitions, nomenclature, diagnostic criteria, and classification systems of FSD that go beyond those provided in the DSM psychiatric compendia.[9] The goal was to provide a common FSD coding in clinical settings worldwide, useful both in research and in practice. The main challenges included the frequent overlap of sexual symptoms, the multitude of causes within the frame of the biopsychosocial model, and the DSM-V redefinition of some disorders (**Box 1**)[1] that may ingenerate confusion in prescribing drugs approved for a specific diagnosis based on the DSM-IV-TR criteria, for instance hypoactive sexual desire disorder (HSDD).[10]

In here, we report key-elements for medical treatment of FSD considering three major areas of intervention: the sex hormonal milieu, the central nervous system (CNS) circuitries, and the neurovascular/neuromuscular system modulating urogenital sexual response.

Therapeutic Options

HCPs can screen for FSD according to their level of expertise and deliver at least basic counseling before eventually referring to sexual medicine specialists for specific care.[4] At the core level, HCPs should be able to identify the most common sexual problems that cause distress, including low sexual desire, difficulty with sexual arousal and with orgasm, sexual pain/genito-pelvic pain, penetration dysfunction, medication-induced symptoms, and relationship conflicts.[4] In addition, basic counseling itself may be a first-line treatment offering emotional relief, education, and empowerment, especially by dispelling myths and providing very simple strategies to cope with symptoms, for instance advice on the use of lubricants.[11,12] The therapeutic algorithm comprises a multidisciplinary approach, including pharmacologic and nonpharmacologic management. It is more likely that acquired, generalized FSD requires a biomedical approach, whereas lifelong or situational FSD needs psychosexual approach.[7,12] In any case, it is essential to address potential biopsychosocial modifiable risk factors (**Fig. 1**) contributing to FSD.

SEX HORMONE MILIEU

Circulating levels of sex steroids (estrogen, testosterone, progesterone), and their metabolites play a fundamental role in linking sexuality to reproduction. They target every tissue involved in the central and peripheral sexual response across the life span of women, and their effects become particularly evident when deprivation of sex steroids occurs.[13–15] Within the CNS, sex steroids prime neural circuitries to be selectively responsive to sexual incentives creating a neurochemical state more likely inducing sexual response.[16] At the urogenital level, sex steroids exert a trophic effect and modulate the threshold of tissue response to external and internal stimuli throughout a neurochemical array regulating genital vasocongestion, vaginal lubrication, and clitoral engorgement.[17,18] That being so, hypoestrogenic and even androgen-insufficient states along with the aging process itself can significantly induce FSD. They may depend on natural (eg, lactational amenorrhea, menopause), pathologic (eg, primary and secondary amenorrhea, premature ovarian insufficiency), and iatrogenic (for instance, surgical menopause and that induced by chemotherapy/radiotherapy, and other hormonal treatments such as hormonal contraception, gonadotropin-releasing hormone analogues, glucocorticoids) causes.[18–20]

At present, hormonal treatments are labeled only for use in postmenopausal women[5,19] to relieve conditions such as HSDD[10] and genitourinary syndrome of menopause (GSM), formerly known as vulvovaginal atrophy (VVA).[21]

Menopause Hormone Therapy

Menopause hormone therapy (MHT) is a therapeutic choice for healthy recently menopausal women reporting moderate to severe vasomotor symptoms and in need of bone loss prevention.[22] It improves several aspects of quality of life, including GSM/VVA and sexual function.[23,24]

Estrogens and progestogens

Impact of systemic MHT on sexual function has been mainly investigated as a secondary end point in clinical trials, with evidence of a small-to-moderate improvement in early menopausal women or in presence of menopausal symptoms, but not in unselected postmenopausal women.[25] Type of molecules and their metabolites, dose, and route of administration should be considered in order to minimize the relative androgen insufficiency induced by exogenous estrogens.[16] Indeed, transdermal estradiol has a lower impact on circulating sex hormone binding globulin (SHBG) and free testosterone.[26] Transdermal administration has been shown to improve sexual function in early postmenopausal women, evaluated through increased total female sexual

Box 1
Main DSM-V changes with respect to DSM-IV-TR

- Sexual response is not always a linear, uniform process; therefore, distinction between certain phases (eg, desire and arousal) may be artificial.

- Sexual desire and arousal disorders are combined into one disorder: female sexual interest/arousal disorder (SIAD) instead of HSDD and female sexual arousal disorder.

- Genito-pelvic pain/penetration disorder is a new DSM-V definition that merges vaginismus and dyspareunia, because they are highly comorbid.

- To make any diagnosis a symptom should be present 75% to 100% of the time and have a minimum duration of approximately 6 months (except substance-/medication-induced sexual dysfunction).

- Only lifelong versus acquired and generalized versus situational subtypes remain.

- Distress should be personal.

function index (FSFI) score, more than oral estrogen formulations.[27] Interestingly, lubrication and pain were the domains mostly influenced by the route of administration, whereas desire did not differ significantly between the two groups.[27] Even the characteristics of combined progestogens in nonhysterectomized women[23,24] and their metabolites may play a role in modulating sexual function due to their different impact on SHBG.[16] However, there is no evidence of well-designed studies showing the superiority of a specific molecule and, therefore, the choice of the progestogens should be based on tolerability and safety.[28]

Tibolone

Tibolone is a selective tissue estrogenic activity regulator approved in many countries, apart the United States, for treatment of menopausal symptoms and for osteoporosis prevention.[29] Because of its multiple endocrine properties (estrogenic, progestogenic, and androgenic), tibolone has been specifically investigated in postmenopausal women with FSD, showing to be superior in improving desire, arousal, and satisfaction as compared with a conventional estro-progestogen combination.[30] Tibolone has been also shown to induce a significant increase of clitoral circulation in postmenopausal women reporting FSD as compared with a combined estro-progestogen preparation.[31]

Transdermal testosterone

Transdermal testosterone treatment at the dose of 300 µg per 24 hours was initially approved in Europe for managing HSDD in surgically menopausal women.[32] Subsequent randomized controlled trials (RCTs) assessed efficacy and short-term safety in naturally menopausal women assuming or not a concomitant estrogen/estro-progestogen treatment.[32] Recently, a systematic review and meta-analysis assessing potential benefits and risks of testosterone for women concluded that testosterone significantly increases sexual function in postmenopausal women with low libido associated with distress, more specifically improving desire, arousal, orgasm, responsiveness to sex stimuli, and increasing the frequency of satisfying sexual events (SSEs), whereas decreasing sexual distress and concerns.[33] Safety profile of transdermal formulation is reassuring at the dose that approximates physiologic testosterone concentration in premenopausal women.[33] Therefore, a global consensus position statement on the use

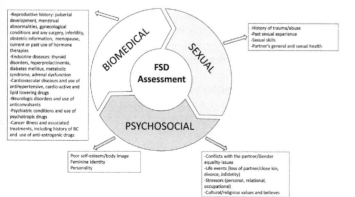

Fig. 1. Biopsychosocial assessment of FSD.

of testosterone therapy in women confirmed HSDD in naturally or surgically menopausal women as the unique evidence-based indication,[34] in particular in women with premature ovarian insufficiency.[35] Clinical and biochemical monitoring should be planned to avoid any supraphysiologic dosage and assess efficacy of transdermal testosterone. If the treatment is not effective following 6 months, then it should be stopped, and indication to its use should be revised.[22,36] Despite agreement of the scientific community, at present, there are not available testosterone products approved for women in most countries, and HCPs are forced to prescribe off-label formulations for men at adjusted doses for women, rising concerns about misuse.[36]

Oral Dehydroepiandrosterone

Cross-sectional studies suggest a positive impact of endogenous dehydroepiandrosterone (DHEA) on several aspects of well-being in women, including sexual function. However, RCTs have failed to demonstrate a significant effect of systemic therapy with DHEA on sexual function in menopausal women with normal adrenal function, whereas it may be beneficial when adrenal insufficiency coexists.[34,37]

Local Hormone Therapy

Systemic MHT improves symptoms associated with GSM/VVA in 75% of postmenopausal women, namely vaginal dryness and dyspareunia, but the risk–benefit profile is acceptable when other symptoms, mainly hot flashes, or prevention of osteoporotic fractures, represent the main indication to treatment.[23,24]

Estrogens

Local estrogen therapy (LET) represents an effective strategy for maintenance of uro-gynecologic and sexual health when GSM/VVA symptoms are the most relevant concern at menopause.[38] Products available include different estrogenic preparations, mainly estradiol, estriol, conjugated equine estrogens, promestriene, delivered through different formulations (cream, gel, pessaries, ring) to be used regularly twice/three times a week and safely up to 1 year.[19,39] A Cochrane review including 30 trials concluded that approved local estrogenic treatments are all similarly effective in relieving vaginal dryness and dyspareunia, thus the choice should consider patient's preference.[40] Even lower urinary tract symptoms, namely recurrent urinary tract infections (rUTI) and urge urinary incontinence, may benefit from LET,[38] which is included as a prophylactic strategy in perimenopausal and postmenopausal women with

uncomplicated rUTI in guidelines for urologists.[41] Moreover, the North American Menopause Society stated that LET can be used for relieving concomitant vulvovaginal and urinary symptoms and in absence of improvement following 3 months should be discontinued.[23] Ultralow dose preparations should be preferred to minimize systemic absorption, with circulating estradiol levels persistently remaining in the postmenopausal range.[23,24,42] The role of minimal estrogenic absorption is still not clear in patients with a history of hormone-sensitive malignancies in terms of recurrence risk, particularly in breast cancer survivors (BCSs), who may present with severe symptoms associated to use of antiestrogenic therapies.[43] However, there is general agreement that ultralow dose vaginal estrogens may be considered in patients with severe symptoms unresponsive to nonhormonal approaches, after careful multidisciplinary evaluation of risks and benefits with the oncologic team, excluding those women assuming aromatase inhibitors (AIs).[43,44] Indeed, recent results from a phase II placebo RCT pointed to efficacy and safety of a 0.005% estriol vaginal gel in BCSs on AIs, with an initial increase in circulating estriol followed by normalization at 12 weeks, and constantly undetectable levels of circulating estradiol and estrone over time.[45]

Dehydroepiandrosterone

DHEA, also known as prasterone, is an inactive precursor converted to estrogens and androgens in the target peripheral tissues, through a mechanism described as intracrinology.[46] Vaginal DHEA formulation represents an innovation in the field of GSM because of its synergistic action of estrogens and androgens on vaginal and vulvar cells while minimizing any systemic absorption.[14,46] RCTs have confirmed the efficacy of daily vaginal administration of prasterone 6.5 mg inserts in significantly improving VVA associated dyspareunia in postmenopausal women and other VVA-associated symptoms.[47,48] A significant improvement of desire, lubrication, orgasm, and sexual satisfaction has also been reported,[49] supporting the crucial role of dyspareunia in driving the vicious circle of postmenopausal FSD.[6] Preliminary data in BCSs on tamoxifen and aromatase AIs are promising but await for further confirmation in order to recommend its use in high-risk populations.[43]

Testosterone cream

A recent expert review concluded that there are still insufficient data to support the use of testosterone for the GSM/VVA treatment, but positive effects are biologically plausible both on genital and urinary health.[14] Local testosterone is promising in

BCSs on AIs, as aromatization to estradiol would be prevented.[50] A double-blind RCT showed efficacy during a 24-week period by comparing an intravaginal T cream 300 mcg to placebo in the treatment of dyspareunia and vaginal dryness. Even sexual function was significantly improved, without significant changes in circulating sex steroids.[51]

Ospemifene

Ospemifene is a selective estrogen receptor modulator with agonist action on vaginal epithelium and bone, partial agonistic action on the endometrium, and a neutral to antagonist effect on breast tissue.[52] It is approved for treating vaginal dryness and dyspareunia and other GSM/VVA associated symptoms, displaying a high rate of clinical relevance.[53] Almost every domain (desire, lubrication, arousal, orgasm, and pain) of sexual function significantly improved following 12 weeks of treatment with 60 mg daily dose of oral Ospemifene 60 mg compared with placebo, when dyspareunia was the most bothersome symptom.[54] Ospemifene represents an interesting alternative for women who do not respond to LET, who are not compliant to vaginal administration, or who present a high-risk profile for conventional estrogen therapy.[55] Preliminary data suggest a potential use to relieve also bladder symptoms at menopause.[56,57]

CENTRAL NERVOUS SYSTEM CIRCUITRIES

CNS circuitries are major targets for sex steroids and mediate instinctual, emotional, and behavioral components of sexual response.[58] Indeed, the neuroendocrine balance of excitatory (dopamine, noradrenaline, and melanocortin receptors [MC3R and MC4R]) and inhibitory (serotonin, the endocannabinoid, and opioid systems) signals modulating sexual desire, arousal, orgasm, and satisfaction is under the influence of the hormonal milieu along with other biopsychosocial inciters and suppressors.[16] It seems likely that HSDD involves either a predisposition toward inhibitory pathways in the brain or a neuroadaptation of structures and functions resulting in a decreased excitation and/or an increased inhibition.[59] This is the theoretic background for investigating psychoactive agents as an effective treatment for desire and arousal disorders, especially in premenopausal women.[5]

Flibanserin

Flibanserin is a centrally acting medication with 5HT1A agonist and 5HT2A antagonist properties leading to an increase of dopamine and norepinephrine within the CNS.[60] Flibanserin is the first drug in its class and has been approved to treat generalized acquired HSDD in premenopausal women.[61] Pivotal phase III trials demonstrated significant efficacy of flibanserin 100 mg once daily at bedtime (qhs) in improving number of SSEs, level of sexual desire, and reduction of distress as compared with placebo after 24 weeks and up to 52 weeks in open arm.[62] Efficacy on number of SSEs, sexual desire, and sexual distress has been proven even in naturally postmenopausal women,[63] but its eventual use is unlabeled. Flibanserin is a chronic drug with a controversial history of approval,[64] and a systematic review and meta-analysis pointed to small clinical efficacy and significant side effects.[65] Following approval, the FDA required a risk evaluation and mitigation strategy, in order to inform women about the risk of hypotension and syncope and further studies to investigate the interaction with alcohol.[61,64] At present, the FDA requires restriction on alcohol consumption with flibanserin with a safety labeling due to its interaction with some liver enzymes.[66]

Bremelanotide

Bremelanotide, a melanocortin receptor agonist that promotes dopamine release because of high affinity for the MC4R in presynaptic neurons of the hypothalamus,[67] has been also recently approved for the treatment of generalized acquired HSDD in premenopausal women.[68] Bremelanotide is a self-administered, subcutaneously on-demand (approximately 45 minutes before anticipated sexual activity) medication marketed at the dose of 1.75 mg following the results of two pivotal phase III trials with an identical design[60] and of a 52-week open label extension study.[70] Primary analyses demonstrated statistically significant and clinically meaningful improvements in sexual desire and related distress with bremelanotide as compared with placebo in premenopausal women with HSDD.[69] Nausea, flushing, and headache were the most common treatment-emergent adverse events and occurred in around 10% of patients taking the active drug. No safety signals emerged during the 52-week open-label extension and benefits were maintained.[70] It is recommended to use no more than one dose of bremelanotide in 24 hours and no more than eight doses per month. However, the drug is safe and has limited interactions with alcohol and with other drugs.[71]

Other Psychoactive Drugs

Patients with mood disorders and those with SSRI-induced HSDD may gain some benefits with the off-label use of psychoactive agents (bupropion and buspirone) acting on the neuroendocrine balance modulating sexual response.[67] Trazodone, another antidepressant with a sedative effect, has been also investigated as an antidote for FSD.[72] Indeed, the positive modulation of the dopamine/serotonin ratio seems the key to help women with sexual desire and arousal disorders.[67,73] That being so, the dopamine agonist apomorphine, approved in men with erectile dysfunction, was tested sublingually (3 mg) in premenopausal women with desire and arousal disorders but side effects and lack of clinical relevance stopped further development.[74]

NEUROVASCULAR/NEUROMUSCULAR SYSTEM

The neurovascular/neuromuscular system is also influenced by sex steroids, which interplay with adrenergic, cholinergic and nonadrenergic, and noncholinergic neurotransmitters and other vasoactive substances, such as vasointestinal peptide and nitric oxide (NO). Coupled to the trophic effect of both estrogens and androgens on urogenital tissues, this array of molecules regulate genital vasocongestion, vaginal lubrication, and clitoral engorgement, as well as pelvic floor function which is critical to achieve orgasm.[16,17]

PD5-inhibitors and other Vasoactive Agents

PDE5-inhibitors, especially sildenafil, have been tested in both premenopausal and postmenopausal women with poor evidence.[75] In women with low desire, there is a discordance between genital and subjective measures of sexual response. Therefore, promoting vasodilation via sustained effects of NO in the vascular system in order to help engorgement of clitoral and vaginal tissues does not translate into an improvement of sexual function.[5,76] Sildenafil may be a potential antidote for women who develop arousal disorder secondary to multiple sclerosis, diabetes, or antidepressant use.[76] Even other vasoactive agents, such as topical NO donors, alprostadil (prostaglandin E1), or oral phentolamine mesylate (a combined α-1 and α-2 adrenergic agonist),[5,74,77,78] were not further investigated.

FUTURE DIRECTIONS

There are not so many new candidate drugs to treat FSD, and the main challenge is to develop psychometrically sounded instruments in order to capture the clinical relevance of specific therapeutic interventions.[79] Moreover, it seems essential to combine different research approaches, ranging from genetic studies[80] to molecular and cellular targets,[74] and including psychosocial approaches, is crucial to obtain meaningful results. An example is given by a personalized approach based on the phenotype prediction score, which included genetic, biological, and psychological markers with the aim to identify different phenotypes of women reporting sexual desire and arousal disorders.[81] According to this model, it is likely that some women display a relatively insensitive excitatory system in the brain for sexual cues, whereas others display a dysfunctional activation of brain mechanisms for sexual inhibition.[81] That being so, different combinations of drugs acting on the sex hormonal milieu, the CNS circuitries, and the neurovascular/neuromuscular system may serve specific therapeutic aims. Even though ongoing phase III clinical study program by using such personalized approach are still lacking,[7,77] an RCT suggested a positive effect of on-demand sublingual sildenafil (50 mg) plus testosterone (0.5 mg) in women with FSIAD due to low sensitivity to sexual cues. Similarly, when testosterone (0.5 mg) was combined with buspirone (10 mg), a meaningful result was observed in women with FSIAD due to high sensitivity to sexual cues.[82] Other drugs remain experimental holding the promise of potential solutions.[77,78,83]

SUMMARY

Medical treatment of FSD is based on interventions that aim, on one hand, to restore the neuroendocrine balance by replacing hormonal deficiencies and, on the other hand, to potentiate the urogenital response to sexual stimulatory clues. Only few evidence-based therapeutic options are, indeed, available to manage HSDD. They include flibanserin and bremelanotide in premenopause and transdermal testosterone in postmenopause. MHT may improve sexual function because of a more general positive effect on health and quality of life of women.

AUTHOR CONTRIBUTIONS

R.E.N. writing, editing, and supervision; L.T. writing and revision of the relevant literature; E.M., D.B., A.R., F.B., revision of the scientific literature and drafting tables and figures; and L.C. writing, editing, and supervision. All authors have read and agreed to the published version of the manuscript.

DISCLOSURE STATEMENT

R.E.N. had past financial relationships (lecturer, member of advisory boards and/or consultant) with Boehringer Ingelheim, Ely Lilly, Endoceutics, Gedeon Richter, HRA Pharma, Merck Sharpe & Dohme, Procter & Gamble Co, TEVA Women's Health Inc, and Zambon SpA. At present, she has ongoing relationship with Astellas, Bayer HealthCare AG, Exceltis, Fidia, Novo Nordisk, Organon & Co, Palatin Technologies, Pfizer Inc, Shionogi Limited, and Theramex. Other authors have nothing to disclose.

REFERENCES

1. American Psychiatric Association. Diagnostic and statistical manual of mental disorders. 5th edition. Washington, DC: American Psychiatric Association; 2014.
2. Nappi RE, Cucinella L, Martella S, et al. Female sexual dysfunction (FSD): Prevalence and impact on quality of life (QoL). Maturitas 2016;94:87–91.
3. Shifren JL, Monz BU, Russo PA, et al. Sexual problems and distress in United States women: prevalence and correlates. Obstet Gynecol 2008;112:970–8.
4. Parish SJ, Hahn SR, Goldstein SW, et al. The International Society for the Study of Women's Sexual Health Process of Care for the Identification of Sexual Concerns and Problems in Women. Mayo Clin Proc 2019;94:842–56.
5. Nappi RE, Cucinella L. Advances in pharmacotherapy for treating female sexual dysfunction. Expert Opin Pharmacother 2015;16:875–87.
6. Simon JA, Davis SR, Althof SE, et al. Sexual well-being after menopause: An International Menopause Society White Paper. Climacteric 2018;21:415–27.
7. Kingsberg SA, Althof S, Simon JA, et al. Female Sexual Dysfunction-Medical and Psychological Treatments, Committee 14. J Sex Med 2017;14:1463–91.
8. Jannini EA, Nappi RE. Couplepause: A New Paradigm in Treating Sexual Dysfunction During Menopause and Andropause. Sex Med Rev 2018;6:384–95.
9. Parish SJ, Cottler-Casanova S, Clayton AH, et al. The Evolution of the Female Sexual Disorder/Dysfunction Definitions, Nomenclature, and Classifications: A Review of DSM, ICSM, ISSWSH, and ICD. Sex Med Rev 2021;9:36–56.
10. Kingsberg SA, Simon JA. Female Hypoactive Sexual Desire Disorder: A Practical Guide to Causes, Clinical Diagnosis, and Treatment. J Womens Health (Larchmt) 2020;29:1101–12.
11. Brandenburg U, Bitzer J. The challenge of talking about sex: the importance of patient-physician interaction. Maturitas 2009;63:124–7.
12. Al-Azzawi F, Bitzer J, Brandenburg U, et al. Therapeutic options for postmenopausal female sexual dysfunction. Climacteric 2010;13:103–20.
13. Lachowsky M, Nappi RE. The effects of oestrogen on urogenital health. Maturitas 2009;63:149–51.
14. Simon JA, Goldstein I, Kim NN, et al. The role of androgens in the treatment of genitourinary syndrome of menopause (GSM): International Society for the Study of Women's Sexual Health (ISSWSH) expert consensus panel review. Menopause 2018;25:837–47.
15. Wierman ME, Nappi RE, Avis N, et al. Endocrine aspects of women's sexual function. J Sex Med 2010;7(1 Pt 2):561–85.
16. Nappi RE, Polatti F. The use of estrogen therapy in women's sexual functioning (CME). J Sex Med 2009;6:603–16.
17. Traish AM, Vignozzi L, Simon JA, et al. Role of Androgens in Female Genitourinary Tissue Structure and Function: Implications in the Genitourinary Syndrome of Menopause. Sex Med Rev 2018;6(4):558–71.
18. Mac Bride MB, Rhodes DJ, Shuster LT. Vulvovaginal atrophy. Mayo Clin Proc 2010;85:87–94.
19. Nappi RE, Cucinella L, Martini E, et al. The role of hormone therapy in urogenital health after menopause. Best Pract Res Clin Endocrinol Metab 2021;35:101595.
20. Davis SR, Wahlin-Jacobsen S. Testosterone in women–the clinical significance. Lancet Diabetes Endocrinol 2015;3:980–92.
21. Nappi RE, Martini E, Cucinella L, et al. Addressing Vulvovaginal Atrophy (VVA)/Genitourinary Syndrome of Menopause (GSM) for Healthy Aging in Women. Front Endocrinol 2019;10:561.
22. Baber RJ, Panay N, Fenton A, IMS Writing Group. IMS Recommendations on women's midlife health and menopause hormone therapy. Climacteric 2016;19:109–50.
23. The 2020 genitourinary syndrome of menopause position statement of The North American Menopause Society. Menopause 2020;27:976–92.
24. Sturdee DW, Panay N, International Menopause Society Writing Group. Recommendations for the management of postmenopausal vaginal atrophy. Climacteric 2010;13:509–22.
25. Nastri CO, Lara LA, Ferriani RA, et al. Hormone therapy for sexual function in perimenopausal and postmenopausal women. Cochrane Database Syst Rev 2013;6:CD009672.
26. Shifren JL, Desindes S, McIlwain M, et al. A randomized, open-label, crossover study comparing the effects of oral versus transdermal estrogen therapy on serum androgens, thyroid hormones, and adrenal hormones in naturally menopausal women. Menopause 2007;14:985–94.
27. Taylor HS, Tal A, Pal L, et al. Effects of Oral vs Transdermal Estrogen Therapy on Sexual Function in Early Postmenopause: Ancillary Study of the Kronos Early Estrogen Prevention Study (KEEPS). JAMA Intern Med 2017;177:1471–9.

28. Liu JH. The Role of Progestogens in Menopausal Hormone Therapy. Clin Obstet Gynecol 2021;64: 772–83.

29. Biglia N, Maffei S, Lello S, et al. Tibolone in postmenopausal women: a review based on recent randomised controlled clinical trials. Gynecol Endocrinol 2010;26:804–14.

30. Nijland EA, Weijmar Schultz WC, Nathorst-Boös J, et al. LISA study investigators. Tibolone and transdermal E2/NETA for the treatment of female sexual dysfunction in naturally menopausal women: results of a randomized active-controlled trial. J Sex Med 2008;5:646–56.

31. Nappi RE, Ferdeghini F, Sampaolo P, et al. Clitoral circulation in postmenopausal women with sexual dysfunction: a pilot randomized study with hormone therapy. Maturitas 2006;55:288–95.

32. Achilli C, Pundir J, Ramanathan P, et al. Efficacy and safety of transdermal testosterone in postmenopausal women with hypoactive sexual desire disorder: a systematic review and meta-analysis. Fertil Steril 2017;107:475–82.e15.

33. Islam RM, Bell RJ, Green S, et al. Safety and efficacy of testosterone for women: a systematic review and meta-analysis of randomised controlled trial data. Lancet Diabetes Endocrinol 2019;7:754–66.

34. Davis SR, Baber R, Panay N, et al. Global Consensus Position Statement on the Use of Testosterone Therapy for Women. Climacteric 2019;22:429–34.

35. Panay N, Anderson RA, Nappi RE, et al. Premature ovarian insufficiency: an International Menopause Society White Paper. Climacteric 2020;23:426–46.

36. Parish SJ, Simon JA, Davis SR, et al. International Society for the Study of Women's Sexual Health Clinical Practice Guideline for the Use of Systemic Testosterone for Hypoactive Sexual Desire Disorder in Women. J Sex Med 2021;18:849–67.

37. Davis SR, Panjari M, Stanczyk FZ. Clinical review: DHEA replacement for postmenopausal women. J Clin Endocrinol Metab 2011;96:1642–53.

38. Nappi RE, Davis SR. The use of hormone therapy for the maintenance of urogynecological and sexual health post WHI. Climacteric 2012;15:267–74.

39. Palacios S, Castelo-Branco C, Currie H, et al. Update on management of genitourinary syndrome of menopause: A practical guide. Maturitas 2015;82: 308–13.

40. Lethaby A, Ayeleke RO, Roberts H. Local oestrogen for vaginal atrophy in postmenopausal women. Cochrane Database Syst Rev 2016;2016(8): CD001500.

41. Anger J, Lee U, Ackerman AL, et al. Recurrent Uncomplicated Urinary Tract Infections in Women: AUA/CUA/SUFU Guideline. J Urol 2019;202:282–9.

42. Santen RJ. Vaginal administration of estradiol: effects of dose, preparation and timing on plasma estradiol levels. Climacteric 2015;18:121–34.

43. Faubion SS, Larkin LC, Stuenkel CA, et al. Management of genitourinary syndrome of menopause in women with or at high risk for breast cancer: consensus recommendations from The North American Menopause Society and The International Society for the Study of Women's Sexual Health. Menopause 2018;25:596–608.

44. Mension E, Alonso I, Castelo-Branco C. Genitourinary Syndrome of Menopause: Current Treatment Options in Breast Cancer Survivors - Systematic Review. Maturitas 2021;143:47–58.

45. Hirschberg AL, Sánchez-Rovira P, Presa-Lorite J, et al. Efficacy and safety of ultra-low dose 0.005% estriol vaginal gel for the treatment of vulvovaginal atrophy in postmenopausal women with early breast cancer treated with nonsteroidal aromatase inhibitors: a phase II, randomized, double-blind, placebo-controlled trial. Menopause 2020;27:526–34.

46. Labrie F. Intracrinology and menopause: the science describing the cell-specific intracellular formation of estrogens and androgens from DHEA and their strictly local action and inactivation in peripheral tissues. Menopause 2019;26:220–4.

47. Labrie F, Archer DF, Martel C, et al. Combined data of intravaginal prasterone against vulvovaginal atrophy of menopause. Menopause 2017;24:1246–56.

48. Holton M, Thorne C, Goldstein AT. An overview of dehydroepiandrosterone (EM-760) as a treatment option for genitourinary syndrome of menopause. Expert Opin Pharmacother 2020;21:409–15.

49. Labrie F, Derogatis L, Archer DF, et al. Effect of Intravaginal Prasterone on Sexual Dysfunction in Postmenopausal Women with Vulvovaginal Atrophy. J Sex Med 2015;12:2401–12.

50. Cox P, Panay N. Vulvovaginal atrophy in women after cancer. Climacteric 2019;22:565–71.

51. Davis SR, Robinson PJ, Jane F, et al. Intravaginal Testosterone Improves Sexual Satisfaction and Vaginal Symptoms Associated With Aromatase Inhibitors. J Clin Endocrinol Metab 2018;103: 4146–54.

52. Archer DF, Simon JA, Portman DJ, et al. Ospemifene for the treatment of menopausal vaginal dryness, a symptom of the genitourinary syndrome of menopause. Expert Rev Endocrinol Metab 2019;14: 301–14.

53. Nappi RE, Panay N, Bruyniks N, et al. The clinical relevance of the effect of ospemifene on symptoms of vulvar and vaginal atrophy. Climacteric 2015;18: 233–40.

54. Constantine G, Graham S, Portman DJ, et al. Female sexual function improved with ospemifene in postmenopausal women with vulvar and vaginal atrophy: results of a randomized, placebo-controlled trial. Climacteric 2015;18:226–32.

55. Nappi RE, Murina F, Perrone G, et al. Clinical profile of women with vulvar and vaginal atrophy who are

not candidates for local vaginal estrogen therapy. Minerva Ginecol 2017;69:370–80.

56. Novara L, Sgro LG, Mancarella M, et al. Potential effectiveness of Ospemifene on Detrusor Overactivity in patients with vaginal atrophy. Maturitas 2020;138:58–61.

57. Schiavi MC, Di Pinto A, Sciuga V, et al. Prevention of recurrent lower urinary tract infections in postmenopausal women with genitourinary syndrome: outcome after 6 months of treatment with ospemifene. Gynecol Endocrinol 2018;34:140–3.

58. Goldstein I, Kim NN, Clayton AH, et al. Hypoactive Sexual Desire Disorder: International Society for the Study of Women's Sexual Health (ISSWSH) Expert Consensus Panel Review. Mayo Clin Proc 2017;92:114–28.

59. Kingsberg SA, Clayton AH, Pfaus JG. The Female Sexual Response: Current Models, Neurobiological Underpinnings and Agents Currently Approved or Under Investigation for the Treatment of Hypoactive Sexual Desire Disorder. CNS Drugs 2015;29: 915–33.

60. Dhanuka I, Simon JA. Flibanserin for the treatment of hypoactive sexual desire disorder in premenopausal women. Expert Opin Pharmacother 2015;16:2523–9.

61. Joffe HV, Chang C, Sewell C, et al. FDA approval of flibanserin – treating hypoactive sexual desire disorder. N Engl J Med 2016;374:101–4.

62. Thorp J, Simon J, Dattani D, et al. Treatment of hypoactive sexual desire disorder in premenopausal women: efficacy of flibanserin in the DAISY study. J Sex Med 2012;9:793–804.

63. Simon JA, Kingsberg SA, Shumel B, et al. Efficacy and safety of flibanserin in postmenopausal women with hypoactive sexual desire disorder: results of the SNOWDROP trial. Menopause 2014;21:633–40.

64. Dooley EM, Miller MK, Clayton AH. Flibanserin: From Bench to Bedside. Sex Med Rev 2017;5.461–9.

65. Jaspers L, Feys F, Bramer WM, et al. Efficacy and safety of flibanserin for the treatment of hypoactive sexual desire disorder in women: a systematic review and meta-analysis. JAMA Intern Med 2016; 176:453–62.

66. Clayton AH, Brown L, Kim NN. Evaluation of safety for flibanserin. Expert Opin Drug Saf 2020;19:1–8.

67. Pfaus JG, Sadiq A, Spana C, et al. The neurobiology of bremelanotide for the treatment of hypoactive sexual desire disorder in premenopausal women. CNS Spectr 2021;1–9. https://doi.org/10.1017/S109285292100002X.

68. Dhillon S, Keam SJ. Bremelanotide: First Approval. Drugs 2019;79:1599–606.

69. Kingsberg SA, Clayton AH, Portman D, et al. Bremelanotide for the Treatment of Hypoactive Sexual Desire Disorder: Two Randomized Phase 3 Trials. Obstet Gynecol 2019;134:899–908.

70. Simon JA, Kingsberg SA, Portman D, et al. Long-Term Safety and Efficacy of Bremelanotide for Hypoactive Sexual Desire Disorder. Obstet Gynecol 2019; 134:909–17.

71. Mayer D, Lynch SE. Bremelanotide: New Drug Approved for Treating Hypoactive Sexual Desire Disorder. Ann Pharmacother 2020;54:684–90.

72. Pyke RE. Trazodone in Sexual Medicine: Underused and Overdosed? Sex Med Rev 2020;8:206–16.

73. Clayton AH, El Haddad S, Iluonakhamhe JP, et al. Sexual dysfunction associated with major depressive disorder and antidepressant treatment. Expert Opin Drug Saf 2014;13:1361–74.

74. Farmer M, Yoon H, Goldstein I. Future Targets for Female Sexual Dysfunction. J Sex Med 2016;13: 1147–65.

75. Schoen C, Bachmann G. Sildenafil citrate for female sexual arousal disorder: a future possibility? Nat Rev Urol 2009;6:216–22.

76. Loddy LS, Yang CC, Stuckey BG, et al. Influence of sildenafil on genital engorgement in women with female sexual arousal disorder. J Sex Med 2012;9:2693–7.

77. Belkin ZR, Krapf JM, Goldstein AT. Drugs in early clinical development for the treatment of female sexual dysfunction. Expert Opin Investig Drugs 2015; 24:159–67.

78. Miller MK, Smith JR, Norman JJ, et al. Expert opinion on existing and developing drugs to treat female sexual dysfunction. Expert Opin Emerg Drugs 2018;23:223–30.

79. Nappi RE, Gardella B. What are the challenges in prescribing pharmacotherapy for female sexual dysfunctions? Expert Opin Pharmacother 2019;20:777-9.

80. Nappi RE, Domoney C. Pharmacogenomics and sexuality: a vision. Climacteric 2013;16(Suppl 1): 25–30.

81. Höhle D, van Rooij K, Bloemers J, et al. A survival of the fittest strategy for the selection of genotypes by which drug responders and non-responders can be predicted in small groups. PLoS One 2021;16: e0246828.

82. Tuiten A, Michiels F, Böcker KB, et al. Genotype scores predict drug efficacy in subtypes of female sexual interest/arousal disorder: A double-blind, randomized, placebo-controlled cross-over trial. Womens Health (Lond) 2018;14. 1745506518788970.

83. Both S. Recent Developments in Psychopharmaceutical Approaches to Treating Female Sexual Interest and Arousal Disorder. Curr Sex Health Rep 2017;9:192–9.

Hormone Treatment of Prostate Cancer:
Evidence for Usage and Safety

Muhieddine Labban, MD[a], Marwan Alkassis, MD[b], Khalid Alkhatib, MD[a],
Logan Briggs, BA[a], Alexander P. Cole, MD[a], Adam S. Kibel, MD[a],
Quoc-Dien Trinh, MD[a],*

KEYWORDS

- Androgen antagonists • Androgen deprivation therapy • Hormonal adverse effects
- Hormone treatment • Prostatic neoplasm

KEY POINTS

- Androgen deprivation therapy (ADT) is effective in reducing testosterone levels to castrate levels in advanced prostate cancers (PCa).
- First-generation antiandrogens are associated with high levels of resistance.
- Second-generation antiandrogens are used for castrate-sensitive and castrate-resistant PCa.
- ADT has an impact on men's quality of life and is associated with endocrine, cardiovascular, sexual, and psychological side effects.
- Intermittent ADT could improve sexual desire and erectile function.

BACKGROUND
History and Epidemiology

Prostate cancer (PCa) is the most common cancer and second most lethal cancer among American men, with 248,530 new cases and 34,130 deaths in 2021.[1] Although the gold-standard treatment of localized PCa is either radical prostatectomy or radiation therapy, patients with more advanced disease benefit from androgen deprivation therapy (ADT). Dr Charles Huggin's Nobel Prize–winning discovery of the antiandrogenic effect of orchiectomy on PCa paved the way for modern day hormonal treatment.[2,3] Since Dr Huggin's discovery, ADT has become the standard of care for advanced PCa,[4] as it is estimated that 50% of men with PCa will eventually need ADT.[5]

Hypothalamic-Pituitary-Adrenal Physiology and Therapeutic Targets

ADT blocks the hypothalamic-pituitary-adrenal (HPA) axis by inhibiting hormone biosynthesis or androgen receptor (AR) activation. Either way, there is decreased activation of AR in prostate cells, preventing the unregulated cell growth and antiapoptotic signals. Thus, the goal of hormonal therapy is to reduce levels of serum testosterone to castrate levels (<50 ng/dL), as its combination with other treatments (ie, radiotherapy or surgery) confers survival benefit and delays disease progression.[4,6–8]

The HPA axis is regulated by the hypothalamus, which releases gonadotropin-releasing hormone (GnRH). In turn, GnRH stimulates luteinizing hormone (LH) and follicle-stimulating hormone (FSH)

---

[a] Division of Urological Surgery, Brigham and Women's Hospital, 45 Francis Street, Boston, MA 02115, USA;
[b] Department of Urology, Hôtel Dieu de France, Université Saint Joseph, Alfred Naccache Boulevard, Beirut, Lebanon
* Corresponding author. Division of Urologic Surgery, Harvard Medical School, Brigham and Women's Hospital, 45 Francis Street, Boston, MA 02115.
E-mail address: qtrinh@bwh.harvard.edu
Twitter: @mdlabban (M.L.); @Mar1K6 (M.A.); @LoganGBriggs1 (L.B.); @Putnam_Cole (A.P.C.); @qdtrinh (Q.-D.T.)

Urol Clin N Am 49 (2022) 309–321
https://doi.org/10.1016/j.ucl.2022.01.001
0094-0143/22/© 2022 Elsevier Inc. All rights reserved.

secretion. LH acts on Leydig cells in the testis to secrete testosterone, and the pathway is regulated through negative feedback inhibition. As such, hormone biosynthesis is targeted either (1) upstream by inhibiting the release of LH from the anterior pituitary gland in such manner that the testes are not stimulated to release testosterone, (2) downstream by inhibiting steroidogenic pathways that produce androgens, or (3) by targeting AR blockade. At the pituitary level, LH-releasing hormone (LHRH) antagonists block GnRH receptors found in the anterior pituitary, thereby inhibiting the release of LH, which results in an immediate suppression of testosterone (Section 2.1). On the other hand, LHRH agonists overstimulate the GnRH receptors at the pituitary level by disrupting the pulsatile release of LH (Section 2.2). Although LHRH agonists cause an initial surge of LH and testosterone, the sustained overstimulation of the pituitary results in cessation of their release.[9] Alternatively, hormone biosynthesis inhibition may be achieved with drugs that inhibit cytochrome P450 17A (CYP17) in the adrenal steroidogenic pathway that produces testosterone, estrogen, progestin, mineralocorticoids, and glucocorticoids (Section 2.3). Finally, AR antagonists are competitive inhibitors of AR in prostate cells (Section 2.4). The choice of pharmacotherapy depends on the stage of the disease as well as the patient's life expectancy, comorbidities, and frailty.[10–12] In this review, the authors explore each of these considerations in relation to hormonal treatment for PCa.

PHARMACOTHERAPY
Luteinizing Hormone–Releasing Hormone Antagonists

LHRH antagonists (ie, degarelix and relugolix) are competitive binders of LHRH receptors in the pituitary, resulting in an LH concentration reduction by 84% within 24 hours of administration.[13] Unlike LHRH agonists (section 2.2), LHRH antagonists are not associated with a testosterone flare; thus, preadministration or coadministration of antiandrogens is not warranted.[14]

Previous-generation LHRH antagonists, such as abarelix, are effective in achieving rapid castrate levels, avoiding testosterone surge, and reducing pain.[15] However, due to serious histamine-mediated systemic allergic and skin reactions (rash and hives),[13] abarelix is now reserved for palliative treatment in select patients. On the other hand, degarelix, a more recent alternative, does not cause systemic allergic reactions.[16,17] In a phase III trials, degarelix was superior to leuprolide in achieving sustained testosterone levels and decreased prostate-specific antigen (PSA) progression-free survival (PFS).[17,18] As such, these findings support the use of degarelix as a first-line ADT. Although degarelix is administered intramuscularly, relugolix is an oral ADT. The HERO trial compared relugolix with leuprolide to evaluate castrate level at 48 weeks after administration. A larger proportion of men who received relugolix maintained castrate levels (96.7%; 95% confidence interval [CI], 94.6–97.6) compared with men who received leuprolide (88.8%; 95% CI, 84.6–91.8; $P < .001$).[19] In addition, relugolix had 54% less risk of major cardiovascular events than leuprolide.[19] Based on the HERO trial, relugolix was approved by the Food and Drug Administration (FDA) in 2020 for the treatment of advanced PCa.[19]

Luteinizing Hormone–Releasing Hormone Agonists

LHRH agonists include leuprolide, goserelin, triptorelin, and histrelin. Depot forms of the LHRH analogues were devised by an amino acid substitution at the sixth position granting it its high potency and longer half-life. In a review of 24 trials, survival analysis of 6,600 patients on LHRH therapy agonists was similar to orchiectomy (hazard ratio [HR] 1.13; 0.92–1.39).[20] However, in men with metastatic disease to the spine or weight-bearing regions, initial exposure to LHRH agonists can result in severe life-threatening exacerbation of symptoms due to the LH and testosterone flare.[21] Associated flares may last between 10 and 20 days and can be associated with up to a 10-fold increase of LH.[13] Concomitant administration of antiandrogen before treatment can functionally block the testosterone surge.[22] Arguably it should be administered at least 1 week in advance of LHRH agonists, but others have found no difference in PSA levels with simultaneous administration of both agents.[23] As such, antiandrogen preadministration or coadministration is required for only 21 to 28 days.

Androgen Synthesis Inhibitors

Although surgical castration prevents androgen production from the testes, other sources of androgen production from the adrenal glands and PCa cells continue to secrete androgens. Therefore, androgen synthesis inhibitors, such as ketoconazole and abiraterone acetate, were developed to inhibit androgens biosynthesis. Both drugs are cytochrome p450 enzyme 17R-hydroxylase-17, 20 lyase (CYP 17A1) inhibitors preventing androgen and glucocorticoid synthesis.[6,24] Accordingly, prednisone is usually administered in combination with ketoconazole or abiraterone to prevent adrenal insufficiency. Per American Urological Association guidelines, ketoconazole may be offered to patients with metastatic castration-resistant prostate cancer (mCRPC) unwilling to receive standard therapy or when therapy is unavailable.[25] However, ketoconazole is not FDA approved for this indication and does not offer survival benefit. In addition, because of its non-selective inhibition, ketoconazole has several side effects (**Table 1**). In contrast, abiraterone acetate has a nonsteroidal core, which increases its selectivity to CYP17, thereby reducing treatment-associated adverse events.[24]

Abiraterone acetate
Abiraterone acetate is the only FDA-approved androgen synthesis inhibitor.[24] Based on the IMAAGEN study, abiraterone acetate plus prednisone and continuous ADT (CADT) demonstrated greater than or equal to 50% reduction in PSA in patients with non-metastatic CRPC (nmCRPC) at high risk for developing metastatic disease.[25,26] These findings are promising especially that abiraterone may be more cost-effective and accessible.[27] Among men with mCRPC, abiraterone with prednisone has been shown to be effective among those who priorly received docetaxel (COU-AA-301)[28,29] and in docetaxel naïve patients (COU-AA-302).[30] Although COU-AA-301 included men with an Eastern Cooperative Oncology Group (ECOG) performance status of less than or equal to 2, COU-AA-302 was restricted to men with ECOG of less than or equal to 1. In patients with mCRPC who received chemotherapy, abiraterone increased overall survival (OS) (14.8 vs 10.9 months), time to PSA progression (10.2 vs 6.6 months), PFS (5.6 months vs 3.6 months), and PSA response rate (29% vs 6%) in comparison to placebo.[29] In patients with docetaxel-naïve mCRPC, abiraterone also improved OS and PFS by 8.3 and 4.4 months, respectively.[30]

More recently, the LATITUDE trial investigated the role of ADT, abiraterone acetate, and prednisone versus ADT alone in newly diagnosed metastatic castration-sensitive prostate cancer (mCSPC). The combination treatment had improved OS (HR 0.62; 95% CI, 0.51–0.76) and radiographic PFS (HR 0.47; 95% CI, 0.39–0.55). Subsequently, abiraterone acetate was FDA approved for patients with high-risk mCSPC.[6,25] On the other hand, the STAMPEDE trial was designed to study the earlier use of abiraterone acetate in men with newly diagnosed PCa, initiating long-term ADT.[31] The cohort included patients with metastatic diseases (52%) and another node-positive or node-indeterminate non-metastatic prostate cancer (20%).[31] Patients were randomized to either ADT or ADT with abiraterone and prednisone. The combination group had improved OS (HR 0.63; 95% CI, 0.52–0.76) and decreased risk of biochemical recurrence (HR 0.29; 95% CI, 0.25–0.34).[31]

Androgen Receptor Blockers

First-generation androgen receptor blockers
Androgens secreted by the testes and the adrenals get converted to dihydrotestosterone (DHT) through the enzyme 5-alpha reductase found in prostate cells. In order to get activated, the AR binds to DHT, resulting in the dissociation of AR chaperons, AR homodimerization, and ultimately translocation of the complex into the nucleus.[24] Once in the nucleus, it acts as a transcription factor to modulate the expression of androgen responsive genes including PSA.[24] Thus, blocking AR is another way to achieve therapeutic castration. When used alone, these agents increase LH and testosterone levels. Although increased testosterone levels might preserve potency, its peripheral aromatization leads to gynecomastia and mastodynia, among other side effects (see **Table 1**).[32]

The first-generation antiandrogens are steroidal analogues that bind to the AR and prevent its translocation to the nucleus.[24] These include bicalutamide, nilutamide, and flutamide. First-generation antiandrogens are associated with increased resistance (Section 3.2). The same phenomenon might also explain the antiandrogen withdrawal syndrome (AWS), which is when the cessation of first-generation antiandrogens in patients whose metastatic cancer has become refractory is associated with decreased PSA levels and clinical improvement.[33] With AWS, PSA drops between 15% and 30%, and the median clinical response lasts between 3 and 6 months.[33,34] Flutamide,[35] bicalutamide,[36] and nilutamide[37] are rarely used in contemporary practice due to discouraging randomized controlled trials (RCTs). Nevertheless, due to increased resistance to first-generation antiandrogens, second-generation antiandrogens with new mode of action were devised.

Second-generation androgen receptor blockers
The second-generation AR blockers include enzalutamide, apalutamide, and darolutamide.[24] Their mode of action is 3-fold: (1) inhibit DHT binding to androgen receptors, (2) prevent translocation of the DHT-AR complex into the nucleus, and (3) inhibit the complex's binding and activation of DNA.[38] In contrast to the first-generation drugs, second-generation antiandrogens have a higher affinity, act solely as antagonists, and are rarely associated with AWS.[24,39] Nevertheless, their

Table 1
Summary of hormone therapy for prostate cancer

ADT Type	Route	Mechanism of Action	Clinical Trial	Treatment Line	Side Effects	Comments	References
LHRH Antagonist							
Degarelix	Injection	Competitive inhibitor of LHRH receptors	17	Advanced PCa	Injection site reactions and chills	No flare, lower CV events than leuprolide with relugolix	17,18,114
Relugolix	Oral		HERO (NCT03085095)		Hot flashes, diarrhea		19
LHRH Agonist							
Leuprolide Goserelin Triptorelin Histrelin	Injection	Desensitization of LHRH receptors after chronic exposure to LHRH agonist	Systematic review of 24 trials		More cardiovascular and cerebrovascular events than LHRH antagonists.	AWS; preadministration or coadministration of antiandrogens	20–23,115
First-Generation Antiandrogens							
Bicalutamide Nilutamide Flutamide	Oral	Bind to AR preventing its translocation to the nucleus	36 37 35	Not used in contemporary practice	Gynecomastia, mastodynia, diarrhea, hepatitis, interstitial pneumonitis; delayed adaption to darkness with nilutamide	Elevated resistance; AWS	32,116–119
Second-Generation Antiandrogens							
Androgen Synthesis Inhibitor							
Abiraterone acetate	Oral	Androgenesis inhibition via CYP17A1 blockade	COU-AA-301 COU-AA-302 LATTITUDE STAMPEDE	CT treated and naive mCRPC mCSPC nmPCa & mPCa	Mineralocorticoid excess, hypokalemia, hypertension, LFT elevation, insulin resistance, hyperglycemia	With prednisone, CI in severe hepatic impairment	24,25,28,30,31,113
Ketoconazole	Oral	Non-selective CYP 450 inhibitor		mCRPC unwilling to receive standard therapy	Neuropathy, ototoxicity, fatigue, grade 3/4 hepatotoxicity	Administered with prednisone	25,120

Androgen Receptor Blockers

Drug	Route	Mechanism	Trials	Indication	Side effects	Notes	References
Enzalutamide	Oral	Inhibits DHT binding to AR, prevents translocation of the DHT AR complex into the nucleus, inhibits the complex's binding and activation of DNA	AFFIRM PREVAIL PROSPER ARCHES—ENZAMET	mCRPC after CT failure mCRPC before CT nmCRPC mCSPC	Hypertension, seizure, fatigue, diarrhea, hot flashes, depression	Seizure risk highest with enzalutamide	38,44,45,112,121
Apalutamide	Oral		SPARTAN TITAN	nmCRPC mCSPC	Hypothyroidism, seizure, skin rash, fatigue		48,49
Darolutamide	Oral		ARAMIS	nmCRPC	fatigue		28

Abbreviations: AWS, androgen withdrawal syndrome; CV, cardiovascular; CT chemotherapy; CI, contraindicated; DHT, dihydrotestosterone; LFT, liver function test.

penetrance through the blood-brain barrier puts the patient at risk of seizure by blocking cerebral gamma-aminobutyric acid (GABA) receptors[40]; this is most notable with enzalutamide, but less common with apalutamide and even less with darolutamide.[24]

Enzalutamide binds to the AR with 5 to 8 times higher affinity than bicalutamide.[41] Combination therapy for ADT and enzalutamide was investigated among men with mCSPC in the ARCHES trial. CADT and enzalutamide compared with CADT and placebo was associated with improved radiographic PFS (HR 0.39; 95% CI, 0.30–0.50; P < .001), time to castration resistance (HR 0.28; 0.22–0.36; P < .001), time to initiation of new antineoplastic therapy (HR 0.28; 0.20–0.40; P < .001), and time to first symptomatic skeletal event (HR 0.52; 0.33–0.80; P = .0026).[42] The ENZAMET trial also showed reduced mortality, improved PSA PFS, and improved clinical PFS with enzalutamide and CADT versus standard non-steroidal antiandrogen therapy.[43]

Among patients with CRPC, the AFFIRM trial has demonstrated improved OS with enzalutamide after chemotherapy failure (HR 0.63; 95% CI, 0.53–0.75; P < .001), whereas the PREVAIL trial confirmed the beneficial role of enzalutamide before chemotherapy administration. The PREVAIL trial also showed improved 12-month radiographic-free survival (HR 0.91; 95% CI, 0.15–0.23) and OS (HR 0.71; 95% CI, 0.60–0.84).[44,45] Enzalutamide has also been shown to be effective for nmCRPC, as it proved to be associated with metastasis-free survival (PROSPER Trial).[46] Side effects of enzalutamide are discussed in **Table 1**.[44,45]

Apalutamide is a nonsteroidal antiandrogen synthetic biaryl thiohydantoin that was discovered when looking for potent molecules with sole antagonistic activity against AR.[47] It is a selective and competitive AR inhibitor with 7 to 10 times bicalutamide's affinity.[47] The SPARTAN and TITAN trials have demonstrated efficacy of apalutamide in nmCRPC and mCSPC, respectively.[10,11] Patients with nmCRPC who received apalutamide had an improved metastasis-free survival compared with 16.2 months in the placebo arm (HR of metastasis or death 0.28; 95% CI, 0.23–0.35).[48] When comparing the AFFIRM and the SPARTAN trials, which both included men with a history of seizure, the risk of seizure with apalutamide was lower than enzalutamide (0.2 vs 0.6%).[44,48] In the TITAN trial, men with mCSPC were randomized to ADT with apalutamide or ADT and placebo. The intervention group had superior 24-month radiographic PFS and decreased mortality (HR 0.48; 95% CI, 0.39–0.60).[49] The side effects were comparable between the 2 arms.[49]

Darolutamide was approved by the FDA in 2019 with fast track designation for use in nmCRPC.[24] It is an AR antagonist for not only the wild-type AR but also for AR mutations known to cause an antagonist-agonist switch with bicalutamide, enzalutamide, and apalutamide.[24,50,51] The ARAMIS trial randomized men with nmCRPC to darolutamide or placebo; the darolutamide arm had a longer median metastasis-free survival (40.4 vs 18.4 months) and reduced metastasis or mortality (HR 0.41; 95% CI, 0.34–0.50).[52] Thanks to its lower penetration through the blood-brain barrier and its lower binding affinity to GABA type A receptors, darolutamide has less neurotoxicity than other antiandrogens, which might explain the lower incidence of falls and fractures (4.2%)[52] compared with apalutamide (15.6%)[48] and enzalutamide (17.0%).[53]

DISCUSSION
Side Effects and Adverse Events

Endocrine

ADT is associated with several adverse events including endocrine, cardiovascular, and sexual side effects among other symptoms affecting men's quality of life (QoL).[54] In fact, the duration of ADT treatment is correlated with decreased bone mineral density (BMD)[55] and an increased risk of bone fracture independently of age, race, and presence of metastasis.[56] Although theoretically a longer exposure to ADT could increase the risk of fractures, intermittent ADT (IADT) did not reduce bone events when compared with CADT but resulted in small improvements in QoL.[57] Multiple strategies are being implemented to reduce BMD loss and bone fractures. Moderate physical activity for at least 150 minutes weekly or vigorous physical activity for 75 minutes is recommended for PCa survivors, as it can mitigate several of the side effects of hormone treatment including skeletal-related events.[58] In addition, to avoid side effects of ADT, urologists should collaborate with primary care providers to obtain the necessary screening. A baseline bone densitometry should be obtained to assess for fracture risk.[58,59] According to the National Comprehensive Cancer Network (NCCN) guidelines, men on ADT would benefit from daily calcium (1000–1200 mg) and vitamin D (400–1000 IU) from food or supplements.[60] In addition, bisphosphonates are efficacious in preserving BMD and decreasing the risk of fractures.[61] In fact, the administration of denosumab (60 mg every 6 months), zoledronic acid (5 mg intravenously annually), and alendronate (70 mg orally weekly) increased BMD in men on ADT at risk of fracture (T-score is between

−1.0 and −2.0 at the femoral neck, total hip, or lumbar spine by DEXA scan or the 10-year fracture risk is >20% for any fracture or >3% for hip fracture).[60]

Metabolic syndrome

The use of ADT increases the risk of metabolic syndrome (risk ratio [RR] 1.75; 95% CI, 1.17–2.41) and non-alcoholic fatty liver disease.[62,63] Men on ADT tend to gain fat mass at the expense of muscle mass[64] due to increase in appetite, insulin levels, and abdominal girth secondary to low testosterone levels.[65] Predictors of weight gain included age younger than 65 years, body mass index less than 30 kg/m^2, and non-diabetic status.[65,66] What is more, ADT decreases insulin sensitivity, leading to diabetes mellitus.[67] These findings are observed with both GnRH agonists (adjusted HR [aHR] 1.44; 95% CI, 1.34–1.55) and orchiectomy (aHR 1.34%; 95% CI, 1.20–1.50).[68] Other studies demonstrated that ADT treatment increases total cholesterol (3.2%–10.6%) and triglycerides (3.8%–46.6%).[09–72] Only one study evaluated the lipid profile according to ADT modality and found no difference between GnRH agonists alone and maximal androgen blockade with bicalutamide.[70] Nevertheless, the incidence of metabolic syndrome was low in patients treated with IADT.[73]

Cardiovascular

Hormone treatment is also associated with cardiovascular diseases (CVD), which could be due to a myriad of causes including (1) large artery stiffening resulting in increase in central arterial pressure,[71] (2) fibrous cap disruption and plaque destabilization by activated T cells that express GnRH receptors,[74] and (3) cardiac receptor stimulation with GnRH agonist activity disrupting the heart's contractility.[75] Other side effects include peripheral artery disease and venous thromboembolism.[76] These changes put patients with PCa at risk of CVD; however, the association between ADT and cardiovascular mortality is still controversial. Keating and colleagues found that men receiving LHRH agonists had a 16% increased risk of coronary heart disease, 11% increased risk of myocardial infarction, and 16% increased risk of sudden cardiac death.[60] There is also evidence that the risk of CVD depends the type of ADT and is most prominent among men older than 74 years, those who received ADT greater than 2 years, and those with history of CVD.[77–80] Nevertheless, a meta-analysis of RCTs in 2011 found no difference between ADT and control (RR 0.93; 95% CI, 0.79–1.10).[81] Similarly, a comparative study between IADT and CADT showed no difference in either cardiovascular events (RR 0.95, 95% CI, 0.83–1.08) or thromboembolic events (RR 1.05, 95% CI, 0.85–1.30); however, patients on IADT had borderline lower cardiovascular-related mortality (RR 0.85, 95% CI, 0.71–1.00).[82]

The NCCN guidelines recommend an ABCDE approach to promote cardiovascular wellness. It encompasses Awareness and Assessment for CVD, Blood pressure monitoring and management, Cholesterol management and Cigarette cessation, Diet and Diabetes management, as well as Exercise and Echocardiogram and/or EKG.[60]

Sexual dysfunction

Sexual dysfunction is seen in up to 90% of men receiving ADT.[83] ADT reduces testosterone levels, significantly leading to a 6-fold decrease in libido and a 3-fold increase in erectile dysfunction.[84] Hormone treatment is also associated with decreased penile length and testicular size, causing more sexual distress.[85] Although low libido treatment is difficult and oral phosphodiesterase-5 inhibitors may not be effective, the use of intraurethral suppositories, intracavernosal injections, or inflatable penile prosthesis can be effective in select patients. In addition, IADT allows testosterone levels recovery between treatment cycles, leading to an improvement in sexual desire and erectile function.[86]

Cognitive dysfunction and quality of life

QoL is severely affected in patients treated with ADT. Men may report alteration in their mental and general health as well as energy, activity, and body image.[87] In fact, the reduction of serum testosterone levels induces vasomotor flushing, fatigue, reduced cognition, mood impairment, insomnia, and anemia.[88] Patients with low testosterone are at increased risk of depression and anxiety,[89–91] and short-term ADT (< 6 months) does not seem to improve the QoL.[92] Moreover, men on ADT are at risk of all-cause dementia (HR 1.17; 95% CI, 1.07–1.27), Alzheimer (HR 1.23; 95% CI, 1.11–1.37), and 10% higher risk of psychiatric services use (HR 1.10; 95% CI, 1.00–1.22).[93–95] Other symptoms such as hot flushes can be bothersome and are mainly managed conservatively.[96] Second-line therapy includes venlafaxine, cyproterone acetate, and medroxyprogesterone, which may reduce the frequency and severity of these symptoms.[97] Lifestyle changes such as dietary corrections and physical exercises are the most studied to improve patient-reported outcomes.[98] In a systematic review including 17 RCTs, Menichetti and colleagues showed that supervised resistance training programs yielded the greatest impact on QoL, followed by dietary interventions combined with lifestyle interventions.[99]

Androgen Deprivation Therapy Resistance

Although most of the patients initially respond to standard ADT (LHRH agonists and antagonist), most will become castrate-resistant within 2 to 3 years.[100] For nmCRPC, the Prostate Cancer Clinical Trial Working Group 3 recommends following PSA doubling time but suggests monitoring PSA increase—PSA increase that is greater than or equal to 25% and more than or equal to 2 ng/mL above the nadir confirmed by a second value more than or equal to 3 weeks later—for mCRPC. One or more mechanisms may be implicated in resistance including AR amplifications, incomplete blockade of AR-ligand signaling, and AR mutations.[101] AR amplification increases the level of AR protein, sensitizing the AR signaling pathway to lower levels of androgens.[102] Alternatively, AR mutations in the ligand-binding domain lead to a decreased specificity of AR–ligand interaction, allowing alternative steroidal molecules (estrogens, corticosteroids, and progesterone) to activate AR.[103,104] This phenomenon explains tumor progression independently of androgen stimulation.

Testosterone Measurement

Although there is no clear consensus, men on ADT could undergo serum testosterone measurements every 3 months to assess the response to ADT and the potential of IADT benefit.[82] In addition, serum testosterone levels during ADT treatment have a prognostic value. In fact, patients with serum testosterone less than or equal to 0.7 nmol/L within the first year of ADT have the best cancer-specific survival, whereas levels greater than or equal to 1.7 nmol/L predicted increased mortality.[105] In another study that examined the prognostic value of baseline testosterone in men with hormone naïve PCa, the investigators found that a lower baseline testosterone level was correlated with improved survival (HR 0.76; 95% CI, 0.63–0.91) in men treated with CADT.[106]

Prostate-Specific Antigen Measurement

PSA, a serine protease, is produced by the epithelial cells of the prostatic gland and is regulated by circulating androgens via AR.[107] Thus, ADT results in decreased PSA levels. PSA can be measured every 6 to 12 months and then annually.[60] More frequent testing could be done in men at high risk of recurrence.[60] PSA levels also have prognostic significance. It was shown that PSA levels less than or equal to 4 ng/mL after 7 months of ADT is a predictor of survival.[108] Nevertheless, relying solely on PSA levels is an inadequate strategy in mCSPC monitoring, as radiographic progression can occur before or even with slight changes in PSA levels.[109]

Drug–Drug Interaction

PCa is a disease of the adults and the elderly who are more likely to be taking medications for other causes. Hence, clinicians administering ADT should be aware of drug–drug interactions. For instance, abiraterone acetate, a CYP17 irreversible blocker, is also a substrate of CYP3A4. Therefore, CYP3A4 inducers (rifampicin) and CYP3A4 inhibitors (erythromycin) would require higher and lower doses of abiraterone, respectively.[110] Moreover, abiraterone acetate inhibits CYP2C8 and CYP2D6, leading to increased plasma levels of amitriptyline, oxycodone, risperidone, amiodarone, and carbamazepine.[111] On the other hand, enzalutamide is a strong CYP3A4 and a moderate CYP2C19 and CYP2C9 inducer.[112] As a result, plasma levels of enzyme substrates such as disopyramide, quetiapine, quinidine, and warfarin would decrease.[111] Moreover, because enzalutamide is metabolized by CYP2C8, its dose should be reduced if coadministered with CYP2C inhibitors (ie, gemfibrozil and pioglitazone).[111] In addition, abiraterone acetate is contraindicated in patients with severe hepatic impairment because it is metabolized by the liver.[113] In contrast, enzalutamide is excreted in the urine, and its clearance is not affected by renal impairment.[112]

DISCLOSURE

Q-D. Trinh reports personal fees from Astellas, Bayer, and Janssen, outside the submitted work. Q-D. Trinh and A.P. Cole report research funding from the American Cancer Society, the Defense Health Agency, Pfizer Global Medical Grants. A. S. Kibel reports advisory board positions on hormone treatment of prostate cancer with Janssen and Myovant and advisory board positions in the realm of prostate cancer with Bayer, Profound, Insightec, and Exlexis. ASK is also part of the Data Safety and Monitoring Committee with Bristol Myers Squibb and Advantage. All other authors report no conflict of interest.

REFERENCES

1. Siegel RL, Miller KD, Fuchs HE, et al. Cancer Statistics, 2021. CA: A Cancer J Clinicians 2021; 71(1):7–33. https://doi.org/10.3322/caac.21654.

2. Huggins C. Prostatic cancer treated by orchiectomy: the five year results. J Am Med Assoc 1946;131(7):576–81.

3. Huggins CB. Nobel Lecture. 23 Apr 2021. Available at: https://www.nobelprize.org/prizes/medicine/1966/huggins/lecture/.

4. Bolla M, Collette L, Blank L, et al. Long-term results with immediate androgen suppression and external irradiation in patients with locally advanced prostate cancer (an EORTC study): a phase III randomised trial. Lancet 2002; 360(9327):103–6.

5. Meng MV, Grossfeld GD, Sadetsky N, et al. Contemporary patterns of androgen deprivation therapy use for newly diagnosed prostate cancer. Urology 2002;60(3 Suppl 1):7–11.

6. Crawford ED, Heidenreich A, Lawrentschuk N, et al. Androgen-targeted therapy in men with prostate cancer: evolving practice and future considerations. Prostate Cancer prostatic Dis 2019;22(1): 24–38.

7. McClintock TR, von Landenberg N, Cole AP, et al. Neoadjuvant Androgen Deprivation Therapy Prior to Radical Prostatectomy: Recent Trends in Utilization and Association with Postoperative Surgical Margin Status. Ann Surg Oncol 2019;26(1): 297–305.

8. Feldman AS, Meyer CP, Sanchez A, et al. Morbidity and Mortality of Locally Advanced Prostate Cancer: A Population Based Analysis Comparing Radical Prostatectomy versus External Beam Radiation. J Urol 2017;198(5):1061–8.

9. Tolkach Y, Joniau S, Van Poppel H. Luteinizing hormone-releasing hormone (LHRH) receptor agonists vs antagonists: a matter of the receptors? BJU Int 2013;111(7):1021–30.

10. Lowrance WT, Breau RH, Chou R, et al. Advanced Prostate Cancer: AUA/ASTRO/SUO Guideline PART I. J Urol 2021;205(1):14–21.

11. Lowrance WT, Breau RH, Chou R, et al. Advanced Prostate Cancer: AUA/ASTRO/SUO Guideline PART II. J Urol 2021;205(1):22–9.

12. Heidenreich A, Bastian PJ, Bellmunt J, et al. EAU guidelines on prostate cancer. Part II: Treatment of advanced, relapsing, and castration-resistant prostate cancer. Eur Urol 2014;65(2):467–79.

13. Weckermann D, Harzmann R. Hormone Therapy in Prostate Cancer: LHRH Antagonists versus LHRH Analogues. Eur Urol 2004;46(3):279–84.

14. Lamharzi N, Halmos G, Jungwirth A, et al. Decrease in the level and mRNA expression of LH-RH and EGF receptors after treatment with LH-RH antagonist cetrorelix in DU-145 prostate tumor xenografts in nude mice. Int J Oncol 1998. https://doi.org/10.3892/ijo.13.3.429.

15. Koch M, Steidle C, Brosman S, et al. An open-label study of abarelix in men with symptomatic prostate cancer at risk of treatment with LHRH agonists. Urology 2003;62(5):877–82.

16. Gittelman M, Pommerville PJ, Persson B-E, et al. A 1-Year, Open Label, Randomized Phase II Dose Finding Study of Degarelix for the Treatment of Prostate Cancer in North America. J Urol 2008; 180(5):1986–92.

17. Klotz L, Boccon-Gibod L, Shore ND, et al. The efficacy and safety of degarelix: a 12-month, comparative, randomized, open-label, parallel-group phase III study in patients with prostate cancer. BJU Int 2008;102(11):1531–8.

18. Crawford ED, Tombal B, Miller K, et al. A Phase III Extension Trial With a 1-Arm Crossover From Leuprolide to Degarelix: Comparison of Gonadotropin-Releasing Hormone Agonist and Antagonist Effect on Prostate Cancer. J Urol 2011;186(3):889–97.

19. Shore ND, Saad F, Cookson MS, et al. Oral Relugolix for Androgen-Deprivation Therapy in Advanced Prostate Cancer. N Engl J Med 2020;382(23): 2187–96.

20. Seidenfeld J, Samson DJ, Hasselblad V, et al. Single-therapy androgen suppression in men with advanced prostate cancer: a systematic review and meta-analysis. Ann Intern Med 2000;132(7): 566–77.

21. Brawer MK. Challenges with luteinizing hormone-releasing hormone agonists: flare and surge. Rev Urol 2004;6(Suppl 7):S12–8.

22. Schulze H, Senge T. Influence of Different Types of Antiandrogens on Luteinizing Hormone-Releasing Hormone Analogue-Induced Testosterone Surge in Patients with Metastatic Carcinoma of the Prostate. J Urol 1990;144(4):934–41.

23. Tsushima T, Nasu Y, Saika T, et al. Optimal Starting Time for Flutamide to Prevent Disease Flare in Prostate Cancer Patients Treated with a Gonadotropin-Releasing Hormone Agonist. Urologia Int 2001;66(3):135–9.

24. Rice MA, Malhotra SV, Stoyanova T. Second-Generation Antiandrogens: From Discovery to Standard of Care in Castration Resistant Prostate Cancer. Review. Front Oncol 2019;9(801).

25. Lowrance WT, Murad MH, Oh WK, et al. Castration-Resistant Prostate Cancer: AUA Guideline Amendment 2018. J Urol 2018;200(6):1264–72.

26. Ryan CJ, Crawford ED, Shore ND, et al. The IMAAGEN Study: Effect of Abiraterone Acetate and Prednisone on Prostate Specific Antigen and Radiographic Disease Progression in Patients with Nonmetastatic Castration Resistant Prostate Cancer. J Urol 2018;200(2):344–52.

27. Klaassen Z, Wallis CJD, Fleshner NE. Abiraterone Acetate for Nonmetastatic Castration-Resistant Prostate Cancer—The Forgotten Dance Partner? JAMA Oncol 2019;5(2):144–5.

28. Fizazi K, Scher HI, Molina A, et al. Abiraterone acetate for treatment of metastatic castration-resistant prostate cancer: final overall survival analysis of the COU-AA-301 randomised, double-blind, placebo-controlled phase 3 study. Lancet Oncol 2012;13(10):983–92.

29. de Bono JS, Logothetis CJ, Molina A, et al. Abiraterone and Increased Survival in Metastatic Prostate Cancer. N Engl J Med 2011;364(21): 1995–2005.

30. Ryan CJ, Smith MR, de Bono JS, et al. Abiraterone in Metastatic Prostate Cancer without Previous Chemotherapy. New Engl J Med 2012;368(2): 138–48.

31. James ND, de Bono JS, Spears MR, et al. Abiraterone for Prostate Cancer Not Previously Treated with Hormone Therapy. New Engl J Med 2017;377(4): 338–51.

32. Knuth UA, Hano R, Nieschlag E. Effect of flutamide or cyproterone acetate on pituitary and testicular hormones in normal men. J Clin Endocrinol Metab 1984;59(5):963–9.

33. Paul R, Breul J. Antiandrogen Withdrawal Syndrome Associated with Prostate Cancer Therapies. Drug Saf 2000;23(5):381–90.

34. Small EJ, Srinivas S. The antiandrogen withdrawal syndrome. Experience in a large cohort of unselected patients with advanced prostate cancer. Cancer 1995;76(8):1428–34. https://doi.org/10. 1002/1097-0142(19951015)76:8<1428::AID-CNCR2 820760820>3.0.CO.

35. Chang A, Yeap B, Davis T, et al. Double-blind, randomized study of primary hormonal treatment of stage D2 prostate carcinoma: flutamide versus diethylstilbestrol. J Clin Oncol 1996;14(8):2250–7.

36. Iversen P, McLeod DG, See WA, et al. Antiandrogen monotherapy in patients with localized or locally advanced prostate cancer: final results from the bicalutamide Early Prostate Cancer programme at a median follow-up of 9.7 years. BJU Int 2010;105(8):1074–81.

37. Mahler C, Verhelst J, Denis L. Clinical pharmacokinetics of the antiandrogens and their efficacy in prostate cancer. Clin Pharm 1998;34(5):405–17.

38. Schalken J, Fitzpatrick JM. Enzalutamide: targeting the androgen signalling pathway in metastatic castration-resistant prostate cancer. BJU Int 2016; 117(2):215–25. https://doi.org/10.1111/bju.13123.

39. Rodriguez-Vida A, Bianchini D, Van Hemelrijck M, et al. Is there an antiandrogen withdrawal syndrome with enzalutamide? BJU Int 2015;115(3): 373–80.

40. Antonarakis ES. Enzalutamide: The emperor of all anti-androgens. Transl Androl Urol 2013;2(2): 119–20.

41. Tran C, Ouk S, Clegg NJ, et al. Development of a second-generation antiandrogen for treatment of

42. Armstrong AJ, Szmulewitz RZ, Petrylak DP, et al. ARCHES: A Randomized, Phase III Study of Androgen Deprivation Therapy With Enzalutamide or Placebo in Men With Metastatic Hormone-Sensitive Prostate Cancer. J Clin Oncol 2019; 37(32):2974–86.

43. Davis ID, Martin AJ, Stockler MR, et al. Enzalutamide with Standard First-Line Therapy in Metastatic Prostate Cancer. New Engl J Med 2019;381(2): 121–31.

44. Scher HI, Fizazi K, Saad F, et al. Increased Survival with Enzalutamide in Prostate Cancer after Chemotherapy. New Engl J Med 2012;367(13):1187–97.

45. Beer TM, Armstrong AJ, Rathkopf DE, et al. Enzalutamide in Metastatic Prostate Cancer before Chemotherapy. New Engl J Med 2014;371(5): 424–33.

46. Tombal B, Saad F, Penson D, et al. Patient-reported outcomes following enzalutamide or placebo in men with non-metastatic, castration-resistant prostate cancer (PROSPER): a multicentre, randomised, double-blind, phase 3 trial. Lancet Oncol 2019;20(4):556–69.

47. Rathkopf DE, Scher HI. Apalutamide for the treatment of prostate cancer. Expert Rev Anticancer Ther 2018;18(9):823–36.

48. Smith MR, Saad F, Chowdhury S, et al. Apalutamide Treatment and Metastasis-free Survival in Prostate Cancer. New Engl J Med 2018;378(15): 1408–18.

49. Chi KN, Agarwal N, Bjartell A, et al. Apalutamide for Metastatic, Castration-Sensitive Prostate Cancer. New Engl J Med 2019;381(1):13–24.

50. Moilanen A-M, Riikonen R, Oksala R, et al. Discovery of ODM-201, a new-generation androgen receptor inhibitor targeting resistance mechanisms to androgen signaling-directed prostate cancer therapies. Scientific Rep 2015;5(1):12007.

51. Fizazi K, Albiges L, Loriot Y, et al. ODM-201: a new-generation androgen receptor inhibitor in castration-resistant prostate cancer. Expert Rev Anticancer Ther 2015;15(9):1007–17.

52. Fizazi K, Shore N, Tammela TL, et al. Darolutamide in Nonmetastatic, Castration-Resistant Prostate Cancer. New Engl J Med 2019;380(13):1235–46.

53. Hussain M, Fizazi K, Saad F, et al. Enzalutamide in Men with Nonmetastatic, Castration-Resistant Prostate Cancer. New Engl J Med 2018;378(26): 2465–74.

54. Perera M, Roberts MJ, Klotz L, et al. Intermittent versus continuous androgen deprivation therapy for advanced prostate cancer. Nat Rev Urol 2020; 17(8):469–81.

55. Berruti A, Dogliotti L, Terrone C, et al. Changes in bone mineral density, lean body mass and fat

advanced prostate cancer. Science 2009; 324(5928):787–90.

content as measured by dual energy x-ray absorptiometry in patients with prostate cancer without apparent bone metastases given androgen deprivation therapy. J Urol 2002;167(6):2361–7.

56. Shahinian VB, Kuo YF, Freeman JL, et al. Risk of fracture after androgen deprivation for prostate cancer. N Engl J Med 2005;352(2):154–64.

57. Hershman DL, Unger JM, Wright JD, et al. Adverse Health Events Following Intermittent and Continuous Androgen Deprivation in Patients With Metastatic Prostate Cancer. JAMA Oncol 2016;2(4):453–61.

58. Gralow JR, Biermann JS, Farooki A, et al. NCCN Task Force Report: Bone Health In Cancer Care. J Natl Compr Canc Netw 2013;11(Suppl 3):S1–50. quiz S51.

59. Shahinian VB, Kuo YF. Patterns of bone mineral density testing in men receiving androgen deprivation for prostate cancer. J Gen Intern Med 2013; 28(11):1440–6.

60. Schaeffer E, Srinivas S, Antonarakis ES, et al. NCCN Guidelines Insights: Prostate Cancer, Version 1.2021. J Natl Compr Canc Netw 2021; 19(2):134–43.

61. Serpa Neto A, Tobias-Machado M, Esteves MA, et al. Bisphosphonate therapy in patients under androgen deprivation therapy for prostate cancer: a systematic review and meta-analysis. Prostate Cancer Prostatic Dis 2012;15(1):36–44.

62. Bosco C, Crawley D, Adolfsson J, et al. Quantifying the Evidence for the Risk of Metabolic Syndrome and Its Components following Androgen Deprivation Therapy for Prostate Cancer: A Meta-Analysis. PLOS ONE 2015;10(3):e0117344.

63. Gild P, Cole AP, Krasnova A, et al. Liver Disease in Men Undergoing Androgen Deprivation Therapy for Prostate Cancer. J Urol 2018;200(3):573–81.

64. van Londen GJ, Levy ME, Perera S, et al. Body composition changes during androgen deprivation therapy for prostate cancer: a 2-year prospective study. Crit Rev Oncol Hematol 2008;68(2):172–7.

65. Seidell JC, Björntorp P, Sjöström L, et al. Visceral fat accumulation in men is positively associated with insulin, glucose, and C-peptide levels, but negatively with testosterone levels. Metabolism 1990;39(9):897–901.

66. Seible DM, Gu X, Hyatt AS, et al. Weight gain on androgen deprivation therapy: which patients are at highest risk? Urology 2014;83(6):1316–21.

67. Smith MR, Lee H, Nathan DM. Insulin sensitivity during combined androgen blockade for prostate cancer. J Clin Endocrinol Metab 2006;91(4):1305–8.

68. Keating NL, O'Malley AJ, Smith MR. Diabetes and cardiovascular disease during androgen deprivation therapy for prostate cancer. J Clin Oncol 2006;24(27):4448–56.

69. Dockery F, Bulpitt CJ, Agarwal S, et al. Testosterone suppression in men with prostate cancer leads to an increase in arterial stiffness and hyperinsulinaemia. Clin Sci (Lond) 2003;104(2):195–201.

70. Salvador C, Planas J, Agreda F, et al. Analysis of the lipid profile and atherogenic risk during androgen deprivation therapy in prostate cancer patients. Urol Int 2013;90(1):41–4.

71. Smith JC, Bennett S, Evans LM, et al. The effects of induced hypogonadism on arterial stiffness, body composition, and metabolic parameters in males with prostate cancer. J Clin Endocrinol Metab 2001;86(9):4261–7.

72. Smith MR, Finkelstein JS, McGovern FJ, et al. Changes in body composition during androgen deprivation therapy for prostate cancer. J Clin Endocrinol Metab 2002;87(2):599–603.

73. Rezaei MM, Rezaei MM, Ghoreifi A, et al. Metabolic syndrome in patients with prostate cancer undergoing intermittent androgen-deprivation therapy. Can Urol Assoc J 2016;10(9–10):E300–5.

74. O'Farrell S, Garmo H, Holmberg L, et al. Risk and timing of cardiovascular disease after androgen-deprivation therapy in men with prostate cancer. J Clin Oncol 2015;33(11):1243–51.

75. Dong F, Skinner DC, Wu TJ, et al. The heart: a novel gonadotrophin-releasing hormone target. J Neuroendocrinol 2011;23(5):456–63.

76. Hu JC, Williams SB, O'Malley AJ, et al. Androgen-deprivation therapy for nonmetastatic prostate cancer is associated with an increased risk of peripheral arterial disease and venous thromboembolism. Eur Urol 2012;61(6):1119–28.

77. Morgans AK, Fan KH, Koyama T, et al. Influence of age on incident diabetes and cardiovascular disease in prostate cancer survivors receiving androgen deprivation therapy. J Urol 2015;193(4):1226–31.

78. Ziehr DR, Chen MH, Zhang D, et al. Association of androgen-deprivation therapy with excess cardiac-specific mortality in men with prostate cancer. BJU Int 2015;116(3):358–65.

79. Schmid M, Sammon JD, Reznor G, et al. Dose-dependent effect of androgen deprivation therapy for localized prostate cancer on adverse cardiac events. BJU Int 2016;118(2):221–9.

80. Cone EB, Marchese M, Reese SW, et al. Lower odds of cardiac events for gonadotrophin-releasing hormone antagonists versus agonists. BJU Int 2020;126(1):9–10.

81. Nguyen PL, Je Y, Schutz FA, et al. Association of androgen deprivation therapy with cardiovascular death in patients with prostate cancer: a meta-analysis of randomized trials. Jama 2011;306(21): 2359–66.

82. Jin C, Fan Y, Meng Y, et al. A meta-analysis of cardiovascular events in intermittent androgen-deprivation therapy versus continuous androgen-deprivation therapy for prostate cancer patients. Prostate Cancer Prostatic Dis 2016;19(4):333–9.

83. Higano CS. Sexuality and intimacy after definitive treatment and subsequent androgen deprivation therapy for prostate cancer. J Clin Oncol 2012; 30(30):3720–5.

84. Corona G, Filippi S, Comelio P, et al. Sexual function in men undergoing androgen deprivation therapy. Int J Impot Res 2021;33(4):439–47.

85. Parekh A, Chen MH, Hoffman KE, et al. Reduced penile size and treatment regret in men with recurrent prostate cancer after surgery, radiotherapy plus androgen deprivation, or radiotherapy alone. Urology 2013;81(1):130–4.

86. Hussain M, Tangen CM, Berry DL, et al. Intermittent versus continuous androgen deprivation in prostate cancer. N Engl J Med 2013;368(14):1314–25.

87. Fowler FJ Jr, McNaughton Collins M, Walker Corkery E, et al. The impact of androgen deprivation on quality of life after radical prostatectomy for prostate carcinoma. Cancer 2002;95(2): 287–95.

88. Teleni L, Chan RJ, Chan A, et al. Exercise improves quality of life in androgen deprivation therapy-treated prostate cancer: systematic review of randomised controlled trials. Endocr Relat Cancer 2016;23(2):101–12.

89. Nead KT, Gaskin G, Chester C, et al. Association Between Androgen Deprivation Therapy and Risk of Dementia. JAMA Oncol 2017;3(1):49–55.

90. Dinh KT, Yang DD, Nead KT, et al. Association between androgen deprivation therapy and anxiety among 78 000 patients with localized prostate cancer. Int J Urol 2017;24(10):743–8.

91. Dinh KT, Reznor G, Muralidhar V, et al. Association of Androgen Deprivation Therapy With Depression in Localized Prostate Cancer. J Clin Oncol 2016; 34(16):1905–12.

92. Dacal K, Sereika SM, Greenspan SL. Quality of life in prostate cancer patients taking androgen deprivation therapy. J Am Geriatr Soc 2006;54(1):85–90.

93. Krasnova A, Epstein M, Marchese M, et al. Risk of dementia following androgen deprivation therapy for treatment of prostate cancer. Prostate Cancer Prostatic Dis 2020;23(3):410–8.

94. Sun M, Cole AP, Hanna N, et al. Cognitive Impairment in Men with Prostate Cancer Treated with Androgen Deprivation Therapy: A Systematic Review and Meta-Analysis. J Urol 2018;199(6): 1417–25.

95. Tully KH, Nguyen DD, Herzog P, et al. Risk of Dementia and Depression in Young and Middle-aged Men Presenting with Nonmetastatic Prostate Cancer Treated with Androgen Deprivation Therapy. Eur Urol Oncol 2021;4(1):66–72.

96. Rhee H, Gunter JH, Heathcote P, et al. Adverse effects of androgen-deprivation therapy in prostate cancer and their management. BJU Int 2015; 115(Suppl 5):3–13.

97. Irani J, Salomon L, Oba R, et al. Efficacy of venlafaxine, medroxyprogesterone acetate, and cyproterone acetate for the treatment of vasomotor hot flushes in men taking gonadotropin-releasing hormone analogues for prostate cancer: a double-blind, randomised trial. Lancet Oncol 2010;11(2): 147–54.

98. Nabi J, Cone EB, Vasavada A, et al. Mobile Health App for Prostate Cancer Patients on Androgen Deprivation Therapy: Qualitative Usability Study. JMIR Mhealth Uhealth 2020;8(11):e20224.

99. Menichetti J, Villa S, Magnani T, et al. Lifestyle interventions to improve the quality of life of men with prostate cancer: A systematic review of randomized controlled trials. Crit Rev Oncol Hematol 2016;108:13–22.

100. Harris WP, Mostaghel EA, Nelson PS, et al. Androgen deprivation therapy: progress in understanding mechanisms of resistance and optimizing androgen depletion. Nat Clin Pract Urol 2009;6(2): 76–85.

101. Scher HI, Sawyers CL. Biology of progressive, castration-resistant prostate cancer: directed therapies targeting the androgen-receptor signaling axis. J Clin Oncol 2005;23(32):8253–61.

102. Edwards J, Krishna NS, Grigor KM, et al. Androgen receptor gene amplification and protein expression in hormone refractory prostate cancer. Br J Cancer 2003;89(3):552–6.

103. Culig Z, Hobisch A, Cronauer MV, et al. Mutant androgen receptor detected in an advanced-stage prostatic carcinoma is activated by adrenal androgens and progesterone. Mol Endocrinol 1993;7(12):1541–50.

104. Zhao XY, Malloy PJ, Krishnan AV, et al. Glucocorticoids can promote androgen-independent growth of prostate cancer cells through a mutated androgen receptor. Nat Med 2000;6(6):703–6.

105. Klotz L, O'Callaghan C, Ding K, et al. Nadir testosterone within first year of androgen-deprivation therapy (ADT) predicts for time to castration-resistant progression: a secondary analysis of the PR-7 trial of intermittent versus continuous ADT. J Clin Oncol 2015;33(10):1151–6.

106. Patel A. Does Baseline Serum Testosterone Influence Androgen Deprivation Therapy Outcomes in Hormone Naïve Patients with Advanced Prostate Cancer? J Urol 2021;205(3):806–11.

107. Sasaki T, Sugimura Y. The Importance of Time to Prostate-Specific Antigen (PSA) Nadir after Primary Androgen Deprivation Therapy in Hormone-Naïve Prostate Cancer Patients. J Clin Med 2018;7(12).

108. Hussain M, Tangen CM, Higano C, et al. Absolute prostate-specific antigen value after androgen deprivation is a strong independent predictor of survival in new metastatic prostate cancer: data

from Southwest Oncology Group Trial 9346 (INT-0162). J Clin Oncol 2006;24(24):3984–90.

109. Bryce AH, Chen YH, Liu G, et al. Patterns of Cancer Progression of Metastatic Hormone-sensitive Prostate Cancer in the ECOG3805 CHAARTED Trial. Eur Urol Oncol 2020;3(6):717–24.

110. Bernard A, Vaccaro N, Acharya M, et al. Impact on abiraterone pharmacokinetics and safety: Open-label drug-drug interaction studies with ketoconazole and rifampicin. Clin Pharmacol Drug Dev 2015;4(1):63–73.

111. Del Re M, Fogli S, Derosa L, et al. The role of drug-drug interactions in prostate cancer treatment: Focus on abiraterone acetate/prednisone and enzalutamide. Cancer Treat Rev 2017;55:71–82.

112. Benoist GE, Hendriks RJ, Mulders PF, et al. Pharmacokinetic Aspects of the Two Novel Oral Drugs Used for Metastatic Castration-Resistant Prostate Cancer: Abiraterone Acetate and Enzalutamide. Clin Pharm 2016;55(11):1369–80.

113. Marbury T, Lawitz E, Stonerock R, et al. Single-dose pharmacokinetic studies of abiraterone acetate in men with hepatic or renal impairment. J Clin Pharmacol 2014;54(7):732–41.

114. Klotz L, Miller K, Crawford ED, et al. Disease Control Outcomes from Analysis of Pooled Individual Patient Data from Five Comparative Randomised Clinical Trials of Degarelix Versus Luteinising Hormone-releasing Hormone Agonists. Eur Urol 2014;66(6):1101–8.

115. Margel D, Peer A, Ber Y, et al. Cardiovascular Morbidity in a Randomized Trial Comparing GnRH Agonist and GnRH Antagonist among Patients with Advanced Prostate Cancer and Preexisting Cardiovascular Disease. J Urol 2019;202(6):1199–208.

116. Bennett CL, Raisch DW, Sartor O. Pneumonitis associated with nonsteroidal antiandrogens: presumptive evidence of a class effect. Ann Intern Med 2002;137(7):625.

117. Han M, Nelson JB. Non-steroidal anti-androgens in prostate cancer–current treatment practice. Expert Opin Pharmacother 2000;1(3):443–9.

118. Thole Z, Manso G, Salgueiro E, et al. Hepatotoxicity Induced by Antiandrogens: A Review of the Literature. Urologia Int 2004;73(4):289–95.

119. Creaven PJ, Pendyala L, Tremblay D. Pharmacokinetics and metabolism of nilutamide. Urology 1991;37(2 Suppl):13–9.

120. Patel V, Liaw B, Oh W. The role of ketoconazole in current prostate cancer care. Nat Rev Urol 2018;15(10):643–51.

121. Batra A, Marchioni M, Hashmi AZ, et al. Cognition and depression effects of androgen receptor axis-targeted drugs in men with prostate cancer: A systematic review. J Geriatr Oncol 2021;12(5):687–95.

Immunotherapy and Checkpoint Inhibitors in Urologic Cancer

Aleksandra Walasek, MD, Dimitar V. Zlatev, MD*

KEYWORDS

- Immunotherapy • Checkpoint inhibitors • Urologic cancer • Monoclonal antibodies
- Drug-antibody conjugates

KEY POINTS

- Pembrolizumab is recommended as an adjuvant treatment option for patients with stage 2 clear cell renal cell carcinoma (with grade 4 or sarcomatoid high-risk features), stage 3 clear cell renal cell carcinoma, or stage 4 clear cell renal cell carcinoma with resection of metastatic lesions.
- Combination therapy currently utilized as first-line for advanced or metastatic clear cell renal cell carcinoma include the checkpoint inhibitors ipilimumab, nivolumab, and pembrolizumab.
- Pembrolizumab is an option for non-muscle invasive bladder cancer that is BCG unresponsive, with a complete response of 20% at 1 year.
- Nivolumab is an option for adjuvant treatment in muscle-invasive non-metastatic bladder cancer patients who had received cisplatin-based neoadjuvant therapy and for whom pathology after cystectomy demonstrated T3, T4, or node positive disease.
- For locally advanced or metastatic bladder cancer, category 1 level evidence supports the use of avelumab as maintenance therapy after first-line platinum-based chemotherapy, pembrolizumab as second-line therapy after platinum-based chemotherapy, and enfortumab vedotin therapy after platinum-based chemotherapy and checkpoint inhibitor immunotherapy.

INTRODUCTION

Major advances have been made in urologic oncology over the past 2 decades.[1–3] A deeper understanding of the cellular and molecular composition of tumor environment, as well as the mechanisms controlling the immune system, has made possible the development and clinical investigation of many innovative cancer therapies.[4] Immunotherapy is defined as a therapeutic approach that targets or manipulates the immune system.[5] Various forms of immune-based therapies have been evaluated, including vaccines, checkpoint inhibitors, monoclonal antibodies, and drug-antibody conjugates. In this review, the authors discuss the major clinical developments in immunotherapy in urothelial, kidney, prostate, testicular, and penile cancer.

Checkpoint Inhibition and Pathophysiology

To understand the mechanism of action of some of the novel immune-based agents, it is important to realize that immune regulation is a complex process that requires its components to act in synergy. Immune cells continuously scan the body to detect abnormal cells. A system of cell interactions is used to target only aberrant cells and prevent erroneous attack on normal cells. T-cell activation is the first step in the immune response and requires the engagement of the T-cell receptor with an antigen on the major histocompatibility

Department of Urology, Massachusetts General Hospital, 55 Fruit Street, Boston, MA 02114, USA
* Corresponding author. Department of Urology, Massachusetts General Hospital, 55 Fruit St, Boston, MA 02114.
E-mail address: dzlatev@mgh.harvard.edu

Urol Clin N Am 49 (2022) 323–334
https://doi.org/10.1016/j.ucl.2022.01.002
0094-0143/22/© 2022 Elsevier Inc. All rights reserved.

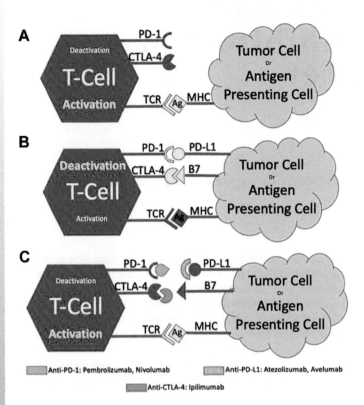

Fig. 1. (*A*) Normal T-cell activation. (*B*) Deactivation of the T-cell via inhibitory signaling. Pathway exploited by cancers to evade immune response. (*C*) Checkpoint inhibitors restore normal immune function and facilitate cancer cell recognition.

complex on an antigen presenting cell or tumor cell. Costimulatory signals such as the binding of CD28 on the T cell with B7 protein on the antigen-presenting cell are also required. During this activating interaction, several inhibitory signals may take place. The 2 most studied inhibitory pathways are programmed cell death protein 1 (PD-1) and cytotoxic T lymphocyte antigen 4 (CTLA-4). PD-1 is a protein on the surface of T cells that can bind with its ligand programmed death-ligand 1 (PD-L1) on tumor cells or normal cells, leading to downregulation of the T-cell response.[6] CTLA-4 is another surface protein on T cells that can bind to B7 on tumor cells or antigen presenting cells, also leading to T-cell inhibition. The PD-1 and CTLA-4 proteins act as checkpoints to prevent immune attack on normal cells but can also be exploited by cancers to evade immune response and remain undetected.[7] Immunotherapy with inhibition of the checkpoint pathways disrupts these inhibitory signals and activates the immune response against cancer cells. **Fig. 1** illustrates checkpoint inhibition.

Immunotherapy in Renal Cell Carcinoma

Surgery has been the cornerstone of treatment of localized or locally advanced renal cell carcinoma (RCC). A proportion of patients nonetheless will experience relapse and require medical management. As RCC is relatively chemotherapy and radiotherapy resistant, patients with advanced disease were initially treated with early immunotherapy consisting of interferon alpha or interleukin-2.[8] An improved understanding of RCC pathways and molecular biology leads to targeted therapies primarily using tyrosine kinase inhibitors.[9] Immunotherapy in renal cancer, similar to other solid cancers, was initially studied for metastatic disease and subsequently implemented in the management of earlier stages of RCC.

Localized Clear Cell Renal Cell Carcinoma

A phase III randomized trial evaluated the efficacy of pembrolizumab, a PD-1 inhibitor, versus placebo in 994 patients with localized clear cell RCC at intermediate or high risk of recurrence after nephrectomy. The study included patients with metastatic involvement before surgery, but with no evidence of disease after nephrectomy and resection of metastatic lesions.[10] At 24-month follow-up, disease-free survival was significantly higher for patients treated with pembrolizumab compared with placebo (77.3% vs 68.1%; 95% confidence interval [CI], 0.53–0.87, $P = .002$). Patients treated with pembrolizumab experienced grade 3 or greater adverse events at a higher rate compared with patients who received placebo (32.4% vs 17.7%). Based on the results from this

Table 1
Systemic immunotherapy for patients with clear cell and non–clear cell renal cell carcinoma

Trial	Regimen	No. of Patients	Patient Characteristics	Follow-up (mo)	Outcomes
Clear cell RCC					
Motzer et al,[11]	Ipilimumab + Nivolumab vs Sunitinib	1096	All risk (but endpoints were for intermediate- and high-risk only), systemic therapy naïve, Karnofsky performance score $\geq$ 70%	25	ORR: Ipi/Nivo 42%, Suni 27%, $P < .001$ CRR: Ipi/Nivo 9%, Suni 1%, $P < .001$ Median PFS (mo): Ipi/Nivo 11.6, Suni 8.4 Median OS (mo): Ipi/Nivo NR, Suni: 26, HR 0.63 (99.8% CI, 0.44–0.89), $P < .001$
Rini et al,[12]	Axitinib + Pembrolizumab vs Sunitinib	861	All risk, systemic therapy naïve, Karnofsky performance score $\geq$ 70%	13	ORR: Axi/Pem 59%, Suni 36%, $P < .001$ Median PFS (mo): Axi/Pem 15.1, Suni 11.1, $P < .001$ Median OS (mo): NR for both, HR 0.53 (95% CI, 0.38–0.74), $P < .0001$
Choueiri et al,[10]	Cabozantinib + Nivolumab vs Sunitinib	979	All risk, systemic therapy naïve, Karnofsky performance score $\geq$ 70%	18	ORR: Cabo/Nivo 56%, Suni 27% $P < .001$ Median PFS (mo): Cabo/Nivo 16.6, Suni 8.3, $P < .001$ Median OS (mo): NR for both, HR 0.60 (98.9% CI, 0.40–0.89), $P = .001$
Motzer et al,[13]	Lenvatinib + Pembrolizumab vs Lenvatinib + Everolimus vs Sunitinib	1069	All risk, systemic therapy naïve, Karnofsky performance score $\geq$ 70%	27	ORR: Len/Pem 71%, Len/Ev 54%, Suni 36% CR: Len/Pem 16%, Len/Ev 10%, Suni 4% Median PFS (mo): Len/Pem 23.9, Len/Ev 14.7, Suni 9.2 Median OS (mo): NR for all, Len/Pem vs Suni HR 0.66 (95% CI, 0.49–0.88), $P = .005$

(continued on next page)

Table 1
(continued)

Trial	Regimen	No. of Patients	Patient Characteristics	Follow-up (mo)	Outcomes
Non–clear cell RCC					
Koshkin et al,[14]	Nivolumab	35	Metastatic non–clear cell RCC	8.5	PR: 20% SD: 29% PFS (mo): 3.5
McKay et al,[15]	Nivolumab	43	Metastatic non–clear cell RCC	11.4	ORR: 19%
McDermott et al,[16]	Pembrolizumab	165	Metastatic non–clear cell RCC		ORR: 27% overall, 29% papillary, 10% chromophobe PFS (mo): 4.2 OS (mo): 28.9

Abbreviations: CR, complete response rate; HR, hazard ratio; mo, months; NR, not reached; ORR, overall response rate; OS, overall survival; PFS, progression free survival; PR, partial response; RCC, renal cell carcinoma; SD, stable disease.

trial, pembrolizumab is recommended as an adjuvant treatment option for patients with stage 2 clear cell RCC with grade 4 or sarcomatoid high-risk features, stage 3 clear cell RCC, or stage 4 clear cell RCC with resection of metastatic lesions and within 1 year of nephrectomy. There is no current evidence to support the role of adjuvant pembrolizumab for patients with non–clear cell RCC.

Recurrent or Metastatic Clear Cell Renal Cell Carcinoma

In the clinical setting of advanced clear cell RCC, checkpoint inhibitors have been studied in large clinical trials and demonstrated promising efficacy, presumably by changing the interaction between tumor cells and immune cells to enhance the antitumor immune response. All checkpoint inhibitors currently used as first-line therapy for advanced or metastatic clear cell RCC are part of combination regimens. A summary of efficacy data for first-line systemic immunotherapy for patients with clear cell RCC is provided in **Table 1**.

The combination of ipilimumab, a monoclonal antibody that inhibits CTLA-4 on activated T cells, and nivolumab, a PD-1 inhibitor, were evaluated against sunitinib, a tyrosine kinase inhibitor, in a landmark randomized phase III trial that included 1096 patients with advanced clear cell RCC.[11] The study initially reported end points for only intermediate- and poor-risk patients, demonstrating higher overall response rates and higher complete response rates in the combination ipilimumab and nivolumab arm (42% and 9%, respectively) compared with sunitinib (27% and 1%, respectively). The results from this trial led to the first Food and Drug Administration (FDA)-approved combination immunotherapy as first-line treatment of patients with intermediate- and poor-risk advanced clear cell RCC.

The combination of cabozantinib, a tyrosine kinase inhibitor, and nivolumab, a PD-1 inhibitor, was subsequently also FDA approved as first-line therapy for advanced clear cell RCC. In a phase III randomized trial of patients with favorable-, intermediate-, or poor-risk advanced clear cell RCC, the combination of cabozantinib and nivolumab demonstrated significantly higher overall response rates and longer progression-free survival (56% and 16.6 months, respectively) compared with sunitinib alone (27% and 8.3 months, respectively).[3] At 19-month median follow-up, the overall survival endpoint was not reached; however, the hazard ratio (HR) significantly favored the cabozantinib and nivolumab group (HR = 0.60; 98.9% CI, 0.40–0.89, P = .001).

The combination of axitinib, a second-generation selective tyrosine kinase inhibitor, and pembrolizumab, a PD-1 inhibitor, is now also FDA approved as first-line therapy for patients with advanced clear cell RCC based on a randomized phase III trial that compared sunitinib monotherapy with the combination of axitinib and pembrolizumab.[12] The trial included 861 patients with favorable-, intermediate-, or poor-risk advanced clear cell RCC. After median follow-up of 13 months, significantly higher overall response rates and longer progression-free survival were observed with the combination regimen of axitinib and pembrolizumab (59% and 15.1 months, respectively) compared with sunitinib (36% and 11.1 months, respectively). The median overall survival endpoint was not reached; however, the HR significantly favored the axitinib and pembrolizumab group (HR = 0.53; 95% CI, 0.38–0.74, P < .0001).

Most recently, the combination of lenvatinib, a multitargeted tyrosine kinase inhibitor, and pembrolizumab, a PD-1 inhibitor, became FDA approved as first-line therapy for patients with advanced clear cell RCC. In a 3-arm, phase III trial of 1069 patients with favorable-, intermediate-, or poor-risk advanced clear cell RCC equally randomized to receive either lenvatinib and pembrolizumab, lenvatinib and everolimus, or sunitinib monotherapy, patients who received lenvatinib and pembrolizumab demonstrated higher overall response rates and longer progression-free survival (71% and 23.9 months, respectively) compared with sunitinib alone (36% and 9.2 months, respectively).[13] At 27-months median follow-up, the overall survival endpoint was not met, but the HR significantly favored lenvatinib and pembrolizumab (HR = 0.66; 95% CI, 0.49–0.88, P = .005). Conversely, overall survival was not significantly different between the lenvatinib and everolimus cohort and the sunitinib group.

Recurrent or Metastatic Non–Clear Cell Renal Cell Carcinoma

Because of the higher prevalence of clear cell RCC, there are fewer clinical trials on immunotherapy for non–clear cell subset of patients with RCC. Similar to the efficacy demonstrated for targeted agents in this space, response rates with immunotherapy agents are significantly lower for non–clear cell RCC than for clear cell RCC. A summary of efficacy data for immunotherapy for patients with non–clear cell RCC is included in **Table 1**.

In a retrospective analysis that evaluated monotherapy with nivolumab, a PD-1 inhibitor, in 35 patients with metastatic non–clear cell RCC, 20% had a partial response and 29% had stable disease at median follow-up of 8.5 months. There was a modest progression-free survival of 3.5 months.[14] Another retrospective analysis of 43 patients with metastatic non–clear cell RCC demonstrated objective responses in 19% of patients treated with checkpoint inhibitors including nivolumab monotherapy.[15]

A phase II trial evaluated the efficacy of pembrolizumab monotherapy in 165 patients with metastatic non–clear cell RCC that included papillary, chromophobe, and unclassified histology.[16] Objective response rates for all histologic subtypes were 27%, with highest response rates for papillary (29%) and lowest for chromophobe histology (10%). Progression-free survival was 4.2 months, and overall survival was 28.9 months.

Immunotherapy in Urothelial Carcinoma

Urothelial carcinoma demonstrates a high mutational burden and is therefore susceptible to treatment with checkpoint inhibitors. Immunotherapy agents have been evaluated in different stages of disease, from nonmuscle invasive bladder cancer to platinum-refractory metastatic urothelial carcinoma.

Non–Muscle Invasive Bladder Cancer

Pembrolizumab, a PD-1 inhibitor, was evaluated in a single-arm phase II trial as treatment of patients with non–muscle invasive bladder cancer with carcinoma in situ (CIS) that is Bacillus Calmette-Guerin (BCG) unresponsive.[1] The trial included 101 patients treated with pembrolizumab for high-risk CIS (with or without solid papillary tumor), who had received intravesical BCG therapy previously and were not able nor willing to proceed with radical cystectomy. A complete response rate of 41% (95% CI, 30.7%–51.1%) was reported at 3 months and the median duration of any treatment response was 16.2 months (95% CI, 6.7–36.2 months). Of the patients who had a complete response, 46% maintained it for at least 1 year. The most common treatment-related adverse effects included hyponatremia and arthralgia. Eight percent of patients had significant treatment-related side effects; however, there were no treatment-related deaths.

Muscle Invasive Nonmetastatic Bladder Cancer

Nivolumab, a PD-1 inhibitor, was evaluated as adjuvant treatment in a phase III study of 709 patients with muscle invasive urothelial carcinoma treated with radical surgery followed by adjuvant nivolumab or placebo.[17] Disease-free survival significantly favored the nivolumab group (20.8 vs 10.8 months; HR 0.70; $P < .001$). In addition, in patients with PD-L1 expression greater than or equal to 1%, disease-free survival was 74% with nivolumab compared with 56% with placebo (HR 0.55; $P < .001$). Long-term follow-up to assess overall survival is ongoing. Based on this promising trial, nivolumab may be considered in the adjuvant setting for patients who had received cisplatin-based neoadjuvant therapy and for whom pathology after cystectomy demonstrated T3, T4, or node positive disease.

Locally Advanced or Metastatic Bladder Cancer

Approximately half of all patients treated with radical cystectomy will relapse after surgery, with distant metastases being more common than local recurrences. The first-line therapy for patients with metastatic bladder cancer is platinum-based chemotherapy.[18] Before immunotherapy, patients who relapsed after platinum-based chemotherapy experienced a reduction in overall survival from 9 to 15 months to 5 to 7 months.[19] Encouragingly, novel immunotherapy agents including checkpoint inhibitors, growth factor receptor inhibitors, and antibody-drug conjugates have demonstrated clinical efficacy for previously treated metastatic urothelial carcinoma and are now FDA approved in this setting. Category 1 level evidence supports the use of pembrolizumab as second-line therapy after platinum-based chemotherapy, enfortumab vedotin treatment after platinum-based chemotherapy and checkpoint inhibitor immunotherapy, and avelumab as maintenance therapy after first-line platinum-based chemotherapy.

Checkpoint Inhibitors

Pembrolizumab, a PD-1 inhibitor, was initially evaluated as second-line therapy and subsequently as first-line therapy for patients with advanced urothelial carcinoma. A randomized phase III trial compared second-line chemotherapy with pembrolizumab in 542 patients with urothelial carcinoma that had progressed after platinum-based chemotherapy.[20] At median follow-up of 14 months, patients treated with pembrolizumab demonstrated a longer median overall survival compared with chemotherapy (10.3 vs 7.4 months; $P = .002$). Follow-up data demonstrated higher median 1- and 2-year progression-free survival with pembrolizumab (44.2% and 26.9%) compared with chemotherapy (29.8% and 14.3%).[2] The side-effect profile also favored pembrolizumab, with fewer long-term grade 3 or greater adverse events (16% vs 50%).

Pembrolizumab is also FDA approved as first-line therapy with restriction to patients who are not eligible for platinum-containing chemotherapy and is not indicated for platinum-eligible patients even with high PD-L1 expression. In a phase II trial that included 370 patients with advanced urothelial carcinoma or those not eligible for cisplatin-based chemotherapy, pembrolizumab demonstrated a 28% long-term objective response rate and a 5% complete response rate. The median overall survival was 11.3 months,[21] and adverse events at approximately 16% were similar to other trials involving pembrolizumab.[22] However, a phase III randomized trial of 1010 patients with unresectable, previously untreated, and advanced or metastatic urothelial carcinoma demonstrated that the addition of pembrolizumab to chemotherapy did not result in significantly prolonged progression-free survival (8.3 vs 7.1 months; $P = .003$) or overall survival (17.0 vs 14.3 months; $P = .04$) compared with platinum-based chemotherapy alone at median follow-up of 31 months.[23] Survival was similar both for the total population as well as those with high PD-L1 expression, leading to the restricted use of pembrolizumab as first-line therapy for metastatic bladder cancer.

Atezolizumab, a PD-L1 inhibitor, is an immunotherapy agent only approved for patients who are not eligible for and have not been previously treated with platinum-based chemotherapy. A phase II trial evaluated atezolizumab in a cohort of 119 patients with locally advanced or metastatic urothelial carcinoma who were not eligible for cisplatin therapy and demonstrated an overall response rate of 23%, complete response rate of 9%, and median overall survival of 16 months.[24] Of note, atezolizumab is not FDA approved nor recommended for patients with locally advanced or metastatic urothelial carcinoma previously treated with platinum-based chemotherapy based on a randomized phase III trial that compared atezolizumab with second-line chemotherapy (docetaxel, paclitaxel, vinflunine) in 931 patients and demonstrated no significant difference in overall response rates or overall survival rates.[25]

Monotherapy with avelumab, a PD-L1 inhibitor, and nivolumab, a PD-1 inhibitor, has demonstrated clinical benefit for advanced or metastatic bladder cancer, with both agents now FDA approved in the setting of metastatic urothelial carcinoma refractory to platinum-based therapy. Avelumab was evaluated in phase I trials consisting of 249 patients with metastatic urothelial carcinoma after platinum-based therapy or patients ineligible for cisplatin-based chemotherapy, demonstrating overall response rates of 17% and a complete response rate of 6%, with acceptable grade 3 or greater treatment-related adverse events of 8%.[26,27] Nivolumab was evaluated in a phase II trial of 270 patients with locally advanced or metastatic urothelial carcinoma who progressed after platinum-based therapy, with an overall response rate of 19% that was independent of PD-1 tumor status.[28] The median overall survival was affected by PD-L1 expression, shorter at 5.9 months for PD-L1 expression less than 1% and longer at 11.3 months for PD-L1 expression greater than or equal to 1%. Longer term data demonstrated a 30-month duration of treatment response and an overall response rate of 25% (95% CI, 16.4%–36.8%).[29]

Antibody-Drug Conjugates

Antibody-drug conjugates deliver therapy by targeting proteins that are highly expressed on tumor cells. These agents have been used in the dual-refractory setting of patients previously treated with platinum-based chemotherapy and checkpoint inhibitor therapy.

Enfortumab vedotin, an anti-nectin-4 antibody conjugated with a drug that disrupts microtubules, is an FDA-approved therapy for refractory metastatic bladder cancer. The initial enfortumab vedotin trial in this setting was a phase II study of 125 patients that demonstrated a robust overall response rate of 44% (95% CI, 35%–53%), as well as a complete response rate of 12%.[30] Of note, treatment-related adverse events were observed in 50% of patients and resulted in dose reductions in one-third of these patients. Subsequently, a phase III randomized trial consisting of 608 patients with urothelial carcinoma refractory to both platinum-based and checkpoint inhibitor therapy randomized patients to enfortumab vedotin and second-line chemotherapy and demonstrated longer progression-free survival (5.6 vs 3.7 months; $P < .001$) and longer overall survival (12.9 vs 9.0 months; $P < .001$) for patients treated with enfortumab vedotin. Treatment-related adverse events were similar (51% for enfortumab vedotin, 50% for chemotherapy).[31]

Sacituzumab govitecan, an antibody for trophoblast cell surface marker 2 conjugated with a topoisomerase inhibitor, was evaluated in a phase II trial of 113 patients who progressed with platinum-based chemotherapy and immunotherapy and demonstrated a 27% overall response rate (95% CI, 20%–36%) and 10.9 months overall survival (95% CI, 9–14 months).[32] **Table 2** provides a summary of immune-based therapy studies in urothelial carcinoma.

Prostate cancer immunotherapy

The main area of interest for immunotherapy in prostate cancer is castrate-resistant metastatic disease. Patients who develop metastatic castrate-resistant prostate cancer (CRPC) will eventually fail traditional treatments. Immunotherapy carries a potential for improved treatment outcomes.

Table 2
Review of immunotherapy in urothelial carcinoma

Trial	Regimen	No. of Patients	Patient Characteristics	Follow-up (mo)	Outcomes
Non–muscle invasive bladder cancer					
Balar et al,[1]	Pembrolizumab	101	Patients with HR, BCG-unresponsive CIS with or without papillary tumors	24	3-mo CRR 41%; median DOR 16.2 mo
Muscle invasive bladder cancer					
Bajorin et al,[17]	Nivolumab	709	MIBC s/p cystectomy	12	DFS 20.8 vs 10.8 mo; DFS with PDL-1 expression 74.5% vs 55.7%
Advanced urothelial carcinoma					
Plimack et al,[20]	Pembrolizumab	543	Patients with urothelial carcinoma that had progressed after platinum-based chemotherapy	14	Median overall survival 10.3 vs 7.4 mo (p 0.002)
Powles et al,[23]	Pembrolizumab	1010	Patients with unresectable, previously untreated and advanced, or metastatic urothelial carcinoma	31	Progression-free survival (8.3 vs 7.1 mo; $P = .003$) or overall survival (17.0 vs 14.3 mo; $P = .04$) compared with platinum-based chemotherapy alone
Apolo et al,[26]	Avelumab	249	Patients with metastatic urothelial carcinoma after platinum-based therapy or patients ineligible for cisplatin-based chemotherapy	16.5	ORR 17%, CR 6%
Sharma et al,[28]	Nivolumab	270	Patients with locally advanced or metastatic urothelial carcinoma who progressed after platinum-based therapy	22	30 mo duration of treatment response and an overall response rate of 25% (95% CI, 16.4%–36.8%)

Abbreviations: CRR, complete response rate; DFS, disease-free survival; ORR, overall response rate; mo, months.

Autologous Vaccine

Sipuleucel-T is an autologous cancer "vaccine" made by the collection of antigen-presenting cells from individual patients and exposure of these cells to prostatic acid phosphatase, an antigen highly expressed by prostate cancer cells, before subsequent reinfusion of the modified cells. It was the first FDA-approved immunotherapy agent for use in prostate cancer based on a phase III trial of 512 patients with minimally symptomatic or asymptomatic metastatic CRPC who were randomized 2:1 to receive either Sipuleucel-T or placebo.[33] The study cohort included patients who had not received systemic therapy and a small proportion of patients who had been treated with chemotherapy but not within 3 months of enrollment. A 4.1-month improvement in median overall survival was observed in the Sipuleucel-T group

(25.8 vs 21.7 months; HR = 0.78; 95% CI, 0.61–0.98, P = .03). Subgroup analysis demonstrated that both patients who did or did not previously receive chemotherapy for prostate cancer benefited from the treatment. The medication was well tolerated, with chills and headache as common and reversible side effects. Sipuleucel-T can be considered as an initial therapy for asymptomatic or minimally symptomatic patients with metastatic CRPC whose disease burden is lower and immune function is presumably more intact. The vaccine can be used in patients with prior treatment with chemotherapy or novel hormonal therapy, however not for patients who have received both. Of note, the benefit of therapy cannot be measured through testing because decline in prostate-specific antigen or objective improvement in imaging has not been demonstrated after treatment with Sipuleucel-T.

Checkpoint Inhibitors

Immune checkpoint inhibitors to the surface protein PD-1 and its ligand PDL-1, as well as monoclonal antibodies targeting CTLA-4, have been evaluated for the treatment of metastatic CRPC with the goal of finding effective treatments for patients with disease that is refractory to other systemic therapies.

Pembrolizumab, an anti-PD1 antibody, was FDA approved in 2017 for treatment of patients with unresectable or metastatic solid tumors that demonstrated high levels of microsatellite instability or deficient mismatch repair based on pooled data from 5 clinical trials on the treatment of 149 colorectal and noncolorectal patients, including 2 patients with prostate cancer, who had progressed on previous treatments and demonstrated objective results in 40% of patients.[34] The indication for the use of pembrolizumab includes several noncolorectal cancer types, but not prostate cancer.

Several trials provided additional information regarding the inhibition of the PD-1 and PD-L1 axis in the treatment of prostate cancer. A nonrandomized phase Ib trial evaluated the use of pembrolizumab in 23 patients with metastatic CRPC who had failed previous therapies and also had PD-L1 expression in at least 1% of stromal cells.[35] Median duration of response was 13.5 month, with objective partial response detected in 4 patients (17%). Eight patients (35%) had stable disease over the course of the study period.[35] The role of pembrolizumab in patients with metastatic CRPC that was refractory to docetaxel chemotherapy and one novel hormonal therapy regardless of microsatellite instability status was further explored in a multicenter phase II study.[36] The cohorts included 133 patients with PD-L1 positive and 66 patients with PD-L1 negative

prostate cancer, as well as 59 patients with bone-predominant disease. The objective response rate in the PD-L1 positive and PD-L1 negative cohorts was 5% (95% CI, 2%–11%) and lower at 3% (95% CI, <1%–11%) in the bone predominant cohort.[36]

A retrospective biomarker analysis from a phase II trial that included 233 patients with high tumor mutational burden ($\geq$10 mutations per megabase) in metastatic or unresectable solid tumors, 6 of which were prostate cancer, treated with pembrolizumab revealed higher objective response rate in the group of patients with high tumor mutational burden (29% vs 6%).[37]

Although the results of prostate cancer treatment with checkpoint inhibitors have thus far been modest, pembrolizumab is an option in the treatment of patients with metastatic CRPC, prior docetaxel therapy, prior treatment with novel hormonal therapy, and high tumor mutational burden.

Cytotoxic T Lymphocyte Antigen 4 Inhibitor

Ipilimumab, a CTLA-4 inhibitor, was studied in 2 phase III trials for patients with metastatic CRPC. In one study, 799 men with disease progression after docetaxel therapy received bone-directed radiotherapy and were randomized to ipilimumab and placebo.[38] Median overall survival was 11.2 months with ipilimumab (95% CI, 9.5–12.7 months) and 10.0 months with placebo (95% CI, 8.3–11.0 months). Another trial that included 598 patients with chemotherapy-naive metastatic CRPC randomized to ipilimumab and placebo demonstrated no significant difference in overall survival.[39]

In an effort to amplify the effects observed with PD-1/PD-L1 inhibitors and CTLA-4 inhibitor monotherapy in men with metastatic CRPC, a phase II trial evaluated the combination on ipilimumab, a CTLA-4 inhibitor, and nivolumab, a PD-1 inhibitor, in metastatic castrate-resistant disease who either had or had not received chemotherapy previously. Preliminary results were promising, with patients who had previously received chemotherapy experiencing higher objective response rates and longer median overall survival (25% and 19.0 months, respectively) compared with patients who had not previously received chemotherapy (10% and 15.2 months, respectively).[40]

Testicular Cancer Immunotherapy

Immune-based therapy in patient with refractory testicular cancer has demonstrated early signs of activity in patients with germ cell tumors who have failed multiple chemotherapy treatments. It is important to note that antitumor activity and reported response rates, although promising, tend to be short lived.

Brentuximab vedotin is an anti-CD30 antibody-drug conjugate studied in refractory CD30-expressing germ cell tumors. A phase II study evaluated the use of brentuximab vedotin in 7 patients with refractory germ cell tumors or metastatic sex cord tumors.[41] Objective response was observed in 2 of these patients. One patient had a complete response after 4 cycles of therapy that persisted for more than 46 months after discontinuation of treatment. Another patient who had a partial response to therapy following 2 cycles of treatment, however, was detected to have disease progression after the fourth cycle of treatment.

At the end of the first stage of a larger phase II trial evaluating the efficacy of brentuximab vedotin in 24 patients with CD30-expressing germ cell tumors, the investigators reported a decrease in levels of serum tumor marker after the first cycle in 7 patients.[42]

PENILE CANCER IMMUNOTHERAPY

Although immunotherapy using checkpoint inhibitors has been established for the treatment of several solid cancers including skin cancers, there are no data on immune-based therapy for patients with penile carcinoma. Treatments currently under investigation include avelumab, a PD-L1 inhibitor, in patients who are unfit for or progressed on platinum-based chemotherapy clinicaltrials.gov; pembrolizumab, a PD-1 inhibitor, in combination with chemotherapy clinicaltrials.gov; atezolizumab, a PD-L1 inhibitor, with and without local radiotherapy clinicaltrials.gov; and maintenance therapy with avelumab, a PD-L1 inhibitor, after response to first-line chemotherapy clinicaltrials.gov.

SUMMARY

Advances in cancer biology and pathogenesis over the last 2 decades have resulted in immunotherapeutic approaches such as vaccines, checkpoint inhibitors, monoclonal antibodies, and combination immunotherapies that have revolutionized the treatment of urologic cancer. These novel targets have a potential to add greatly to existing therapies. We trust that the many combination immunotherapy studies involving checkpoint inhibitors and other agents will provide much needed insight into the molecular mechanisms of resistances and toxicity associated with immune-based therapy and subsequently improve urologic cancer treatment outcomes.

ACKNOWLEDGMENTS

The authors acknowledge Tatiana Zlateva for her assistance with the design and construction of the figure used in the text.

DISCLOSURE

The authors have no commercial or financial conflict of interest to disclose.

RESOURCES

1. Balar AV, Kamat AM, Kulkarni GS, et al. Pembrolizumab monotherapy for the treatment of high-risk non-muscle-invasive bladder cancer unresponsive to BCG (KEYNOTE-057): an open-label, single-arm, multicentre, phase 2 study. Lancet Oncol 2021; 22(7):919–30.
2. Fradet Y, Bellmunt J, Vaughn DJ, et al. Randomized phase III KEYNOTE-045 trial of pembrolizumab versus paclitaxel, docetaxel, or vinflunine in recurrent advanced urothelial cancer: results of >2 years of follow-up. Ann Oncol 2019;30(6):970–6.
3. Choueiri TK, Powles T, Burotto M, et al. Nivolumab plus Cabozantinib versus Sunitinib for Advanced Renal-Cell Carcinoma. N Engl J Med 2021;384(9):829–41.
4. Ratta R, Zappasodi R, Raggi D, et al. Immunotherapy advances in uro-genital malignancies. Crit Rev Oncol Hematol 2016;105:52–64.
5. Papaioannou NE, Beniata OV, Vitsos P, et al. Harnessing the immune system to improve cancer therapy. Ann Transl Med 2016;4(14):261.
6. Sharpe AH, Wherry EJ, Ahmed R, et al. The function of programmed cell death 1 and its ligands in regulating autoimmunity and infection. Nat Immunol 2007;8(3):239–45.
7. Donin NM, Lenis AT, Holden S, et al. Immunotherapy for the Treatment of Urothelial Carcinoma. J Urol 2017;197(1):14–22.
8. Koneru R, Hotte SJ. Role of cytokine therapy for renal cell carcinoma in the era of targeted agents. Curr Oncol 2009;16(Suppl 1):S40–4.
9. Motzer RJ, Hutson TE, Tomczak P, et al. Sunitinib versus interferon alfa in metastatic renal-cell carcinoma. N Engl J Med 2007;356(2):115–24.
10. Choueiri TK, Tomczak P, Park SH, et al. Adjuvant Pembrolizumab after Nephrectomy in Renal-Cell Carcinoma. N Engl J Med 2021;385(8):683–94.
11. Motzer RJ, Tannir NM, McDermott DF, et al. Nivolumab plus Ipilimumab versus Sunitinib in Advanced Renal-Cell Carcinoma. N Engl J Med 2018;378(14): 1277–90.
12. Rini BI, Plimack ER, Stus V, et al. Pembrolizumab plus Axitinib versus Sunitinib for Advanced Renal-Cell Carcinoma. N Engl J Med 2019;380(12):1116–27.
13. Motzer R, Alekseev B, Rha SY, et al. Lenvatinib plus Pembrolizumab or Everolimus for Advanced Renal

Cell Carcinoma. N Engl J Med 2021;384(14): 1289–300.

14. Koshkin VS, Barata PC, Zhang T, et al. Clinical activity of nivolumab in patients with non-clear cell renal cell carcinoma. J Immunother Cancer 2018; 6(1):9.

15. McKay RR, Bossé D, Xie W, et al. The Clinical Activity of PD-1/PD-L1 Inhibitors in Metastatic Non-Clear Cell Renal Cell Carcinoma. Cancer Immunol Res 2018;6(7):758–65.

16. McDermott DF, Lee JL, Ziobro M, et al. Open-Label, Single-Arm, Phase II Study of Pembrolizumab Monotherapy as First-Line Therapy in Patients With Advanced Non-Clear Cell Renal Cell Carcinoma. J Clin Oncol 2021;39(9):1029–39.

17. Bajorin DF, Witjes JA, Gschwend JE, et al. Adjuvant Nivolumab versus Placebo in Muscle-Invasive Urothelial Carcinoma. N Engl J Med 2021;384(22): 2102–14.

18. De Santis M, Bellmunt J, Mead G, et al. Randomized phase II/III trial assessing gemcitabine/carboplatin and methotrexate/carboplatin/vinblastine in patients with advanced urothelial cancer who are unfit for cisplatin-based chemotherapy: EORTC study 30986. J Clin Oncol 2012;30(2):191–9.

19. Bellmunt J, Théodore C, Demkov T, et al. Phase III trial of vinflunine plus best supportive care compared with best supportive care alone after a platinum-containing regimen in patients with advanced transitional cell carcinoma of the urothelial tract. J Clin Oncol 2009;27(27):4454–61.

20. Plimack ER, Bellmunt J, Gupta S, et al. Safety and activity of pembrolizumab in patients with locally advanced or metastatic urothelial cancer (KEYNOTE-012): a non-randomised, open-label, phase 1b study. Lancet Oncol 2017;18(2):212–20.

21. Vuky J, Balar AV, Castellano D, et al. Long-Term Outcomes in KEYNOTE-052: Phase II Study Investigating First-Line Pembrolizumab in Cisplatin-Ineligible Patients With Locally Advanced or Metastatic Urothelial Cancer. J Clin Oncol 2020; 38(23):2658–66.

22. Balar AV, Castellano D, O'Donnell PH, et al. First-line pembrolizumab in cisplatin-ineligible patients with locally advanced and unresectable or metastatic urothelial cancer (KEYNOTE-052): a multicentre, single-arm, phase 2 study. Lancet Oncol 2017; 18(11):1483–92.

23. Powles T, Csőszi T, Özgüroğlu M, et al. Pembrolizumab alone or combined with chemotherapy versus chemotherapy as first-line therapy for advanced urothelial carcinoma (KEYNOTE-361): a randomised, open-label, phase 3 trial. Lancet Oncol 2021;22(7): 931–45.

24. Balar AV, Galsky MD, Rosenberg JE, et al. Atezolizumab as first-line treatment in cisplatin-ineligible patients with locally advanced and metastatic

urothelial carcinoma: a single-arm, multicentre, phase 2 trial. Lancet 2017;389(10064):67–76.

25. Powles T, Durán I, van der Heijden MS, et al. Atezolizumab versus chemotherapy in patients with platinum-treated locally advanced or metastatic urothelial carcinoma (IMvigor211): a multicentre, open-label, phase 3 randomised controlled trial. Lancet 2018;391(10122):748–57.

26. Apolo AB, Infante JR, Balmanoukian A, et al. Avelumab, an Anti-Programmed Death-Ligand 1 Antibody, In Patients With Refractory Metastatic Urothelial Carcinoma: Results From a Multicenter, Phase Ib Study. J Clin Oncol 2017;35(19):2117–24.

27. Patel MR, Ellerton J, Infante JR, et al. Avelumab in metastatic urothelial carcinoma after platinum failure (JAVELIN Solid Tumor): pooled results from two expansion cohorts of an open-label, phase 1 trial. Lancet Oncol 2018;19(1):51–64.

28. Sharma P, Retz M, Siefker-Radtke A, et al. Nivolumab in metastatic urothelial carcinoma after platinum therapy (CheckMate 275): a multicentre, single-arm, phase 2 trial. Lancet Oncol 2017;18(3). 312–22.

29. Sharma P, Siefker-Radtke A, de Braud F, et al. Nivolumab Alone and With Ipilimumab in Previously Treated Metastatic Urothelial Carcinoma: CheckMate 032 Nivolumab 1 mg/kg Plus Ipilimumab 3 mg/kg Expansion Cohort Results. J Clin Oncol 2019;37(19):1608–16.

30. Rosenberg JE, O'Donnell PH, Balar AV, et al. Pivotal Trial of Enfortumab Vedotin in Urothelial Carcinoma After Platinum and Anti-Programmed Death 1/Programmed Death Ligand 1 Therapy. J Clin Oncol 2019;37(29):2592–600.

31. Powles T, Rosenberg JE, Sonpavde GP, et al. Enfortumab Vedotin in Previously Treated Advanced Urothelial Carcinoma. N Engl J Med 2021;384(12):1125-35.

32. Tagawa ST, Balar AV, Petrylak DP, et al. TROPHY-U-01: A Phase II Open-Label Study of Sacituzumab Govitecan in Patients With Metastatic Urothelial Carcinoma Progressing After Platinum-Based Chemotherapy and Checkpoint Inhibitors. J Clin Oncol 2021;39(22):2474–85.

33. Kantoff PW, Higano CS, Shore ND, et al. Sipuleucel-T immunotherapy for castration-resistant prostate cancer. N Engl J Med 2010;363(5):411–22.

34. Marcus L, Lemery SJ, Keegan P, et al. FDA Approval Summary: Pembrolizumab for the Treatment of Microsatellite Instability-High Solid Tumors. Clin Cancer Res 2019;25(13):3753–8.

35. Hansen AR, Massard C, Ott PA, et al. Pembrolizumab for advanced prostate adenocarcinoma: findings of the KEYNOTE-028 study. Ann Oncol 2018; 29(8):1807–13.

36. Antonarakis ES, Piulats JM, Gross-Goupil M, et al. Pembrolizumab for Treatment-Refractory Metastatic Castration-Resistant Prostate Cancer: Multicohort,

Open-Label Phase II KEYNOTE-199 Study. J Clin Oncol 2020;38(5):395–405.

37. Marabelle A, Fakih M, Lopez J, et al. Association of tumour mutational burden with outcomes in patients with advanced solid tumours treated with pembrolizumab: prospective biomarker analysis of the multicohort, open-label, phase 2 KEYNOTE-158 study. Lancet Oncol 2020;21(10):1353–65.

38. Kwon ED, Drake CG, Scher HI, et al. Ipilimumab versus placebo after radiotherapy in patients with metastatic castration-resistant prostate cancer that had progressed after docetaxel chemotherapy (CA184-043): a multicentre, randomised, double-blind, phase 3 trial. Lancet Oncol 2014;15(7): 700–12.

39. Morris MJ, Pouliot F, Saperstein L, et al. A phase III, multicenter study to assess the diagnostic performance and clinical impact of 18F-DCFPyL PET/CT in men with suspected recurrence of prostate cancer (CONDOR). J Clin Oncol 2019;37(15_suppl):TPS5093.

40. Sharma P, Pachynski RK, Narayan V, et al. Nivolumab Plus Ipilimumab for Metastatic Castration-Resistant Prostate Cancer: Preliminary Analysis of Patients in the CheckMate 650 Trial. Cancer Cell 2020;38(4):489–99.e3.

41. Albany C, Einhorn L, Garbo L, et al. Treatment of CD30-Expressing Germ Cell Tumors and Sex Cord Stromal Tumors with Brentuximab Vedotin: Identification and Report of Seven Cases. Oncologist 2018;23(3):316–23.

42. Necchi A, Magazzu D, Anichini A, et al. An open-label, single-group, phase 2 study of brentuximab vedotin as salvage therapy for males with relapsed germ-cell tumors (GCT): Results at the end of first stage (FM12GCT01). J Clin Oncol 2016;34(2_suppl):480.

Medical Treatment and Prevention of Urinary Stone Disease

Kyle Spradling, MD[a],*, Calyani Ganesan, MD[b], Simon Conti, MD, MEd[a]

KEYWORDS

- Urolithiasis • Thiazide • Alkali therapy • Medical expulsive therapy

KEY POINTS

- Pathophysiology underlying urolithiasis remains an area of active investigation.
- Medical treatment of urolithiasis is primarily aimed at optimizing metabolic factors and reducing urinary supersaturation of stone components.
- Medical expulsive therapy for ureteral stones may be an effective treatment tool in certain patients, particularly those with larger distal ureteral stones.
- Medical dissolution therapy is a helpful tool that can be used alongside surgical treatment in the management of uric acid urinary stones.

BACKGROUND

Urinary stone disease is one of the most commonly treated urologic conditions, and the prevalence of urinary stone disease has been increasing in recent decades.[1–5] Between 1994 and 2010, prevalence rates of urinary stone disease increased from 5.2% to 8.8% worldwide.[6,7] In the United States, lifetime prevalence rates of urinary stone disease are 7% and 11% for women and men, respectively.[7] In Europe, an estimated 25 to 50 million people are living with symptomatic urinary stone disease.[8] In Asia, prevalence rates have grown rapidly in the last 2 decades, particularly in Japan and Korea.[9,10] As the burden of urinary stone disease increases around the world, the economic burden also increases. In 2000, the annual cost of urinary stone disease in the United States was $2.1 billion[5]; however, an additional $1.2 billion in costs per year is expected by 2030.[11]

Numerous epidemiologic and ecologic studies have revealed other trends in the prevalence of urinary stone disease. Urinary stones are more common in men than in women with a peak in prevalence between age 40 and 59 years.[12,13] In the United States, urinary stone disease is less common in African Americans and Hispanic Caucasians when compared with non-Hispanic Caucasians.[6,14] Prevalence rates are higher in residents of the southern United States compared with those living in other geographic locations.[12,15] Those living in warmer and wetter climates have higher rates of urinary stone disease likely due to dehydration and lower urine volumes associated with greater insensible fluid losses.[16,17]

Urinary stone disease is associated with significant morbidity and is a common cause of acute and chronic kidney disease. An estimated 3% of renal failure cases are a result of urinary stone disease.[18] In patients with ureteral stones, around 20% require surgical intervention by 4 weeks.[19] Although surgical techniques and technology continue to advance in the field of endourology and surgical management of urinary stone disease, recurrence rates of urinary stones after treatment remain high, with 20% of stone formers developing a recurrence within 5 years and nearly

[a] Department of Urology, Stanford University School of Medicine, Stanford, CA, USA; [b] Division of Nephrology, Stanford University School of Medicine, Stanford, CA, USA
* Corresponding author. Department of Urology, Stanford University School of Medicine, 300 Pasteur Drive MC 5118, Stanford, CA 94305.
E-mail address: spradlkd@stanford.edu

Urol Clin N Am 49 (2022) 335–344
https://doi.org/10.1016/j.ucl.2021.12.007
0094-0143/22/© 2021 Elsevier Inc. All rights reserved.

40% developing recurrence within 15 years.[20] As such, metabolic evaluation is often indicated in patients with recurrent urinary stone disease in order to identify metabolic abnormalities and provide targeted medical treatment in order to prevent growth of existing stones and formation of new urinary stones. Herein, the authors review the pathophysiology of urinary stone formation and discuss current pharmacotherapies used in the prevention and treatment of urinary stone disease.

PATHOPHYSIOLOGY

Despite its growing prevalence, economic burden, and associated morbidity, the underlying mechanism behind urinary stone formation remains largely unclear. Nearly 80% of all stones are calcium-based stones (calcium oxalate or calcium phosphate); 10% are magnesium ammonium phosphate hexahydrate (struvite) stones; 9% uric acid stones; and 1% are rarer stones such as cystine, ammonium acid urate, or drug-related stones.[21] Although there are different types of stone compositions, a common requirement for stone formation and propagation seems to be the presence of urinary supersaturation of the mineral components.[22] The pathway to urinary supersaturation is likely multifactorial. Dietary, environmental, and genetic factors seem to play a role. Low urine volume or excessive urinary excretion of calcium, for example, has been shown to increase calcium oxalate supersaturation, leading to higher rates of calcium stone formation.[23] In contrast, genetic disorders such as primary hyperoxaluria type 1 or type 2 lead to higher urinary oxalate levels and increased calcium oxalate supersaturation.[24]

Multiple hypotheses have been proposed to explain the pathophysiology of urinary stone formation and are under active investigation. The free particle hypothesis, first described by Vermeulen and colleagues in 1968, suggests that a nucleus of stone crystals forms freely in urine in the setting of increased supersaturation (homogeneous nucleation).[25] The fixed particle hypothesis states that crystal nuclei form when a nephron injury occurs and crystal nuclei form within a lumen of the nephron and become fixed, or adhere, to the lumen epithelium at the site of injury. This model, suggested by Verkoelen and colleagues in 2007, requires a crystal-cell attachment where crystal growth can occur only if the crystal nucleus is fixed in position within a lumen.[26] Finally, the Randall's plaque hypothesis for urinary stone formation, described in a historical paper by Randall in 1940, suggests that interstitial calcium phosphate deposits located at the renal papilla become a nidus for urinary crystals to attach and grow (heterogenous nucleation). These deposits (called Randall plaques) cause a loss of the urothelial layer at the renal papilla, which in turn allows the calcium deposits to be in direct contact with urine within the renal calyx.[27]

Recent studies using endoscopic technology and microscopic examination of renal papillary biopsies support the Randall plaque hypothesis for urinary stone formation. Evan and colleagues found that urinary stones seemed to originate from Randall plaques in most of the patients with idiopathic calcium oxalate urinary stones. In other types of stone formers (calcium phosphate, cystine, and so forth) their findings supported a fixed particle model in which stone crystals originated within the medullary collecting ducts or ducts of Bellini.[22] More recently, novel imaging technologies such as electron microscopy have further delineated the pathogenetic sequence of events, referred to as Anderson-Carr-Randall progression, leading to Randall plaque deposits at the renal papilla, suggesting that the additional event of proximal intratubular mineralization may proceed the interstitial calcification of the renal papilla. Further investigation is ongoing, but these precursors to Randall plaques could represent a future target for pharmacologic treatment of urinary stone disease.[28]

Building on these earlier investigations into the cause of urinary stone formation, Chi and colleagues discovered a potential role of zinc in the initiation of urinary stone formation. Using a *Drosophila* fly model, they found that a decrease of zinc levels through dietary changes or pharmacologic interventions led to a reduction in stone formation in flies.[29] Furthermore, Randall plaques contain high levels of zinc, which may play an important role in the Randall plaque mineralization pathway. As such, pharmacologic therapy aimed at regulating zinc levels in humans may be a promising prophylactic medical treatment of urinary stone formers, but further investigation is this area is ongoing.

MEDICAL THERAPIES FOR STONE PREVENTION

Given that the pathophysiologic mechanisms underlying urinary stone formation remain unclear, contemporary pharmacologic therapies used in the prevention of urinary stone disease primarily focus on optimizing mineral components of the urine to reduce urinary supersaturation. **Table 1** summarizes current pharmacotherapies used for prevention of stone disease and lists their typical dosages, mechanisms of action, as well as

Table 1
Pharmacotherapies for the prevention of urinary stone disease

Name	Dose	Indication	Mechanism of Action	Adverse Effects
Thiazide and Thiazide-Type Diuretics				
Chlorthalidone	50 mg daily and titrate up as tolerated	Hypercalciuria	Blocks the Na^+/Cl^- channel in the distal convoluted tubule cells of the kidney; promotes the release of sodium into the urine and the reabsorption of calcium	Hypokalemia, hypomagnesemia, hyponatremia, hypercalcemia
Hydrochlorothiazide	50 mg daily and titrate up as tolerated			Increases uric acid, glucose, low-density lipoprotein, and triglycerides
Indapamide	2.5–5 mg daily			
Alkali Therapy				
Potassium citrate	10–20 meq two to three times daily	Low urine pH in the setting of uric acid stones	Provides an alkali load; raises urine citrate excretion and urine pH	Hyperkalemia Abdominal discomfort, diarrhea, nausea, and vomiting
Sodium bicarbonate	650 mg three times daily and titrate up as tolerated	Hypocitraturia in the setting of calcium oxalate stones		Hypernatremia, hypocalcemia Edema Abdominal distention, eructation, and flatulence Metabolic alkalosis
Sodium citrate (490 mg/ 5 mL) and citric acid solution (640 mg/5 mL)	10–30 mL three to four times daily			Diarrhea, nausea. and vomiting
Other Therapies				
Allopurinol	100 mg daily and titrate up as tolerated to 300 mg daily	Hyperuricosuria in the setting of calcium oxalate stones	Xanthine oxidase inhibitor; lowers serum and urine uric acid	Acute gout attack Hepatotoxicity Delayed hypersensitivity reactions including rash and Steven-Johnson syndrome Neutropenia Abdominal pain and dyspepsia

(continued on next page)

Table 1
(continued)

Name	Dose	Indication	Mechanism of Action	Adverse Effects
Alpha-mercaptopropionyl glycine (tiopronin)	800 mg split into 3 doses daily; titrate to 1000 mg/daily total as tolerated	Cystinuria	Increases solubility of cystine	Fatigue, rash Nausea, oral mucosal ulcer, and diarrhea Arthralgia
Calcium citrate	200 mg to 1 g/daily as tolerated; doses can be divided	Enteric hyperoxaluria	Decreases intestinal oxalate absorption	Headache Hypercalcemia and hypophosphatemia Constipation, eructation, and flatulence
Pyridoxine	5mg/kg and titrate as tolerated; max dose 20 mg/kg daily	Primary hyperoxaluria type 1 (PH1)	Cofactor for enzyme liver-specific alanine glyoxylate aminotransferase, the enzyme deficient in patients with PH1	Ataxia, drowsiness, headache, nausea Acidosis, folate deficiency, increase in aspartate aminotransferase Hypersensitivity reaction

Of note, antibiotics that can be used in the setting of struvite stones to treat urinary tract infections caused by urease producing bacteria may be treated with antibiotics specific to urine culture results.

common adverse effects associated with each therapy. Pharmacologic therapies and dietary recommendations (increasing fluid intake, maintenance of normal calcium diet, reduction of sodium and oxalate-rich foods) can be based on metabolic evaluation and 24-hour urine assessment (selective therapy) or empirical therapy.[30] Because pharmacotherapy for urinary stone prevention is largely specific to stone type, urinary stone analysis data are often used in conjunction with 24-hour urine testing to guide selective therapy.[30] Although both the American Urologic Association (AUA) and European Association of Urology (EAU) guidelines on urinary stone disease recommend the use of 24-hour urine assessment in high-risk or recurrent urinary stone formers,[31,32] there remains a lack of evidence in the current literature to support the routine use of 24-hour urine assessment to improve clinical outcomes for patients with urinary stone disease, and little data exist to show that targeted therapy based on metabolic evaluation improves stone recurrence rates compared with empirical therapy.[33] Only one randomized controlled trial has been performed comparing urinary stone recurrence rates between first-time calcium stone formers receiving empirical dietary recommendations versus selective dietary measures based on 24-hour urine collection data. In this study, the selective therapy group was favored to have lower recurrence rates (7% vs 23%, *P* < .01); however, there were numerous issues with the study design, including poor follow-up in the empirical treatment group.[34] Additional clinical trials are needed to clarify which patients may benefit from selective therapy based on metabolic evaluation for urinary stone disease. For now, the use of 24-hour urine assessment to guide selective pharmacotherapy in urinary stone formers remains controversial, and the 2014 American College of Physicians Guidelines on calcium urinary stone prevention recommends empirical therapy with thiazides, alkali therapy, and allopurinol in patients with urinary stone disease refractory to dietary interventions.[35]

Thiazides

In patients with calcium-based urinary stones, hypercalciuria, and normal serum calcium levels, thiazide diuretics are recommended by the AUA and are one of the most commonly prescribed pharmacologic therapies for recurrent stone formers.[31] Before starting a thiazide, a trial of sodium restriction can be implemented and hyperparathyroidism should be excluded. Thiazides work by increasing renal calcium reabsorption at the level of both proximal and distal convoluted tubules, effectively reducing excretion of urinary calcium. A meta-analysis of 6 randomized controlled trials in patients with hypercalciuria determined that thiazide use was associated with nearly a 50% risk reduction in stone recurrence rates (risk ratio [RR] 0.53, 95% confidence interval [CI]: 0.41–0.68) over a 3-year follow-up period.[36] Typical dosages of thiazide-like diuretics include chlorthalidone, 50 mg, daily or indapamide, 2.5 mg, daily. Common side effects include hypokalemia, gastrointestinal symptoms, rash, hypotension, and hyperglycemia. Hypokalemia has been reportedly seen in 13% to 50% of patients on thiazide diuretics,[36] so monitoring of serum potassium levels is important and some patients may require potassium supplementation in conjunction with thiazide therapy.

Alkali Therapy

Alkali therapy is commonly prescribed for urinary stone disease to increase urinary citrate levels and urinary pH. It is indicated for calcium oxalate stone formers with hypocitraturia. In addition, alkali therapy plays an important role in prevention of uric acid stone disease by raising urinary pH.[37] There are multiple forms of alkali therapy that can be used including, but not limited to, potassium citrate, sodium bicarbonate, and sodium citrate/citric acid (Shohl's) solution.

The most commonly used form of alkali therapy is potassium citrate. Multiple randomized controlled trials have shown potassium citrate effectively reduces stone recurrence rates in patients with history of calcium stones and hypocitraturia, with a decrease in stone recurrence from 72% to 20% in patients treated with potassium citrate and placebo, respectively.[37,38] Treatment dosage is 10 mEq three times daily or 20mEq twice daily, with a maximum daily dose of 100 mEq per day, and the most common side effect is gastrointestinal symptoms such as diarrhea. Hyperkalemia can occur with potassium citrate supplementation, so monitoring of serum potassium is recommended. In patients at risk for hyperkalemia, such as those with reduced kidney function, sodium bicarbonate can be used to raise urine citrate levels and urine pH. It is commonly prescribed as 650 mg (7.8 mEq of alkali) three times daily, and the dose is titrated up as tolerated. The most common side effects include abdominal discomfort and an increase in edema due to the sodium load. Lastly, sodium citrate and citric acid solution is another medication that can be used to raise both urine citrate and urine pH. It is commonly prescribed as 10 to 30 mL four times daily.

Allopurinol

Patients with a history of calcium oxalate stones who have normal urinary calcium levels and hyperuricosuria on 24-hour urine testing may benefit from allopurinol therapy.[39] Allopurinol works as a competitive and noncompetitive inhibitor of xanthine oxidase at low and high concentrations, respectively, to lower serum and urinary uric acid levels.[40] The typical dosage is 200 to 300 mg daily (sometimes divided into 2 doses), and common side effects include rash and gastrointestinal symptoms. Rare, more serious side adverse reactions may include neutropenia, abnormal liver function, leukocytosis, fever, Stevens-Johnson syndrome, or progressive kidney failure.[40,41] A double-blind, randomized controlled trial including 60 patients with hyperuricosuria and normocalciuria and recurrent calcium oxalate calculi showed a significant decrease in the frequency of stone events in patients treated with allopurinol compared with placebo. The allopurinol group additionally had a significantly longer time until stone recurrence.[38]

Oxalate-Reducing Therapies

Dietary modification consisting of a reduction in oxalate-rich foods is the primary treatment approach for calcium oxalate stone formers with hyperoxaluria. However, in certain patient populations, dietary modification alone cannot achieve the necessary reduction in urinary oxalate excretion. Patients with malabsorptive conditions such as inflammatory bowel disease and those who have undergone gastric surgeries such as a Roux-en-Y gastric bypass surgery have enteric hyperoxaluria. In these cases, enhanced intestinal absorption of free oxalate is caused by increased binding of diet calcium by free fatty acids, which reduces the calcium available to bind dietary oxalate in gut. Oral calcium citrate supplementation binds oxalate within the gastrointestinal tract and decreases intestinal absorption of oxalate and reduces urinary oxalate excretion.[42]

Another important patient population that exhibits high levels of urinary oxalate excretion are those with primary hyperoxaluria. Primary hyperoxaluria is a rare autosomal recessive condition of which there are 3 main types, each associated with a specific metabolic defect. Primary hyperoxaluria type I is the most common and severe form, and it is caused by a deficiency of the liver-specific enzyme alanine-glyoxylate aminotransferase (AGT).[42] In patients with primary hyperoxaluria type 1 pyridoxine supplementation was associated with a 25% reduction in urinary oxalate levels.[43,44] Pyridoxine's efficacy is attributed to its role as a cofactor for AGT; however, the molecular basis and precise mechanism for pyridoxine's effects on urinary oxalate excretion remain unclear. The side-effect profile of pyridoxine is minimal, but sensory neuropathy has been noted at high doses.

Probiotics

Newer pharmacologic therapies for the treatment of hyperoxaluria are under investigation. Recent studies have found that the large intestine plays a role in oxalate homeostasis, with oxalate-degrading microorganisms, such as *Oxalobacter formigenes*, playing an important role in oxalate absorption and secretion pathways in the intestines.[45] For example, studies in children with cystic fibrosis have demonstrated very low colonization levels of Oxalobacter in the gut compared with healthy children, and these patients were found to be at an increased risk of calcium oxalate stone disease (3.5% vs 0.2%).[46] Although animal model studies have shown some promising findings for the use of Oxalobacter probiotics to treat hyperoxaluria, human studies have not demonstrated consistent results.[47] More recently, Lingeman and colleagues trialed an oral nonabsorbable crystalline form, oxalate decarboxylase (the enzyme naturally found in Oxalobacter), in a small group of patients with urinary stone and noted a significant decrease in calcium oxalate supersaturation levels with treatment.[48] Certainly, therapies focused on the gastrointestinal microbiome may prove to be useful and safe therapies for patients with recurrent calcium oxalate stones.

MEDICAL THERAPIES FOR STONE TREATMENT
Medical Expulsive Therapy

Medical dissolution therapy has not been shown to be effective against calcium stones, and thus, the mainstay for treatment of large calcium-based urinary stones is surgical removal. However, smaller ureteral stones (<1 cm) may be managed with expectant management and a trial of spontaneous passage.[49] For smaller ureteral stones, the use of medical expulsive therapy is commonly used to facilitate the passage of stones. Multiple medical management therapies have been described including α-blockers, corticosteroids, and calcium channel blockers.[50] α-blockers have been well described in the literature as an effective agent for medical expulsive therapy and are included in both AUA and EAU guidelines as an option for patients for whom surgical intervention is not initially recommended.[31,32] Tamsulosin, the most studied α-blocker, has been shown to increase stone expulsion rates for ureteral stones in multiple randomized controlled trials.[51–53] However, in a large randomized placebo-controlled trial including more than 1100 patients, Pickard and colleagues found no difference in stone clearance at 4 weeks with tamsulosin therapy compared with placebo.[19] Subgroup analyses in patients with distal ureteral stones greater than 5 mm, however, did see a benefit of tamsulosin, and according to the results of a more recent meta-analysis in 2019, the use of tamsulosin was associated with improved stone expulsion rates for ureteral stones 5 mm to 10 mm but was not effective for stones less than 5 mm in size.[54] Tamsulosin was also associated with significantly lower rates of surgical intervention compared with placebo (RR 0.68%, 95% CI: 0.50–0.93), suggesting there may still be a role for tamsulosin use in medical expulsive therapy, particularly in patients with larger distal ureteral stones. Typical dose is 0.4 mg daily and common side effects of tamsulosin include dizziness, anejaculation, and postural hypotension.

The use of corticosteroids for medical expulsive therapy has been described in smaller prospective studies. Although there are some data to suggest that combination therapy with corticosteroids and α-blocker therapy may lead to higher stone expulsion rates and faster time to stone passage compared with control or α-blocker alone, the evidence is not strong, and there is insignificant evidence to suggest a benefit of corticosteroids as a monotherapy for medical expulsive therapy.[55,56]

Calcium channel blockers have been previously described to play a role in medical expulsive therapy, with nifedipine demonstrating some benefit in facilitating stone passage and reduction of renal colic.[56] However, multiple randomized controlled trials comparing nifedipine with tamsulosin have consistently shown significantly better rates of stone expulsion with tamsulosin,[57] and a systematic review including 7 studies comparing α-blockers and calcium channel blockers for distal ureteral stones found that alpha blockade was associated with significantly higher expulsion rates with an RR of 0.81 ($P < .00001$).[58] For this reason, EAU guidelines do not include calcium blocker therapy as a recommended monotherapy for medical expulsive therapy.[32]

Uric Acid

Approximately 10% of kidney stones are composed of uric acid, and in this subset of urinary stone patients, medical dissolution therapy can be an effective noninvasive treatment option. Medical dissolution therapy is achieved by increasing the urinary pH (goal >6) with potassium citrate or sodium bicarbonate supplementation. Although the use of medical dissolution therapy is endorsed by the AUA and EAU, there is a relative paucity of randomized controlled trials existing on this subject. A recent retrospective review found complete resolution rates of uric acid stones can be as high as 67% with relatively low rates of adverse reactions.[59] Elbaset and colleagues designed a randomized controlled trial comparing shock wave lithotripsy with medical dissolution therapy with potassium citrate for uric acid stones, and they found better stone free rates in patients undergoing both treatments compared with patients receiving only shockwave lithotripsy.[60] As mentioned earlier, the most common side effects associated with potassium citrate are gastrointestinal symptoms (nausea, bloating, diarrhea).

Struvite

Magnesium ammonium phosphate hexahydrate (struvite) stones arise in the setting of ureaseproducing bacterial urinary tract infections, and treatment consists of the surgical removal of the stone and antibiotic therapy to treat the infection. In patients who are not surgical candidates, Renacidin (hemiacidrin) and acetohydroxamic acid are 2 historical examples of alternative treatment of struvite stones. Although rarely used today due to the complexity of its irrigation protocol, irrigation of the renal collecting system with Renacidin solution through a nephrostomy tube after percutaneous struvite stone surgery was shown to effectively reduce struvite stone recurrence rates.[61] By chemically dissolving remnant stone fragments with Renacidin, the nidus for recurrent infection is removed and struvite stones are, in theory, less likely to recur. In addition, in a small randomized controlled trial, acetohydroxamic acid, which acts as a urease inhibitor, was shown to effectively inhibit growth of existing struvite stones compared with placebo.[62] Of note, however, the side effects profile of acetohydroxamic acid is high and often not well tolerated. Nearly 50% of patients undergoing treatment require a decrease in dosage or cessation of treatment due to adverse reactions such as anemia, headache, and/or gastrointestinal symptoms.[62]

Cystinuria

Cystine urinary stones are rare (1%–2%) and occur in patients with cystinuria, an inherited autosomal recessive disorder leading to a deficiency in the reabsorption of cystine at the proximal convoluted tubule, high levels of cystine in urine, and the frequent formation of urinary stones. The mainstay of cystinuria treatment is hydration and urine alkalinization therapy; however, some patients require additional pharmacotherapy with alpha mercapto-propionyl glycine (Thiola).[63] The mechanism of action involves promotion of cystine binding to decrease the amount of soluble cystine in urine. Because thiol medications have significant adverse effect profiles and low patient compliance rates, novel treatments are under investigation. One treatment, alpha-llpoic acid, has shown early promise in animal studies for protection against cystine stone formation. Using a mouse model, Zee and colleagues demonstrated that oral alpha-lipoic acid supplementation leads to increased urinary cystine solubility and thus lower rates of cystine stone formation with very low adverse side effects.[64] Human trials are currently underway and alpha-lipoic acid may ultimately become a useful and safe novel medical therapy for patients with cystinuria and recurrent stone disease.

SUMMARY

The pathophysiology underlying urinary stone formation remains an area of active investigation. There are many pharmacotherapies aimed at optimizing metabolic factors and reducing urinary supersaturation of stone components that play an important role in urinary stone prevention. In addition, medical expulsive therapy for ureteral stones and medical dissolution therapy for uric acid–based urinary stones are helpful treatment tools and are used alongside surgical treatments in the management of urinary stones.

DISCLOSURE

The authors have nothing to disclose.

REFERENCES

1. Johnson CM, Wilson DM, O'Fallon WM, et al. Renal stone epidemiology: A 25-year study in Rochester Minnesota. Kidney Int 1979;16:624–31.
2. Yoshida O, Okada Y. Epidemiology of urolithiasis in Japan: A chronological and geographical study. Urol Int 1990;45:104–11.
3. Serio A, Fraioli A. Epidemiology of nephrolithiasis. Nephron 1999;81:26–30.
4. Trinchieri A, Coppi F, Montanari E, et al. Increase in the prevalence of symptomatic upper urinary track stones during the past ten years. Eur Urol 2000;37:23–32.
5. Pearle MS, Calhoun EA, Gurhan GC. Urologic diseases in American project: Urolithiasis. J Urol 2005;173(3):848–57.
6. Stamatelou KK, Francis ME, Jones CA, et al. Time trends in reported prevalence of kidney stones in the United States: 1976-1994. Kidney Int 2003;63:1817–23.
7. Scales CD, Smith AC, Hanley JM, et al. Prevalence of kidney stones in the United States. Eur Urol 2012;62:160–5.
8. Osther PJS. Epidemiology of kidney stones in the European Union Urolithiasis: basic science and clinical practice. London, UK: Springer; 2012. p. 3–12.
9. Iguchi M, Umekawa T, Katoh Y, et al. Prevalence of urolithiasis in Kaizuka City, Japan—an epidemiologic study of urinary stones. Int J Urol 1996;3:175–9.
10. Bae SR, Seong JM, Kim LY, et al. The epidemiology of reno-ureteral stone disease in Koreans: a nationwide population-based study. Urolithiasis 2014;42:109–14.
11. Antonelli JA, Maalouf NM, Pearle MS, et al. Use of the National Health and Nutrition Examination Survey to calculate the impact of obesity and diabetes on cost and prevalence of urolithiasis in 2030. Eur Urol 2014;66:724–9.
12. Curhan GC, Rimm EB, Willett WC, et al. Regional variation in nephrolithiasis incidence and prevalence among United States men. J Urol 1994;151:838–41.
13. Hiatt RA, Dales LG, Friedman GD, et al. Frequency of urolithiasis in a prepaid medical care program. Am J Epidemiol 1982;115:255–65.
14. Sarmina I, Spirnak JP. Urinary lithiasis in the black population: An epidemiological study and review of the literature. J Urol 1987;138:14–7.
15. Soucie JM, Coates RJ, McClellan W, et al. Relation between geographic variability in kidney stones prevalence and risk factors for stones. Am J Epidemiol 1996;143:487–95.
16. Geraghty RM, Proietti S, Traxer O, et al. Worldwide Impact of Warmer Seasons on the Incidence of Renal Colic and Kidney Stone Disease: Evidence from a Systematic Review of Literature. J Endourol 2017;(8):729–35.
17. Dallas KB, Conti S, Liao JC, et al. Redefining the Stone Belt: Precipitation Is Associated with Increased Risk of Urinary Stone Disease. J Endourol 2017;31(11):1203–10.
18. Jungers P, Joly D, Barbey F, et al. ESRD caused by nephrolithiasis: prevalence, mechanisms, and prevention. Am J Kidney Dis 2004;44(5):799–805.
19. Pickard R, Starr K, MacLennan G, et al. Medical expulsive therapy in adults with ureteric colic: a multicentre, randomised, placebo-controlled trial. Lancet 2015;386:341–9.
20. Rule AD, Lieske JC, Li X, et al. The ROKS nomogram for predicting a second symptomatic stone episode. J Am Soc Nephrol 2014;25(12):2878–86.
21. Coe FL, Evan A, Worcester E. Kidney stone disease. J Clin Invest 2005;115(10):2598–608.
22. Evan AP. Physiopathology and etiology of stone formation in the kidney and the urinary tract. Pediatr Nephrol 2010;25(5):831–41.

23. Curhan GC, Willett WC, Speizer FE, et al. Twenty-four-hour urine chemistries and the risk of kidney stones among women and men. Kidney Int 2001; 59(6):2290–8.

24. Bouzidi H, Majdoub A, Daudon M, et al. Primary hyperoxaluria: A review. Nephrol Ther 2016;12(6): 431–6.

25. Vermeulen CW, Lyon ES. Mechanisms of genesis and growth of calculi. Am J Med 1968;45(5):684–92.

26. Verkoelen CF, Verhulst A. Proposed mechanisms in renal tubular crystal retention. Kidney Int 2007; 72(1):13–8.

27. Randall A. The etiology of primary renal calculus. Int Abstr Surg 1940;71:209–40.

28. Wiener SV, Ho SP, Stoller ML. Beginnings of nephrolithiasis: insights into the past, present and future of Randall's plaque formation research. Curr Opin Nephrol Hypertens 2018;27(4):236–42.

29. Chi T, Kim MS, Lang S, et al. A Drosophila Model Identifies a Critical Role for Zinc in Mineralization for Kidney Stone Disease. PLoS One 2015;10(5): e0124150.

30. Frassetto L, Kohlstadt I. Treatment and prevention of kidney stones: An update. Am Fam Physician 2011; 84(11):1234–42.

31. Pearle MS, Goldfarb DS, et al. Medical management of kidney stones: AUA Guideline. J Urol 2014;192(2): 316–24.

32. Tiselius HG, Ackermann D, Alken P, et al. Guidelines on urolithiasis. Arnhem. The Netherlands: European Association of Urology; 2006.

33. Hsi RS, Sanford T, Goldfarb DS, et al. The Role of the 24-Hour Urine Collection in the Prevention of Kidney Stone Recurrence. J Urol 2017;197(4):1084–9.

34. Kocvara R, Plasgura P, Petrik A, et al. A prospective study of nonmedical prophylaxis after a first kidney stone. BJU Int 1999;84(4):393–8.

35. American College of Physicians (ACP). Dietary and pharmacologic management to prevent recurrent nephrolithiasis in adults: A clinical practice guideline from the American College of Physicians. Ann Intern Med 2014;161(9):659–67.

36. Morgan MS, Pearle MS. Medical management of renal stones. BMJ 2016;352. i52.

37. Ettinger B, Pak CY, Citron JT, et al. Potassium-magnesium citrate is an effective prophylaxis against recurrent calcium oxalate nephrolithiasis. J Urol 1997;158:2069–73.

38. Barcelo P, Wuhl O, Servitge E, et al. Randomized double blind study of potassium citrate in idiopathic hypocitraturic calcium nephrolithiasis. J Urol 1993; 150:1761–4.

39. Pak CY. Etiology and treatment of urolithiasis. Am J Kidney Dis 1991;18:624–37.

40. Ettinger B, Tang A, Citron JT, et al. Randomized trial of allopurinol in the prevention of calcium oxalate calculi. N Engl J Med 1986;315:1386–9.

41. Stamp LK, Day RO, Yun J. Allopurinol hypersensitivity: investigating the cause and minimizing the risk. Nat Rev Rheumatol 2016;12(4):235–42.

42. Hoyer-Kuhn H, Kohbrok S, Volland R, et al. Vitamin B6 in primary hyperoxaluria I: first prospective trial after 40 years of practice. Clin J Am Soc Nephrol 2014;9:468–77.

43. Coe FL, Parks JH, Asplin JR. The pathogenesis and treatment of kidney stones. N Engl J Med 1992; 327(16):1141–52.

44. Buno Soto A, Torres Jimenez R, Olveira A, et al. Lithogenic risk factors for renal stones in patients with Crohn's disease. Arch Esp Urol 2001;54(3): 282–92.

45. Peck AB, Canales BK, Nguyen CQ. Oxalate-degrading microorganisms or oxalate-degrading enzymes: which is the future therapy for enzymatic dissolution of calcium-oxalate uroliths in recurrent stone disease? Urolithiasis 2016;44:45–50.

46. Strandvik B, Hjelte L. Nephrolithiasis in cystic fibrosis. Acta Paediatr 1993;82(3):306–7.

47. Jairath A, Parekh N, Otano N, et al. Oxalobacter formigenes: opening the door to probiotic therapy for the treatment of hyperoxaluria. Scand J Urol 2015; 49(4):334–7.

48. Lingeman JE, Pareek G, Easter L, et al. ALLN-177, oral enzyme therapy for hyperoxaluria. Int Urol Nephrol 2019;51:601–8.

49. Fink HA, Wilt TJ, Eidman KE, et al. Medical management to prevent recurrent nephrolithiasis in adults: a systematic review for an American College of Physicians clinical guideline. Ann Intern Med 2013;158: 535–43.

50. Zerwekh JE, Holt K, Pak CY. Natural urinary macromolecular inhibitors: attenuation of inhibitory activity by urate salts. Kidney Int 1983;23:838–41.

51. Bos D, Kapoor A. Update on medical expulsive therapy for distal ureteral stones: Beyond alpha-blockers. Can Urol Assoc J 2014;8(11–12):442–5.

52. Al-Ansari A, Al-Naimi A, Alobaidy A, et al. Efficacy of tamsulosin in the management of lower ureteral stones: a randomized double-blind placebo-controlled study of 100 patients. Urology 2010; 75(1):4–7.

53. Kaneko T, Matsushima H, Morimoto H, et al. Efficacy of low dose tamsulosin in medical expulsive therapy for ureteral stones in Japanese male patients: a randomized controlled study. Int J Urol 2010;17(5): 462–5.

54. Tamsulosin as a Medical Expulsive Therapy for Ureteral Stones: A Systematic Review and Meta-Analysis of Randomized Controlled Trials. J Urol 2019;201(5):950–5.

55. Porpiglia F, Vaccino D, Billia M. Corticosteroids and tamsulosin in the medical expulsive therapy for symptomatic distal ureter stones: Single drug or association? Eur Urol 2006;50:339–44.

56. Dellabella M, Milanese G, Muzzonigro G. Randomized trial of the efficacy of tamsulosin, nifedipine and phloroglucinol in medical expulsive therapy for distal ureteral calculi. J Urol 2005;174:167–72.

57. Seitz C, Liatsikos E, Porpiglia F, et al. Medical therapy to facilitate the passage of stones: what is the evidence? Eur Urol 2009;56(3):455–71.

58. Cao D, Yang L, Liu L, et al. A comparison of nifedipine and tamsulosin as medical expulsive therapy for the management of lower ureteral stones without. ESWL Sci Rep 2014;(4):5254.

59. Gridley CM, Sourial MW, Lehman A, et al. Medical dissolution therapy for the treatment of uric acid nephrolithiasis. World J Urol 2019;37:2509–15.

60. Elbaset MA, Hashem A, Eraky A, et al. Optimal noninvasive treatment of 1-2.5cm radiolucent renal stones: oral dissolution therapy, shock wave lithotripsy or combined treatment-a randomized controlled trial. World J Urol 2020;38:207–12.

61. Gonzalez RD, Whiting BM, Canales BK. The history of kidney stone dissolution therapy: 50 years of optimism and frustration with renacidin. J Endourol 2012;26(2):110–8.

62. Williams JJ, Rodman JS, Peterson CM. A randomized double-blind study of acetohydroxamic acid in struvite nephrolithiasis. N Engl J Med 1984;311(12):760–4.

63. Remien A, Kallistratos G, Purchardt P. Eur Urol 1975; 1(5):227–8.

64. Zee T, Bose N, Zee J, et al. a-Lipoic acid treatment prevents cystine urolithiasis in a mouse model of cystinuria. Nat Med 2017;23(3):288–90.

Immunosuppression Therapy in Kidney Transplantation

Oshorenua Aiyegbusi, MBChB, Ellon McGregor, MBChB, MD,
Siobhan K. McManus, MBChB, PhD, Kate I. Stevens, MBChB, PhD*

KEYWORDS

- Immunosuppression • Kidney transplant • Immunology

KEY POINTS

- Immunosuppression strategies in kidney transplantation have evolved significantly.
  Standard immunosuppression now includes T cell depleting therapy and steroids at induction, followed by tacrolimus and mycophenolate with or without oral steroids as maintenance therapy.
- Immunosuppression carries unwanted side effects
  Kidney transplant improves mortality and quality of life for the recipient. These improved outcomes run parallel with unwanted side effects including increased risk of infection and malignancy.
- Effective immunosuppression strategies are key in kidney transplantation.
  The Holy Grail is a strategy that prevents rejection while minimizing toxic side effects. Novel pharmacologic approaches, a better understanding of immune tolerance, epigenetics, and genomics should make this possible.

INTRODUCTION

The idea of replacing diseased organs has been around since the 18th century .[1] In 1933, the first recorded human cadaveric transplant was performed in Russia by Yurii Voronoy.[2] Unrecognised blood group incompatibility resulted in the death of the patient 2 days later. The discovery of immunologic tolerance by Billingham, Brent, Simonsen, and Medawar in the 1950s raised hope in the field of transplantation that there might be a way of manipulating allogenic immunologic response.[1,3] In 1954, the first successful kidney transplant occurred between identical twins, performed by Joseph.E. Murray and J.Hartwell Harrison in Boston, USA.[4] By 1959, experimental research from Robert Schwartz and William Dameshek showed mercaptopurine (used in leukemia) could induce immunologic tolerance by reducing antibody response.[5] Roy Calne tested the effect of mercaptopurine on the rejection of dog kidney homografts and found that it prolonged their survival.[6] 1962 was an explosive year in the world of transplantation. With the help of Calne, Murray went on to demonstrate the ground-breaking potential of immunosuppressive drugs. Murray achieved success in prolonging human-kidney graft survival using mercaptopurine and azathioprine instead of irradiation.[7] Tom Starzl also showed incredible graft survival of greater than 70% at 1 year with the addition of prednisolone to azathioprine.[8]

The development of the first effective drugs in kidney transplantation transformed the field. Newer more effective drugs have continued to improve graft and patient survival after kidney transplantation over subsequent decades.[9] Between 2010 and 2020, the graft survival in the

The Authors have nothing to disclose.
The Glasgow Renal and Transplant Unit, Queen Elizabeth University Hospital, Glasgow, UK
* Corresponding author.
E-mail address: Kate.stevens@glasgow.ac.uk
Twitter: @kateisabelle24 (K.I.S.)

0094-0143/22/© 2021 Elsevier Inc. All rights reserved.

UK for deceased donors was 94% and 86% at one and 5 years, respectively.[10] One and 5-year patient survival was 97% and 88%, respectively. For living donors, graft survival is 98% and 93% at one and 5 years with patient survival 99% and 95% at one and 5 years, respectively. Similar survival benefits associated with kidney transplantation are seen globally.[11]

In the last 20 years, the evolution of immunosuppression drugs and improved organ matching has contributed to better clinical outcomes. In the modern era, the goal remains to limit complications while maximizing graft survival and patient quality of life. This review provides a brief overview of the current pharmacologic agents commonly used in kidney transplantation.

EPIDEMIOLOGY OF KIDNEY TRANSPLANTATION

The number of people with end-stage kidney disease (ESKD) is rapidly increasing, with diabetes and hypertension the 2 leading causes of kidney disease.[12] Over 2.5 million people worldwide currently receive renal replacement therapy, and this is projected to double to 5.4 million by 2030.[13]

Since the 1990s, it has been recognized that a successful kidney transplant offers survival advantage and improves the quality of life and mortality compared with maintenance dialysis.[14,15] In 2014, there were about 80,000 kidney transplants from living and deceased donors globally.[16] In the UK, whereby universal health care is standard, roughly 4000 transplants occur each year, with another 5000 patients waiting for a transplant (6% of the UK population had CKD in 2014).[17,18]

Worldwide, there are inequalities in access to transplantation, with transplant rates of more than 30 per million population in 2010 restricted to Western Europe, USA, and Australia.[11] As hemodialysis is costly, low-middle income countries are encouraged to develop living donor kidney transplantation.[19] Several strategies involving key stakeholders have been designed and implemented to reduce disparities in transplantation among disadvantaged nations.[11] Kidney transplantation remains the preferred choice of treatment of ESKD in patients who are suitable.

TRANSPLANT IMMUNOLOGY – THE ALLOIMMUNE RESPONSE

The immune response of the recipient to the allograft is termed an alloimmune response. It is important to appreciate the alloimmune response to understand how immunosuppression agents exert their actions in kidney transplantation. Without immunosuppression agents, the transplant recipient's immune system recognizes the grafted tissue (allograft) as foreign and sets out to attack and destroy it (**Fig. 1**).

The immune response develops in response to donor tissue interacting with the major histocompatibility complex (MHC) proteins. These MHC molecules are called human leukocyte antigens (HLA), and the genetic region is located on the short arm of chromosome 6. The degree of HLA mismatch between donor and recipient plays a role in determining the risk of chronic rejection and graft loss. MHC molecules provide the means for displaying antigenic peptides to T cells. Antigen-presenting cells (APCs) express HLA molecules. They engage with the recipient's T cells to create the alloimmune response.

Allorecognition can occur by one of the 3 pathways: direct, indirect, and semi-direct. In the direct pathway, recipient's T cells recognize intact allogeneic HLAs expressed on the surface of donor cells.[20] Direct recognition is essential in acute rejection. Without appropriate immunosuppression, an alloresponse would follow due to the high number of recipient T-cells stimulated by

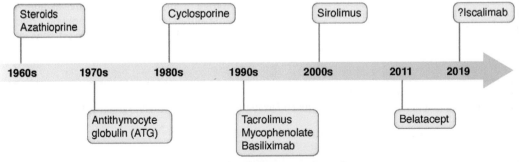

Fig. 1. Timeline of immunosuppression agents used in kidney transplantation.

the graft antigens and cause acute cellular rejection.

In the indirect pathway, T cells recognize peptides derived from donor HLAs presented by recipient APC.[21] Allopeptides are present during acute and chronic rejection. The indirect pathway is especially relevant in chronic or late acute rejection.[20] As long as the allograft is present in the host, the recipient APCs can pick up the alloantigen shed from the graft, present to T cells, and commence an alloimmune response. Therefore, maintenance immunosuppression is required for the lifetime of the allograft to prevent late rejection and chronic rejection.

The role of the third pathway (semi-direct) in transplantation is less well understood.

T cell recognition of alloantigen is central to the cascade of events that result in the rejection of a transplanted organ (**Fig. 2**). T cell recognizes alloantigen through T cell receptors (TCR) through a 3-signal process. An antigen triggers T cells transduced through the TCR-MHC complex (signal 1). A second costimulatory signal (signal 2) is provided via interaction with molecules and T cells.[20] Delivery of signals 1 and 2 activate several pathways including the calcium-calcineurin pathway and expression of cytokines, for example, interleukin-2 (IL-2). These pathways and cytokines interact leading to the activation of "target of rapamycin" pathway to provide signal 3, which subsequently triggers T cell proliferation. The result is fully activated T cells (CD4+ and CD8+T cells) that destroy and kill foreign cells.

In addition to T cells, other immune interactions contribute to graft rejection. Activated B cells lead to producing alloantibody against donor HLA antigens. Chemokines recruit the innate immune system. Innate immunity refers to the nonspecific natural immune system that involves macrophages, neutrophils, natural killer (NK) cells, cytokines, and complement components.

Immunosuppression agents disrupt the processes that play key roles in allograft rejection and rejection-associated tissue damage.

Immunosuppression Strategies

Kidney recipients require immunosuppression to prevent rejection. Many factors such as immunologic risk, comorbidities, clinical efficacy, and adverse effects may influence the selection of agents. Infection, malignancies (especially skin cancers), and cardiovascular disease are the principal complications postkidney transplantation. Inadvertently, the chronic use of immunosuppressive agents increases the long-term risk of these complications. The goal in immunosuppressive therapy is

to balance graft survival and the effects of over immunosuppression while considering the patients' individual needs. Immunosuppressive therapy in kidney transplantation falls into 2 broad categories: induction therapy and maintenance therapy.

Induction Therapy

Induction therapy is the immunosuppression treatment given at the time of kidney transplantation. Induction therapy aims to modulate T cell responses at the time of antigen presentation, thereby reducing early graft injury. Kidney Disease Improving Global Outcomes (KDIGO) guidelines favor using a T lymphocyte depleting agent or an interleukin 2 receptor blocking antibody (IL2-Ra) for induction, with lymphocyte-depleting induction reserved for high immunologic risk recipients (**Table 1**). There is variability geographically in the choice of agent. In Europe and Australia, IL2-Ra is used widely. In contrast, antithymocyte globulin (ATG) is used more frequently in the United States.[22–24] A more potent induction agent is the monoclonal antibody alemtuzumab (Campath).

Interleukin 2 receptors

Basiliximab (Simulect) is a chimeric monoclonal antibody against the α-chain of the interleukin-2 receptor (IL-2Ra).[25] Daclizumab (Zenapax), a humanized monoclonal antibody, is no longer in production due to reported cases of autoimmune encephalitis.[26]

CD25 is the alpha chain of the IL-2 receptor, normally expressed only by activated T-cells and important in the cellular response association with rejection.[27] Basiliximab competitively inhibits the alpha subunit of IL-2a. The terminal half-life is 7 days and no significant drug interactions reported.[27,28]

Basiliximab reduces the incidence of acute rejection when compared with placebo.[29] From the 2010 Cochrane meta-analysis, IL2-RA is comparable to ATG. There was no difference for biopsy-proven rejection at 3 or 6 months; however, there was a benefit of ATG therapy over IL-2Ra at 1 year (30% increase in rejection with IL-2Ra). When compared with placebo in this review, IL-2Ra consistently reduced the incidence of biopsy-proven biopsy results (69% at 3 months, 32% at 6 months, and 28% at 1-year post-transplantation). There was no difference in mortality; however, graft loss including death with a function allograft was reduced. IL2-Ra did not affect malignancy or cytomegalovirus (CMV) rates of infection.

Polyclonal antibodies

Polyclonal antibodies were the first biological immunosuppressive agent introduced into clinical

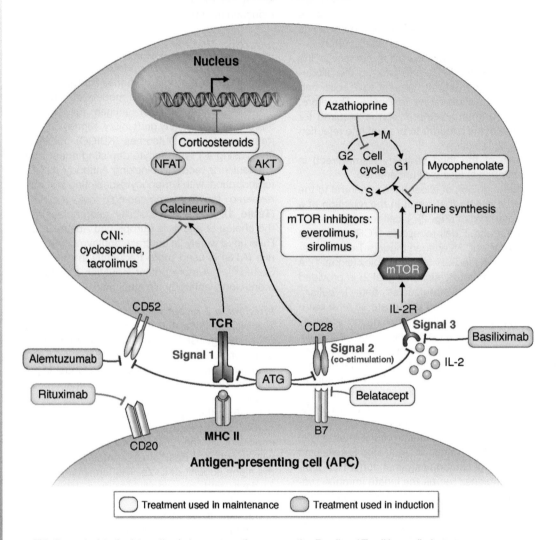

Fig. 2. T cell activation pathways and mechanisms of immunosuppression T cell. This figure depicts the interaction between an antigen-presenting B-cell and T-cell in an allo-immune response. Targets for immunosuppression are also shown (rituximab is a useful desensitization strategy in kidney transplantation). *Abbreviations:* NFAT, nuclear of activated T cell; AKT, protein kinase B, serine/threonine-specific protein kinase; CNI, calcineurin inhibitor; TCR, T-cell receptor; MHC, major histocompatibility complex; ATG, antithymocyte globulin; mTOR, mammalian target of rapamycin; IL-2, interleukin-2; IL-2R, IL-2 receptor.

transplantation. ATG (Thymoglobulin) is a polyclonal antibody derived from the immunization of rabbits with human thymocytes. The resulting IgG fraction from sera is then purified and pasteurized for use. Thymoglobulin consists of antibodies specific for T cell epitopes. Although the IgGs are anti–T-cell predominant, they also have activity against B cells, monocytes and neutrophils.[30] The mechanism of action of ATG is lymphocyte depletion, predominantly complement-mediated

Table 1
Induction immunosuppressive agents

Drug	Mechanism of Action	Common Side Effects	Common Drug Interactions
Basiliximab (Simulect)	Monoclonal antibodies against IL-2Ra (interleukin 2 receptor alpha)	Infusion reactions Gastrointestinal symptoms; abdominal pain. Diarrhea, nausea Leukopenia	No significant drug interactions Risk/Severity of infection increased with live vaccinations
Antithymocyte Globulin (ATG)	Polyclonal antibody with antilymphocyte actions (especially T-cells).	Infusion reactions Leukopenia Reactivation of infection	Risk/Severity of infection increased with live vaccinations
Alemtuzumab (Campath)	Anti-CD52 monoclonal antibody. Targets T, B lymphocytes, and other immune cells	Infusion reactions Leukopenia	No significant drug interactions

lysis of peripheral lymphocytes, and T-cell activation-induced apoptosis. The plasma half-life is 2 to 4 days with a terminal half-life of 13 days.[31] Adverse effects include leukopenia, systemic reactions from cytokine release (fever, chills, hypotension, and pulmonary edema), and infections.[32,33] Other reactions include skin rash, pruritis, thrombocytopenia and rarely anaphylaxis. To minimize these reactions, a combination of steroids, antihistamines, and paracetamol are given routinely 30 to 60 minutes before starting therapy.

Early trials in the 1970s showed efficacy for ATG when compared with a combination of corticosteroid and azathioprine, improving graft survival by 20%.[34] Later studies confirm induction therapy with ATG is superior to noninduction in tacrolimus-based regimens in preventing acute rejection (15% vs 30% in induction vs noninduction arms).[35] When compared with cyclosporine based treatment, the rate of acute rejection was lower in those treated with ATG-Tacrolimus (15%) compared with ATG-cyclosporine (21%) and tacrolimus based triple therapy (25%).[36]

Monoclonal antibodies – anti-CD52 (alemtuzumab)

Alemtuzumab is a monoclonal antibody against the CD52 antigen which is present on all peripheral blood lymphocytes. The evidence for alemtuzumab, when compared with ATG or IL2-Ra, is heterogeneous. In one study, patients in a low immunologic risk group had a lower rate of acute rejection at 1-year posttransplant (3% vs 20% in alemtuzumab and basiliximab, respectively).[37] There was no difference in patient or graft survival. In the higher risk group, alemtuzumab was compared with ATG, and there was no difference in acute rejection in both groups. Another study showed inferiority in graft and patient survival, particularly in the higher risk group.[38] However, late rejection is more likely to occur with alemtuzumab.[37,39] Another concern with alemtuzumab is that the perceived increased risk of infection as B and T depletion persists longer than with ATG.[40] However, meta-analysis has shown inconsistent results, reporting no significant differences between alemtuzumab and ATG for infection, graft failure, biopsy-proven acute rejection, and chronic allograft infection.[41] The majority of published studies in which alemtuzumab was used induction therapy are nonrandomized. However, it remains a valuable induction agent. Currently, it is unlicensed for use in organ transplantation in any market, and its use in this setting remains off-label. It is now only registered for multiple sclerosis and B-cell chronic lymphocytic leukemia.

Maintenance Therapy

The purpose of maintenance immunosuppression is to dampen the alloimmune response by using a combination of agents targeting different pathways. Treatment is commenced before or at the time of transplantation. Current KDIGO guidelines recommend a combination of calcineurin inhibitor and antiproliferative with or without corticosteroid. Higher doses of immunosuppression are used in the first 3 months when the risk of rejection is highest. Gradually immunosuppression is tapered to maintain sufficient immunosuppression. In this section, commonly used agents for maintenance therapy following kidney transplantation are described.

Calcineurin inhibitors

Calcineurin inhibitors (CNI) remain the cornerstone of immunosuppression for kidney transplantation. The 2 commonly used calcineurin inhibitors are cyclosporine and tacrolimus. Both agents act on

T lymphocytes by selectively inhibiting intracellular calcineurin, thereby suppressing the transcription of interleukin (IL)-2 and other cytokines.

Cyclosporine

In the 1980s, cyclosporine transformed organ transplantation by significantly reducing rejection rates.[42] Cyclosporine is a neutral lipophilic cyclic peptide isolated from the fungus *Hypocladium inflatum gams*.[43]

Cyclosporine is an inhibitor of calcineurin, a phosphatase enzyme that regulates numerous cellular processes, and that is involved in calcium-dependent signal transduction. Typically, in T cells, activation of T cell receptors increases intracellular calcium and thereby the activation of calcium responsive proteins such as calmodulin. The activation of calmodulin leads to the dephosphorylation of the nuclear transcription factor of activated T cells (NFAT).[44]

By preventing the calcineurin-mediated dephosphorylation, cyclosporine inhibits the nuclear translocation of the NFAT family thus reducing gene expression in activated T cells.[45]

Oral and intravenous formulations are available for cyclosporine. It is widely distributed into cells and plasma due to its lipophilic characteristics. Metabolism is extensively by the hepatic cytochrome P-450 CYP3A enzyme, thus prone to significant drug interactions in patients with hepatic dysfunction.[46] Some metabolism also occurs in the gut mucosa. Although cyclosporine is excreted in the bile, dose adjusting may be required in the presence of kidney dysfunction.

Close monitoring of cyclosporine levels is mandatory due to its pharmacokinetic profile, having a narrow therapeutic index. Hepatic metabolism via the cytochrome enzyme plays a role in the bioavailability and drug interactions. Several clinically relevant drug interactions are recognized (**Table 2**). Inducers or inhibitors of the cytochrome P450 enzyme result in decrease or increase in cyclosporine levels.

Target concentration levels vary on immunologic risk, choice of induction therapy, stage of kidney transplantation, and other patient factors. Typically, higher targets are aimed in the first year posttransplant, gradually reducing to avoid rejection while minimizing adverse effects. Immediately posttransplantation, levels are measured as frequently as daily. After discharge from the hospital, levels are monitored routinely.

The most common side effect of cyclosporine is nephrotoxicity (acute and chronic).[47] Cyclosporine (and tacrolimus) induce dose-dependent and reversible renal vasoconstriction to the afferent arterioles.[47] Cyclosporine induced renal vasoconstriction can delay the recovery from AKI. Clinically this may be difficult to differentiate from other causes of graft dysfunction. Though renal vasoconstriction is reversible in the short term, repeated renal ischemia from cyclosporine contributes to chronic interstitial fibrosis that occurs in long-term cyclosporine use. Other adverse effects include hyperkalemia, hypomagnesemia, hyperuricemia, hyperchloremic acidosis, hypertension, thrombotic microangiopathy, hyperlipidemia, gingival hyperplasia, and neurotoxicity.[48]

Tacrolimus

Tacrolimus, a macrolide agent derived from the fungus *Streptomyces tsukubaensis,* was introduced in kidney transplantation in the late 1990s.[49] Early results indicated tacrolimus was a more potent immunosuppressant than cyclosporin in reducing the rate of rejection.[50] Several studies have confirmed the superiority of tacrolimus in preventing graft loss by rejection.[51]

Although tacrolimus is structurally unrelated to cyclosporine, its mode of action is similar. It binds to an immunophilin, FK-binding protein (FKBP) in T lymphocytes creating a drug–receptor complex and subsequently inhibiting calcium-dependent activity. Tacrolimus also potentiates the actions of glucocorticoids and progesterone by binding to FKBPs contained within the hormone–receptor complex, preventing degradation.[52]

Tacrolimus is highly lipophilic and undergoes extensive tissue distribution; it is available in both oral and intravenous formulation. Complete metabolism occurs in the liver and gut through cytochrome P450 CYP3A enzymatic activity with excretion via the biliary system.

The approach to monitoring drug levels is similar to cyclosporine, as described. The side effect profile is comparable to that of cyclosporine; nephrotoxicity, neurotoxicity, hypertension, hyperlipidemia, diabetes, hyperkalemia, and hypomagnesemia. Tacrolimus is more diabetogenic than cyclosporine. Hypertension and hyperlipidemia are less likely to occur with tacrolimus while neurologic side effects more likely.[53,54] Tremors are a common neurologic side effect of tacrolimus. Gastrointestinal adverse effects occur more frequently with tacrolimus than cyclosporine.[53] Cosmetic side effects (gingival hyperplasia and hirsutism) are seen with cyclosporine therapy and less frequently with tacrolimus.

Tacrolimus is the preferred calcineurin inhibitor in most transplant centers worldwide. This is largely because tacrolimus is more potent and associated with less rejection and nephrotoxicity. In a meta-analysis, the benefit from tacrolimus diminished when used at higher doses, likely due to dose-related calcineurin toxicity and infection.[51]

Table 2
Maintenance immunosuppressive agents

Drug	Mechanism of Action	Common Side Effects*	Common Drug Interactions
Cyclosporine	Binds to cyclophilin: complex inhibits calcineurin phosphatase and T-cell activation. Suppress synthesis of IL-2 and other cytokines	Nephrotoxicity Hypertension Neurotoxicity Gingival hyperplasia Hirsutism Diabetes Mellitus Dyslipidaemia Hyperkalemia	Increased levels with: Erythromycin, clarithromycin Antifungals (particularly azoles) Verapamil, diltiazem, amlodipine Grapefruit Decreased levels with: Phenytoin, carbamazepine Isoniazid, rifampicin
Tacrolimus	Binds to FKBP12; similar mechanism of action to cyclosporine. Drug-receptor complex inhibits calcineurin phosphatase, T-cell activation, and other cytokines.	Similar to cyclosporine TREMOR	Similar to cyclosporine
Sirolimus/Everolimus	Binds to FKBP12; complex inhibits target of rapamycin and IL-2 mediated T-cell proliferation	Pneumonitis Poor wound healing Mouth ulcers Dyslipidaemia Thrombocytopenia Peripheral edema Proteinuria	Increased levels with: Erythromycin, clarithromycin Antifungals (particularly azoles) Fusidic acid Increased toxicity with calcineurin inhibitors.
Mycophenolate mofetil	Blocks purine synthesis, preventing the proliferation of T and B cells	Gastrointestinal symptoms; abdominal pain, nausea, vomiting, diarrhea (mainly), constipation Anemia Leukopenia	Increased levels with: Acyclovir, valganciclovir Decreased levels with: Proton pump inhibitors Quinolone antibiotics Absorption reduced by cyclosporine
Azathioprine	Interferes with DNA synthesis	Bone marrow suppression Leukopenia Hepatotoxicity	Increased levels with: Allopurinol Febuxostat Warfarin (decreased anticoagulant effect)
Corticosteroids	Antiinflammatory, immunosuppressive, and lymphocytic effects.	Diabetes Mellitus Hypertension 8 gain Osteoporosis Mood changes Sleep disturbance	Low-grade interactions
Belatacept (Nulojix)	T-lymphocyte antigen 4 (CTLA-4). Interferes with costimulatory pathway	Leukopenia Posttransplant lymphoproliferative disorder	No significant drug interactions

* Immunosuppressive agents are associated with an increased risk of infection including infection from for example, Cytomegalovirus (CMV) and BK virus which are only a concern in those who are immunocompromised and malignancy (in particular skin malignancies).

Tacrolimus association with the induction of hypertension and hyperlipidemia are significant concerns as the main cause of death among transplant recipients with a functioning graft is cardiovascular disease. Nevertheless, calcineurin inhibitors remain an essential class of immunosuppressive therapy in maintaining graft function.

Due to the hepatic CYP3A enzyme metabolism of CNI, consideration to prescribing practices is important. Coadministration of certain drugs can have led to life-threatening adverse effects. For example, clarithromycin should be avoided in patients on tacrolimus due to the risk of tacrolimus toxicity (see **Table 2**).

Mammalian target of rapamycin inhibitors

Sirolimus is a macrolide antibiotic produced from *Streptomyces hygroscopicus* which is structurally related to tacrolimus. Everolimus is a derivative of sirolimus with increased bioavailability.

These two agents are the mammalian target of rapamycin inhibitors (mTORi) and are approved for kidney transplantation. The main rationale for using these drugs is to avoid the adverse effects of calcineurin inhibitors, particularly nephrotoxicity and neurotoxicity. Due to its antitumoral effects, it is also used in kidney recipients with skin cancers.

Sirolimus and everolimus bind to the intracellular immunophilin FK-binding protein 12 (FKBP-12), however unlike tacrolimus, do not inhibit calcineurin activity.[55] Instead, they are highly specific inhibitors of mammalian target of rapamycin. mTOR inhibitors have antiproliferative effects. In contrast to CNI, mTORi does not affect the early changes of T-cell activation. Instead, they act late in the cell cycle, preventing IL2 mediated T-cell (and B cell) proliferation. Sirolimus also inhibits smooth muscle cell proliferation and may promote immune responses to cancer (approved as a treatment of lymphangioleiomyomatosis and renal cell carcinoma).

Both sirolimus and everolimus are metabolized via the cytochrome P450 system and excreted via the GI tract.[25] Therapeutic monitoring is advisable with target trough concentration for kidney recipients.

As both agents are substrates for cytochrome P450, inducers and inhibitors of this system can result in significant drug interactions. Coadministration of sirolimus and cyclosporine results in higher peak levels of sirolimus. Major adverse events include hematological effects (leukopenia, thrombotic microangiopathy is reported in combination with cyclosporin), metabolic effects (hyperlipidemia, hypercholesterolemia), dermatologic effects (mucositis, acne, poor wound healing).

Peripheral edema, proteinuria, and lymphocele formation post kidney transplantation are also recognized complications.[56]

mTORi have been shown to be effective immunosuppressive agents in kidney transplantation. Regimens using mTORi as a replacement for either calcineurin inhibitors or antimetabolite agents have been studied. Overall, patient and graft survival are comparable[57,58] In a systemic review of 33 RCTs evaluating mTORi (either sirolimus or everolimus) as a replacement for CNIs, there was no difference in graft survival, and patients had higher glomerular filtration rate (GFR) at 1 year.[57] However, there was a higher risk of acute rejection (RR 1.72, 95% CI (1.34–2.22) and increased risk of dyslipidemia and bone marrow suppression. In a meta-analysis of 11 RCTs examining the use of mTORi as a replacement for azathioprine or MMF, there were no differences in graft function or patient survival, and mTORi seemed to reduce the risk of acute rejection (RR 0.84, 95% CI 0.71–0.99).[58] Longer term outcomes are lacking from these studies.

Translating to clinical practice, mTORi are used as a CNI sparing strategy individualized to patients' specific clinical needs, balancing risks of benefit and adverse effects. Its use is significantly limited by the high incidence of side effects.[57]

Antiproliferative immunosuppressants

Mycophenolate Mycophenolate mofetil (MMF) is a prodrug of mycophenolic acid (MPA) that inhibits purine synthesis.[59] Proliferating T cells and B cells are dependent on DNA synthesis and mycophenolate inhibits this process. MPAs also reduce proliferative responses to allogenic stimulation.[59]

MMF is well absorbed after oral administration and rapidly metabolized by the liver to its active form, MPA. Plasma concentrations peak within 1 to 3 hours, with secondary peaks occurring at 6 to 12 hours due to enterohepatic circulation.[60] Active MPA undergoes glucuronidation to mycophenolic acid glucuronide which is primarily eliminated in the urine. No dose adjustment is required in hepatic dysfunction, although MPA is extensively bound to albumin.[61]

Gastrointestinal adverse events are prevalent with MMF and seem to be dose related.[62] Bone marrow suppression and consequently infection (particularly opportunistic) is a concern with MMF.[63] Posttransplantation, patients are monitored closely as concurrent use of other bone marrow suppression medication (such as valganciclovir) can predispose to leukopenia. MMF is also contraindicated in pregnancy due to the increased risk of birth defects and miscarriage in the first trimester. Women of childbearing age have prepregnancy counseling and are switched to azathioprine before conception.

MPA is available as enteric-coated mycophenolate sodium. The mechanism of action is similar to MMF; however, the enteric coating allows the delayed release of mycophenolic acid into the small intestine and may reduce gastrointestinal side effects, improving tolerabilty.[64]

Three large multi-centre double-blind randomized controlled trials from the 1990s revolutionized the use of MMF in kidney transplantation.[65–67] Two compared MMF to azathioprine and the third to placebo in patients taking cyclosporine and corticosteroids. Meta-analysis of these pivotal studies showed the incidence of graft loss at 1-year posttransplant was 2.6% in patients taking MMF compared with 6.3% for patients taking azathioprine or placebo.[68] Following this, most transplant centers favor MMF over azathioprine as the primary antimetabolite and adopt a 2g per day protocol.

Azathioprine Azathioprine (AZA) was the first immunosuppressive agent to achieve widespread use in kidney and other organ transplantation.[69] Nowadays, it is seldom used in kidney transplantation, reserved for cases of MMF intolerance and patients planning to become pregnant. The introduction and efficacy of mycophenolate mofetil and tacrolimus in the early and late 1990s, respectively, led to replacing of azathioprine as the predominant antimetabolite agent in kidney transplantation.[51,68]

Azathioprine is a prodrug of 6-mercaptopurine, a purine antagonist. Inhibition of cell proliferation is the main immunosuppressive effect of azathioprine on lymphocytes. After the oral ingestion of azathioprine, it is absorbed from the gastrointestinal tract and has a serum half-life of 0.2 to 0.5 hours.[70] In the GI system and red blood cells, AZA is converted to 6-mercaptopurine via the action of glutathione 6-mercaptopurine. It is further metabolized to active (6-thioguanosine nucleotides) and inactive metabolites (6-thiouric acid and 6-methylmercaptopurine).[71] Thioguanosine nucleotides interfere with purine synthesis and result in the inhibition of lymphocyte proliferation. In addition to the effects on DNA synthesis, azathioprine also inhibits the CD28 costimulation signal pathway and directly promotes apoptosis.[72]

Drug interaction with AZA is principally related to the enzymatic effect of xanthine oxidase and thiopurine S-methyltransferase (TPMT). Both enzymes are involved in the metabolism of 6-mercaptopurine into nontoxic metabolites. Purine analogs such as allopurinol inhibit xanthine oxidase, thereby increasing the toxicity of AZA.[73]

Some individuals have deficiency in TPMT increases the risk of myelosuppression from AZA.[71] For this reason, TPMT activity is checked prior starting treatment and xanthine oxidase inhibitors are generally avoided. Adverse effects are related to the gastrointestinal system including nausea, vomiting, and hepatitis.

Corticosteroids Corticosteroids were one of the first classes of drugs used in solid organ transplantation to prevent rejection. In the early 1960s, the "almost miracle" effect of corticosteroids was noted by Goodwin and Mims and 3 years later confirmed by Starzl and colleagues in kidney transplantation.[8,74] Transplant clinicians quickly adopted the routine use of corticosteroids (in combination with azathioprine) as maintenance therapy.[75]

Intracellularly, corticosteroids bind to the glucocorticoid receptor and generate a cascade of interactions leading to antiinflammatory, immunosuppressive, and lymphocytic effects. The net result is the depletion of T cells as a consequence of inhibition of IL-2, proinflammatory markers, and induction of apoptosis.[76,77]

A common practice in kidney transplantation is to administer a large dose of methylprednisolone perioperatively, tapering to a small dose (such as 5 mg daily) long-term posttransplantation. It is also used to treat acute rejection as a pulsed dose.

The side effects and morbidity associated with chronic steroid use are a concern in kidney transplantation. Chronic corticosteroid use contributes to insulin-resistant diabetes, weight gain, osteoporosis, hypertension, hyperlipidemia, and other systemic and cosmetic effects well known with its use. In pediatric kidney recipients, steroid avoidance is not associated with an increased risk of rejection.[78,79] In the adult recipient, steroid minimization strategies have gained popularity to mitigate adverse effects. Different strategies include complete withdrawal early after transplantation, lower cumulative dose, or complete avoidance.[80]

Generally, in clinical practice, patients with low immunologic risk (therefore, lower risk of rejection) are the preferred group for steroid withdrawal. Higher rates of acute rejection are seen with steroid free.[81–84]

Costimulation blocker Belatacept was approved as the first costimulation blocker in transplantation in 2011. It is also the first biological therapy used for maintenance therapy for transplant recipients. Belatacept is a T-lymphocyte antigen 4 (CTLA-4) fusion protein that binds CD80/86 on APCs to CD28 on T cells selectively interfering with the costimulatory pathway.[85] Available only as an intravenous infusion, belatacept has a mean half-life of about 7 days after a single-dose infusion.[86] It is given on the day of transplant and then monthly IV infusions posttransplantation. Its use is limited to transplant recipients who are Epstein–Barr Virus (EBV) seronegative or those with unknown EBV status due to the increased risk of developing posttransplant lymphoproliferative disorder (PTLD) evident in phase III studies.[87]

The BENEFIT and BENEFIT-EXT trials compared cyclosporine and belatacept in kidney recipients and extended criteria donor kidney recipients, respectively. Both results showed similar graft function at 12 months posttransplant in the belatacept group with superiority in kidney function due to the absence of nephrotoxicity.[88,89] Longer term analysis confirmed comparable graft survival despite an increased occurrence of acute rejection and PTLD.[90–92] Additionally, belatacept avoids the cardiovascular side effects seen with a CNI-based regimen. A limitation of the BENEFIT studies is that belatacept therapy was compared with cyclosporine. There is no large RCT that have been performed that compared outcomes of patients treated with either belatacept or tacrolimus. Most transplant centers use tacrolimus as the preferred antimetabolite. A limitation of the BENEFIT studies is that belatacept therapy was compared with ciclosporin therapy. Currently, the CNI of choice in most transplant centers is tacrolimus. No large, head-to-head, randomized controlled trials have been performed that compared the outcomes of patients treated with either belatacept or tacrolimus.

Two newer agents namely CFZ533 (iscalimab) and ASKP1240 (bleselumab) are currently being investigated for immunosuppressive therapy in kidney transplant recipients. These agents target the CD40/CD154 costimulatory pathway. The subcutaneous delivery of iscalimab offers a promising alternative to belatacept.

Bleselumab is a fully human anti-CD40 monoclonal antibody that prevents costimulatory signals required for T cell activation. It inhibits both humoral and cellular immune responses by blocking the interaction of the cell surface receptor CD40 and its ligand (CD154) between T cells, B cells, and antigen-presenting cells.[93] Recent phase II trials compared bleselumab/MMF and bleselumab/Tac to the standard of care (Tacrolimus, mycophenolate mofetil based regimen).[94] Results showed a noninferiority in the bleselumab/Tac group but not the bleselumab/MMF group compared with standard care. Similarly, drug-related side effects were higher in the bleselumab/MMF arm than in others.

Iscalimab another non–B-cell depleting fully human anti-CD40 antibody interfering with the CD40/CD154 pathway. Recently presented histologic data demonstrated benefit reducing chronic allograft changes.[95] These findings, albeit limited, are to be confirmed in ongoing Phase 2b trials.[96]

AGING AND IMMUNOSUPPRESSION

Many patients once considered high risk due to increasing age, are now routinely transplanted. Older patients also exhibit less immunogenicity as aging is thought to dampen the innate immune system.[97] Increasing recipient age (>65 years) is associated with lower rates of rejection; however, the impact of acute rejection may be more significant in this age group. Often these patients are age matched with older donors which are associated with poorer graft outcomes.[98] Elderly recipients are more likely to have multiple comorbidities at the time of transplant than younger patients.[99] Physiologic changes that occur in aging may alter drug pharmacokinetics. Individual tailoring of immunosuppressive therapy is, therefore, crucial in the elderly population due to altered immune response, increased risk of drug toxicity, infections, malignancy, and cardiovascular diseases. Some transplant centers use a reduced dose of MMF (reduction by 50%) and avoid corticosteroids due to the increased risk of delirium postoperatively. Other options include lower target concentration of CNIs and minimal induction agents.

Other Considerations

Various other immunosuppressive drugs (such as rituximab) interfere with immune pathways involved in allograft recognition and rejection. As the population lives longer, individuals require more than one kidney transplant in their lifetime. Sensitization in kidney transplantation refers to patients with detectable anti-HLA antibodies. Sensitization to HLA antigens occurs mainly through blood transfusion, pregnancy, and previous organ transplantation. Sensitized patients have high titers of preformed circulating anti-HLA antibodies. Desensitization lowers immunogenicity, thereby allowing transplantation with induction and maintenance therapy as previously discussed. Rituximab is a CD20 monoclonal antibody used in many desensitization protocols across transplant centers. An in-depth discussion of desensitization strategies is beyond the scope of this review.

In addition to immunosuppressive therapy, kidney transplant recipients require coadministration of chemoprophylaxis. While immunosuppressive medication prevents graft rejection, it increases the risk of developing infection especially opportunistic infections such as cytomegalovirus (CMV) infection. Both the donor and recipient are tested for cytomegalovirus preceding transplantation.

Valganciclovir or ganciclovir is used as primary prophylaxis therapy in patients at risk for CMV infection for at least 3 months after transplantation.[100] CMV donor-positive/recipient-negative (D+/R-) patients are at the highest risk of developing CMV infection and disease. Without preventive treatment, CMV infection and disease occurs in about 70% and 56% of patients.[101] With prophylactic treatment, CMV disease falls by a third.[101,102] In patients who are CMV D-/R+ and D+/R+, the risk of CMV infection remains as high as 70%; however, the risk of CMV disease falls to 20%. CMV D-/R has the lowest risk of CMV infection and disease (5%) and do not need prophylactic treatment.[103] The safety profile of valganciclovir is similar to ganciclovir. Leukopenia is a concern with both agents.

Prophylactic cotrimoxazole (trimethoprim-sulfamethoxazole) is also administered after kidney transplantation to prevent *Pneumocystis jirovecii* pneumonia, PCP (formerly known as *Pneumocystis carinii* pneumonia). PCP is an opportunistic fungal pathogen known to cause life-threatening pneumonia in immunocompromised patients, including kidney transplant recipients. About 5% of patients who do not take prophylaxis develop PCP.[104] Current guidelines recommend 3 to 6 months for PCP prophylactic treatment following kidney transplantation.[100] Alternatives include dapsone, pentamidine, and atovaquone. Adverse effects of cotrimoxazole include GI disturbances, skin disorders (including Stevens–Johnson syndrome), and leukopenia.

The combination of mediations used in kidney recipients has synergistic adverse effects. MMF, cotrimoxazole, and valganciclovir in combination potentiate the risk of myelosuppression and thus opportunistic infection. CNIs, cotrimoxazole and renal angiotensin aldosterone inhibitors (RAASi) can lead to hyperkalemia and graft dysfunction. Generally, angiotensin-converting enzyme inhibitors and angiotensin receptor blockers are avoided posttransplant, unless clinically indicated. Kidney recipients are also closely monitored for new-onset diabetes after transplantation (NODAT) due to the use of tacrolimus and steroids in maintenance therapy.

SUMMARY

Kidney transplantation has advanced significantly since the early days of Voronoy in the 1930s. Standard immunosuppression now includes T cell depleting therapy and steroids at induction, followed by tacrolimus and mycophenolate with or without oral steroids as maintenance therapy. This "gold-standard" therapy has led to the impressive outcomes we now see in kidney transplantation. The average life span of a kidney transplant is 15 years with improved mortality and quality of life for the recipient. Unfortunately, these improved outcomes run parallel with unwanted side effects associated with immunosuppression agents as well as longer-term complications including higher rates of malignancy. While cardiovascular risk is improved compared with patients on dialysis, it is still higher in kidney transplant recipients than in matched controls in the general population.[105] As the population lives longer, an increasing number of older patients with ESKD are receiving kidney transplants. Older patients (>65 years) are at a higher risk of complications including infection and malignancy.

Although pharmacologic immunosuppression is the mainstay of therapeutic strategies, establishing tolerance to an allograft has become an area of interest in kidney transplantation. The therapeutic potential of regulatory T cells (T regs) in promoting transplant tolerance is a growing field.

The future aims to individualize immunosuppression such that a patient is maintained on a dose adequate to prevent the rejection of the transplanted organ while minimizing toxic side effects. Novel pharmacologic approaches, reperfusion techniques, a better understanding of immune tolerance, epigenetics, and genomics should make this possible.

REFERENCES

1. Barker CF, Markmann JF. Historical overview of transplantation. Cold Spring Harb Perspect Med 2013; 3(4):a014977. https://doi.org/10.1101/cshperspect. a014977.

2. Matevossian E, Kern H, Hüser N, et al. Surgeon Yurii Voronoy (1895–1961) – a pioneer in the history of clinical transplantation: in Memoriam at the 75th Anniversary of the First Human Kidney Transplantation. Transpl Int 2009;22:1132–9. https://doi.org/10. 1111/j.1432-2277.2009.00986.x.

3. Calne RY, Shackman R, Nolan B, et al. Results of kidney transplantation. Lancet 1970;1(7648):671–2. https://doi.org/10.1016/s0140-6736(70)90901-3.

4. Harrison JH, Merrill JP, Murray JE. Renal homotransplantation in identical twins. 1955. J Am Soc Nephrol 2001;12(1):201–4. https://doi.org/10.1681/ ASN.V121201.

5. Schwartz R, Dameshek W. Drug-induced immunological tolerance. Nature 1959;183(4676):1682–3. https://doi.org/10.1038/1831682a0.

6. Calne RY. The rejection of renal homografts. Inhibition in dogs by 6-mercaptopurine. Lancet 1960; 1(7121):417–8. https://doi.org/10.1016/s0140-6736 (60)90343-3.

7. Murray JE, Merrill JP, Harrison JH, et al. Prolonged survival of human-kidney homografts by immuno-suppressive drug therapy. Ann Plast Surg 1984; 12(1):70–83. https://doi.org/10.1097/00000637-198401000-00010.

8. Starzl TE, Marchioro TL, Waddell WR. The reversal of rejection in human renal homografts with subsequent development of homograft tolerance. Surg Gynecol Obstet 1963;117:385–95.

9. Meier-Kriesche HU, Ojo AO, Port FK, et al. Survival improvement among patients with end-stage renal disease: trends over time for transplant recipients and wait-listed patients. J Am Soc Nephrol 2001;12(6):1293–6. https://doi.org/10.1681/ASN.V1261293.

10. NHS Blood and Transplant. Annual report on kidney transplantation 2020. Available at: https://nhsbtdbe.blob.core.windows.net/umbraco-assets-corp/25574/kidney-annual-report-2020-21.pdf. Accessed July 13, 2021.

11. Garcia GG, Harden P, Chapman J. The global role of kidney transplantation. Am J Nephrol 2012. https://doi.org/10.1159/000336371.

12. Couser WG, Remuzzi G, Mendis S, et al. The contribution of chronic kidney disease to the global burden of major noncommunicable diseases. Kidney Int 2011;80(12):1258–70. https://doi.org/10.1038/ki.2011.368.

13. Liyanage T, Ninomiya T, Jha V, et al. Worldwide access to treatment for end-stage kidney disease: a systematic review. Lancet 2015;385(9981):1975–82. https://doi.org/10.1016/S0140-6736(14)61601-9.

14. Schnuelle P, Lorenz D, Trede M, et al. Impact of renal cadaveric transplantation on survival in end-stage renal failure: evidence for reduced mortality risk compared with hemodialysis during long-term follow-up. J Am Soc Nephrol 1998;9(11):2135–41.

15. Port FK, Wolfe RA, Mauger EA, et al. Comparison of survival probabilities for dialysis patients vs cadaveric renal transplant recipients. JAMA 1993; 270(11):1339–43.

16. Mahillo B, Carmona M, Alvarez M, et al. Worldwide distribution of solid organ transplantation and access of population to those practices. Transplantation 2018;102:S71–2. https://doi.org/10.1097/01.tp.0000542650.33995.b3.

17. Barron E. Chronic kidney disease prevalence model. Public Heal Engl 2014. Available at: https://assets.publishing.service.gov.uk/government/uploads/system/uploads/attachment_data/file/612303/ChronickidneydiseaseCKDprevalencemodelbriefing.pdf. July 17, 2021.

18. Transplant Actvity. NHS Blood and Transplant. Annual Report on Kidney Transplantation. Available at: https://nhsbtdbe.blob.core.windows.net/umbraco-assets-corp/16778/nhsbt-kidney-transplantation-annual-report-2018-19.pdf. July 18, 2021.

19. Himmelfarb J, Vanholder R, Mehrotra R, et al. The current and future landscape of dialysis. Nat Rev Nephrol 2020;16(10):573–85. https://doi.org/10.1038/s41581-020-0315-4.

20. Kumbala D, Zhang R. Essential concept of transplant immunology for clinical practice. World J Transpl 2013;3(4):113–8. https://doi.org/10.5500/wjt.v3.i4.113.

21. Vella JP, Spadafora-Ferreira M, Murphy B, et al. Indirect allorecognition of major histocompatibility complex allopeptides in human renal transplant recipients with chronic graft dysfunction. Transplantation 1997;64(6):795–800. https://doi.org/10.1097/00007890-199709270-00001.

22. Campbell S, McDobald S, Excell L, et al. ANZDATA registry report. 2008. Available at: https://www.anzdata.org.au/report/anzdata-31st-annual-report-2008/. July 24, 2021.

23. Matas AJ, Smith JM, Skeans MA, et al. OPTN/SRTR 2012 annual data report: kidney. Am J Transpl 2014;14(Suppl 1):11–44. https://doi.org/10.1111/ajt.12579.

24. Opelz G, Döhler B, Collaborative Transplant Study. Influence of immunosuppressive regimens on graft survival and secondary outcomes after kidney transplantation. Transplantation 2009;87(6):795–802. https://doi.org/10.1097/TP.0b013e318199c1c7.

25. Taylor AL, Watson CJ, Bradley JA. Immunosuppressive agents in solid organ transplantation: Mechanisms of action and therapeutic efficacy. Crit Rev Oncol Hematol 2005;56(1):23–46. https://doi.org/10.1016/j.critrevonc.2005.03.012.

26. ▼ Daclizumab withdrawn from the market worldwide. Drug Ther Bull 2018;56(4):38. https://doi.org/10.1136/dtb.2018.4.0604.

27. Berard JL, Velez RL, Freeman RB, et al. A review of interleukin-2 receptor antagonists in solid organ transplantation. Pharmacotherapy 1999;19(10):1127–37. https://doi.org/10.1592/phco.19.15.1127.30582.

28. Van Gelder T, Warlé M, Ter Meulen RG. Anti-interleukin-2 receptor antibodies in transplantation: what is the basis for choice? Drugs 2004;64(16):1737–41. https://doi.org/10.2165/00003495-200464160-00001.

29. Webster AC, Playford EG, Higgins G, et al. Interleukin 2 receptor antagonists for renal transplant recipients: a meta-analysis of randomized trials. Transplantation 2004;77(2):166–76. https://doi.org/10.1097/01.TP.0000109643.32659.C4.

30. Hardinger KL. Rabbit antithymocyte globulin induction therapy in adult renal transplantation. Pharmacotherapy 2006;26(12):1771–83. https://doi.org/10.1592/phco.26.12.1771.

31. Deeks ED, Keating GM. Rabbit antithymocyte globulin (thymoglobulin): a review of its use in the prevention and treatment of acute renal allograft rejection. Drugs 2009;69(11):1483–512. https://doi.org/10.2165/00003495-200969110-00007.

32. Taniguchi Y, Frickhofen N, Raghavachar A, et al. Antilymphocyte immunoglobulins stimulate peripheral blood lymphocytes to proliferate and release lymphokines. Eur J Haematol 1990;44(4):244–51. https://doi.org/10.1111/j.1600-0609.1990.tb00387.x.

33. Merion RM, Howell T, Bromberg JS. Partial T-cell activation and anergy induction by polyclonal antithymocyte globulin. Transplantation 1998;65(11):1481–9. https://doi.org/10.1097/00007890-199806150-00013.

34. Cosimi AB, Wortis HH, Delmonico FL, et al. Randomized clinical trial of antithymocyte globulin in cadaver renal allograft recipients: importance of T cell monitoring. Surgery 1976;80(2):155–63.

35. Mourad G, Garrigue V, Squifflet JP, et al. Induction versus noninduction in renal transplant recipients with tacrolimus-based immunosuppression. Transplantation 2001;72(6):1050–5. https://doi.org/10.1097/00007890-200109270-00012.

36. Charpentier B, Rostaing L, Berthoux F, et al. A three-arm study comparing immediate tacrolimus therapy with antithymocyte globulin induction therapy followed by tacrolimus or cyclosporine A in adult renal transplant recipients. Transplantation 2003;75(6):844–51. https://doi.org/10.1097/01.TP.0000056635.59888.EF.

37. Hanaway MJ, Woodle ES, Mulgaonkar S, et al. Alemtuzumab induction in renal transplantation. N Engl J Med 2011;364(20):1909–19. https://doi.org/10.1056/NEJMoa1009546.

38. Sureshkumar KK, Thai NL, Hussain SM, et al. Influence of induction modality on the outcome of deceased donor kidney transplant recipients discharged on steroid-free maintenance immunosuppression. Transplantation 2012;93(8):799–805. https://doi.org/10.1097/TP.0b013e3182472898.

39. Watson CJ, Bradley JA, Friend PJ, et al. Alemtuzumab (CAMPATH 1H) induction therapy in cadaveric kidney transplantation–efficacy and safety at five years. Am J Transpl 2005;5(6):1347–53. https://doi.org/10.1111/j.1600-6143.2005.00822.x.

40. Clatworthy MR, Friend PJ, Calne RY, et al. Alemtuzumab (CAMPATH-1H) for the treatment of acute rejection in kidney transplant recipients: long-term follow-up. Transplantation 2009;87(7):1092–5. https://doi.org/10.1097/TP.0b013e31819d3353.

41. Zheng J, Song W. Alemtuzumab versus antithymocyte globulin induction therapies in kidney transplantation patients: a systematic review and meta-analysis of randomized controlled trials. Medicine (Baltimore) 2017;96(28):e7151. https://doi.org/10.1097/MD.0000000000007151.

42. Gordon RD, Iwatsuki S, Shaw BW Jr, et al. Cyclosporine-steroid combination therapy in 84 cadaveric renal transplants. Am J Kidney Dis 1985;5(6):307–12. https://doi.org/10.1016/s0272-6386(85)80159-1.

43. Matsuda S, Koyasu S. Mechanisms of action of cyclosporine. Immunopharmacology 2000;47(2–3):119–25. https://doi.org/10.1016/s0162-3109(00)00192-2.

44. Baksh S, Burakoff SJ. The role of calcineurin in lymphocyte activation. Semin Immunol 2000;12(4):405–15. https://doi.org/10.1006/smim.2000.0221.

45. Schreiber SL, Crabtree GR. The mechanism of action of cyclosporin A and FK506. Immunol Today 1992;13(4):136–42. https://doi.org/10.1016/0167-5699(92)90111-J.

46. Christians U, Sewing KF. Cyclosporin metabolism in transplant patients. Pharmacol Ther 1993;57(2–3):291–345. https://doi.org/10.1016/0163-7258(93)90059-m.

47. Shah MB, Martin JE, Schroeder TJ, et al. The evaluation of the safety and tolerability of two formulations of cyclosporine: neoral and sandimmune. A meta-analysis. Transplantation 1999;67(11):1411–7. https://doi.org/10.1097/00007890-199906150-00004.

48. Kahan BD. Cyclosporine. N Engl J Med 1989;321(25):1725–38. https://doi.org/10.1056/NEJM198912213212507.

49. Wallemacq PE, Reding R. FK506 (tacrolimus), a novel immunosuppressant in organ transplantation: clinical, biomedical, and analytical aspects. Clin Chem 1993;39(11):2219–28. https://doi.org/10.1093/clinchem/39.11.2219.

50. Pirsch JD, Miller J, Deierhoi MH, et al. A comparison of tacrolimus (FK506) and cyclosporine for immunosuppression after cadaveric renal transplantation. FK506 Kidney Transplant Study Group. Transplantation 1997;63(7):977–83. https://doi.org/10.1097/00007890-199704150-00013.

51. Webster AC, Woodroffe RC, Taylor RS, et al. Tacrolimus versus ciclosporin as primary immunosuppression for kidney transplant recipients: meta-analysis and meta-regression of randomised trial data. BMJ 2005;331(7520):810. https://doi.org/10.1136/bmj.38569.471007.AE.

52. Thomson AW, Bonham CA, Zeevi A. Mode of action of tacrolimus (FK506): molecular and cellular mechanisms. Ther Drug Monit 1995;17(6):584–91. https://doi.org/10.1097/00007691-199512000-00007.

53. U.S. Multicenter FK506 Liver Study Group. A comparison of tacrolimus (FK 506) and cyclosporine for immunosuppression in liver transplantation. N Engl J Med 1994;331(17):1110–5. https://doi.org/10.1056/NEJM199410273311702.

54. Randomised trial comparing tacrolimus (FK506) and cyclosporin in prevention of liver allograft rejection. European FK506 Multicentre Liver Study Group. Lancet 1994;344(8920):423–8.

55. Mita MM, Mita A, Rowinsky EK. The molecular target of rapamycin (mTOR) as a therapeutic target against cancer. Cancer Biol Ther 2003;2(4 Suppl 1):S169–77.

56. Valente JF, Hricik D, Weigel K, et al. Comparison of sirolimus vs. mycophenolate mofetil on surgical complications and wound healing in adult kidney transplantation. Am J Transpl 2003;3(9):1128–34. https://doi.org/10.1034/j.1600-6143.2003.00185.x.

57. Lim WH, Eris J, Kanellis J, et al. A systematic review of conversion from calcineurin inhibitor to mammalian target of rapamycin inhibitors for maintenance immunosuppression in kidney transplant recipients. Am J Transpl 2014;14(9):2106–19. https://doi.org/10.1111/ajt.12795.

58. Webster AC, Lee VW, Chapman JR, et al. Target of rapamycin inhibitors (sirolimus and everolimus) for primary immunosuppression of kidney transplant recipients: a systematic review and meta-analysis of randomized trials. Transplantation 2006;81(9):1234–48. https://doi.org/10.1097/01.tp.0000219703.39149.85.

59. Allison AC, Eugui EM. Mycophenolate mofetil and its mechanisms of action. Immunopharmacology 2000;47(2–3):85–118. https://doi.org/10.1016/s0162-3109(00)00188-0.

60. Bullingham RE, Nicholls AJ, Kamm BR. Clinical pharmacokinetics of mycophenolate mofetil. Clin Pharmacokinet 1998;34(6):429–55. https://doi.org/10.2165/00003088-199834060-00002.

61. Parker G, Bullingham R, Kamm B, et al. Pharmacokinetics of oral mycophenolate mofetil in volunteer subjects with varying degrees of hepatic oxidative impairment. J Clin Pharmacol 1996;36(4):332–44. https://doi.org/10.1002/j.1552-4604.1996.tb04209.x.

62. Fulton B, Markham A. Mycophenolate mofetil. A review of its pharmacodynamic and pharmacokinetic properties and clinical efficacy in renal transplantation. Drugs 1996;51(2):278–98. https://doi.org/10.2165/00003495-199651020-00007.

63. Sollinger HW. Mycophenolates in transplantation. Clin Transpl 2004;18(5):485–92. https://doi.org/10.1111/j.1399-0012.2004.00203.x.

64. Budde K, Dürr M, Liefeldt L, et al. Enteric-coated mycophenolate sodium. Expert Opin Drug Saf 2010;9(6):981–94. https://doi.org/10.1517/14740338.2010.513379.

65. Mathew TH. A blinded, long-term, randomized multicenter study of mycophenolate mofetil in cadaveric renal transplantation: results at three years. Tricontinental Mycophenolate Mofetil Renal Transplantation Study Group [published correction appears in Transplantation 1998 Sep 27;66(6):817]. Transplantation 1998;65(11):1450–4. https://doi.org/10.1097/00007890-199806150-00007.

66. A blinded, randomized clinical trial of mycophenolate mofetil for the prevention of acute rejection in cadaveric renal transplantation. The Tricontinental Mycophenolate Mofetil Renal Transplantation Study Group. Transplantation 1996;61(7):1029–37.

67. Sollinger HW. Mycophenolate mofetil for the prevention of acute rejection in primary cadaveric renal allograft recipients. U.S. Renal Transplant Mycophenolate Mofetil Study Group. Transplantation 1995;60(3):225–32. https://doi.org/10.1097/00007890-199508000-00003.

68. Halloran P, Mathew T, Tomlanovich S, et al. Mycophenolate mofetil in renal allograft recipients: a pooled efficacy analysis of three randomized, double-blind, clinical studies in prevention of rejection. The International Mycophenolate Mofetil Renal Transplant Study Groups [published correction appears in Transplantation 1997 Feb 27;63(4):618]. Transplantation 1997;63(1):39–47. https://doi.org/10.1097/00007890-199701150-00008.

69. Murray JE, Merrill JP, Dammin GJ, et al. Kidney transplantation in modified recipients. Ann Surg 1962;156(3):337–55. https://doi.org/10.1097/00000658-196209000-00002.

70. Huskisson EC. Azathioprine. Clin Rheum Dis 1984;10(2):325–32.

71. Van Scoik KG, Johnson CA, Porter WR. The pharmacology and metabolism of the thiopurine drugs 6-mercaptopurine and azathioprine. Drug Metab Rev 1985;16(1–2):157–74. https://doi.org/10.3109/03602538508991433.

72. Tiede I, Fritz G, Strand S, et al. CD28-dependent Rac1 activation is the molecular target of azathioprine in primary human CD4+ T lymphocytes. J Clin Invest 2003;111(8):1133–45. https://doi.org/10.1172/JCI16432.

73. Sahasranaman S, Howard D, Roy S. Clinical pharmacology and pharmacogenetics of thiopurines. Eur J Clin Pharmacol 2008;64(8):753–67. https://doi.org/10.1007/s00228-008-0478-6.

74. Goodwin WE, Mims MM, Kaufman JJ. Human renal transplantation III. Technical problems encountered in six cases of kidney homotransplantation. Trans Am Assoc Genitourin Surg 1962;54:116–25.

75. Curtis J. Corticosteroids and kidney transplantation. Clin J Am Soc Nephrol 2006;1(5):907–8. https://doi.org/10.2215/CJN.02340706.

76. De Lucena DD, Rangel ÉB. Glucocorticoids use in kidney transplant setting. Expert Opin Drug Metab Toxicol 2018;14(10):1023–41. https://doi.org/10.1080/17425255.2018.1530214.

77. Fauci AS, Dale DC, Balow JE. Glucocorticosteroid therapy: mechanisms of action and clinical

considerations. Ann Intern Med 1976;84(3): 304–15. https://doi.org/10.7326/0003-4819-84-3-304.

78. Sarwal MM, Ettenger RB, Dharnidharka V, et al. Complete steroid avoidance is effective and safe in children with renal transplants: a multicenter randomized trial with three-year follow-up. Am J Transpl 2012;12(10):2719–29. https://doi.org/10.1111/j.1600-6143.2012.04145.x.

79. Naesens M, Salvatierra O, Benfield M, et al. Subclinical inflammation and chronic renal allograft injury in a randomized trial on steroid avoidance in pediatric kidney transplantation. Am J Transpl 2012;12(10):2730–43. https://doi.org/10.1111/j.1600-6143.2012.04144.x.

80. Banerjee A, Julie BM, Sharma A, et al. Steroid withdrawal protocols in renal transplantation. Arch Clin Nephrol 2017;4(1):001–8. https://doi.org/10.17352/acn.000029.

81. Krämer BK, Klinger M, Vítko Š, et al. Tacrolimus-based, steroid-free regimens in renal transplantation: 3-year follow-up of the ATLAS trial. Transplantation 2012;94(5):492–8. https://doi.org/10.1097/TP.0b013e31825c1d6c.

82. Vincenti F, Schena FP, Paraskevas S, et al. A randomized, multicenter study of steroid avoidance, early steroid withdrawal or standard steroid therapy in kidney transplant recipients [published correction appears in Am J Transplant.2008 May; 8(5):1080]. Am J Transpl 2008;8(2):307–16.

83. Matas AJ, Ramcharan T, Paraskevas S, et al. Rapid discontinuation of steroids in living donor kidney transplantation: a pilot study. Am J Transpl 2001; 1(3):278–83. https://doi.org/10.1034/j.1600-6143.2001.001003278.x.

84. Woodle ES, First MR, Pirsch J, et al. A prospective, randomized, double-blind, placebo-controlled multicenter trial comparing early (7 day) corticosteroid cessation versus long-term, low-dose corticosteroid therapy. Ann Surg 2008;248(4):564–77. https://doi.org/10.1097/SLA.0b013e318187d1da.

85. Noble J, Jouve T, Janbon B, et al. Belatacept in kidney transplantation and its limitations. Expert Rev Clin Immunol 2019;15(4):359–67. https://doi.org/10.1080/1744666X.2019.1574570.

86. Moudgil A, Dharnidharka VR, Feig DI, et al. Phase I study of single-dose pharmacokinetics and pharmacodynamics of belatacept in adolescent kidney transplant recipients. Am J Transpl 2019;19(4): 1218–23. https://doi.org/10.1111/ajt.15236.

87. Grinyó J, Charpentier B, Pestana JM, et al. An integrated safety profile analysis of belatacept in kidney transplant recipients. Transplantation 2010; 90(12):1521–7. https://doi.org/10.1097/TP.0b013e3182007b95.

88. Vincenti F, Charpentier B, Vanrenterghem Y, et al. A phase III study of belatacept-based immunosuppression regimens versus cyclosporine in renal transplant recipients (BENEFIT study). Am J Transpl 2010;10(3):535–46. https://doi.org/10.1111/j.1600-6143.2009.03005.x.

89. Durrbach A, Pestana JM, Pearson T, et al. A phase III study of belatacept versus cyclosporine in kidney transplants from extended criteria donors (BENEFIT-EXT study). Am J Transpl 2010;10(3): 547–57. https://doi.org/10.1111/j.1600-6143.2010.03016.x.

90. Vincenti F, Larsen CP, Alberu J, et al. Three-year outcomes from BENEFIT, a randomized, active-controlled, parallel-group study in adult kidney transplant recipients. Am J Transpl 2012;12(1): 210–7. https://doi.org/10.1111/j.1600-6143.2011.03785.x.

91. Pestana JO, Grinyo JM, Vanrenterghem Y, et al. Three-year outcomes from BENEFIT-EXT: a phase III study of belatacept versus cyclosporine in recipients of extended criteria donor kidneys. Am J Transpl 2012;12(3):630–9. https://doi.org/10.1111/j.1600-6143.2011.03914.x.

92. Vincenti F, Rostaing L, Grinyo J, et al. Belatacept and long-term outcomes in kidney transplantation [published correction appears in N Engl J Med. 2016 Feb 18;374(7):698]. N Engl J Med 2016;374(4): 333–43. https://doi.org/10.1056/NEJMoa1506027.

93. Okimura K, Maeta K, Kobayashi N, et al. Characterization of ASKP1240, a fully human antibody targeting human CD40 with potent immunosuppressive effects. Am J Transpl 2014;14(6):1290–9. https://doi.org/10.1111/ajt.12678.

94. Harland RC, Klintmalm G, Jensik S, et al. Efficacy and safety of bleselumab in kidney transplant recipients: a phase 2, randomized, open-label, non-inferiority study. Am J Transpl 2020;20(1):159–71. https://doi.org/10.1111/ajt.15591.

95. Farkash E, Naik A, Tedesco-Silva H, et al. CNI-Free Therapy with Iscalimab (anti-CD40 mAb) preserves allograft histology compared to standard of care after kidney transplantation [abstract]. Am J Transpl 2019;19(suppl 3). Available at: https://atcmeetingabstracts.com/abstract/cni-free-therapy-with-iscalimab-anti-cd40-mab-preserves-allograft-histology-compared-to-standard-of-care-after-kidney-transplantation/. August 5, 2021.

96. Study of efficacy, safety, tolerability, pharmacokinetic (PK) and Pharmacodynamic (PD) of an anti-CD40 monoclonal antibody, CFZ533, in kidney transplant recipients (CIRRUS I). Available at: https://www.clinicaltrials.gov/ct2/show/NCT03663335. August 5, 2021.

97. Colvin MM, Smith CA, Tullius SG, et al. Aging and the immune response to organ transplantation.

J Clin Invest 2017;127(7):2523–9. https://doi.org/10.1172/JCI90601.

98. Meier-Kriesche HU, Cibrik DM, Ojo AO, et al. Interaction between donor and recipient age in determining the risk of chronic renal allograft failure. J Am Geriatr Soc 2002;50(1):14–7. https://doi.org/10.1046/j.1532-5415.2002.50002.x.

99. Kauffman HM, McBride MA, Cors CS, et al. Early mortality rates in older kidney recipients with comorbid risk factors. Transplantation 2007;83(4):404–10. https://doi.org/10.1097/01.tp.0000251780.01031.81.

100. Kidney Disease: Improving Global Outcomes (KDIGO) Transplant Work Group. KDIGO clinical practice guideline for the care of kidney transplant recipients. Am J Transpl 2009;9(Suppl 3):S1–155. https://doi.org/10.1111/j.1600-6143.2009.02834.x.

101. Hartmann A, Sagedal S, Hjelmesaeth J. The natural course of cytomegalovirus infection and disease in renal transplant recipients. Transplantation 2006;82(2 Suppl):S15–7. https://doi.org/10.1097/01.tp.0000230460.42558.b0.

102. Harvala H, Stewart C, Muller K, et al. High risk of cytomegalovirus infection following solid organ transplantation despite prophylactic therapy. J Med Virol 2013;85(5):893–8. https://doi.org/10.1002/jmv.23539.

103. Hodson EM, Jones CA, Strippoli GF, et al. Immunoglobulins, vaccines or interferon for preventing cytomegalovirus disease in solid organ transplant recipients. Cochrane Database Syst Rev 2007;(2):CD005129. https://doi.org/10.1002/14651858.CD005129.pub2.

104. Gerrard JG. Pneumocystis carinii pneumonia in HIV-negative immunocompromised adults. Med J Aust 1995;162(5):233–5. https://doi.org/10.5694/j.1326-5377.1995.tb139873.x.

105. Foley RN, Murray AM, Li S, et al. Chronic kidney disease and the risk for cardiovascular disease, renal replacement, and death in the United States Medicare population, 1998 to 1999. J Am Soc Nephrol 2005;16(2):489–95. https://doi.org/10.1681/ASN.2004030203.